MAGNETIC RESONANCE
BIOEFFECTS, SAFETY, AND PATIENT MANAGEMENT

SECOND EDITION

Provided as an educational service by

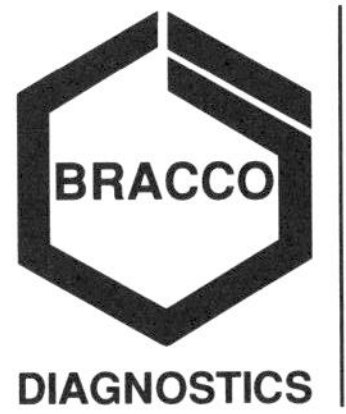

MAGNETIC RESONANCE
BIOEFFECTS, SAFETY, AND PATIENT MANAGEMENT

SECOND EDITION

FRANK G. SHELLOCK, Ph.D.
Director
Research and Development
Future Diagnostics, Inc.
RadNet Management, Inc.
and
Clinical Professor of Radiology
University of Southern California, School of Medicine
Los Angeles, California

EMANUEL KANAL, M.D.
Associate Professor
Director of Magnetic Resonance Services
University of Pittsburgh Medical Center
Pittsburgh, Pennsylvania

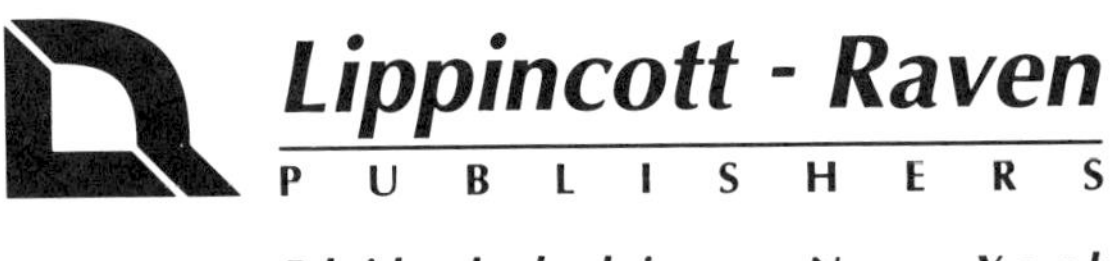
Lippincott - Raven
PUBLISHERS
Philadelphia • New York

Printed in the United States of America

Shellock, Frank G.

Magnetic resonance: bioeffects, safety, and patient management/ Frank G. Shellock, Emanuel Kanal—2nd ed.

p. cm.

Includes bibliographical references and index.

ISBN 0-397-58437-7

1. Magnetic resonance imaging—Safety measures. 2. Magnetic resonance imaging—Physiological effect. I. Kanal, Emanuel. II. Title.

[DNLM: 1. Magnetic Resonance Imaging—adverse effects. 2. Magnetic Resonance Imaging—standards. 3. Equipment Safety. WN 445 S545m 1996]

RC78.7.N83S53 1996

616.07′548—dc21

DNLM/DLC

for Library of Congress

96–46644

CIP

9 8 7 6 5 4 3 2 1

TO JAANA K. SALLINEN-COHAN,
Minä rakastan sinua . . . and I'm as serious as a heart attack!

To MY WIFE
—my Eishes Chayil—my everything. I love you past where the numbers stop.

And to MY PARENTS,
with eternal love, appreciation, respect, and gratitude. You were right.
EK

Contents

Preface

Clinical magnetic resonance (MR) procedures including imaging, angiography, and spectroscopy have now been performed for over a decade. As this technology continues to evolve, innovative MR system designs and techniques have been created that require higher static magnetic fields, higher and faster gradient magnetic fields, stronger radiofrequency (RF) transmitters, and new RF receiver coils. These developments have improved and contributed to the capabilities and utilization of clinical MR procedures. Not surprisingly, the evolution of MR technology has been unprecedented among radiologic modalities.

Unfortunately, the advances in MR procedures have occurred so rapidly that there are often gaps in the level of understanding of the MR practitioner. These deficiencies include unanswered questions regarding the important issues of MR bioeffects, safety, and patient management. The purpose of the new edition of this book is to provide an updated timely, sophisticated, and complete source of information and reference material for radiologists, technologists, and others concerned with various aspects of MR that potentially present a hazard or risk to the patient or health care worker. In addition, practical guidelines and recommendations are included that assist in the daily management of patients in the MR environment. We hope that the content of this book will serve as a means of continuing to ensure the safe, effective, and appropriate use of MR technology.

Frank G. Shellock
Emanuel Kanal

Acknowledgments

Many individuals have encouraged and supported me in my pursuit of a career as a scientist involved in MR bioeffects and safety research, including Drs. Thomas Budinger, John V. Crues III, and S. Morry Blumenfeld. I am grateful for their guidance and support.

Special thanks to Drs. Daniel (Joe) Schaefer (General Electric Company), Christopher Gordon (U.S. Environmental Protection Agency), and Ralph Schuping (U.S. Food and Drug Administration). These are colleagues who have provided me with crucial scientific input and, more importantly, their friendship.

I am especially grateful for the support that I received for my bioeffects research initially from the General Electric Company and, on a more extensive basis, from the National Cancer Institute, National Institutes of Health.

Finally, I am grateful to my co-author, Dr. Emanuel Kanal, for his commitment to produce a second edition of this book and for his good-natured ability to adhere to my taskmaster tactics. Manny, it's always a pleasure to work with you!

FGS

I would like to acknowlegde and recognize Frank: the ideal—and patient!—co-author, perfect gentleman, and true friend. I'd do it all again for you! (What am I saying? . . .)

EK

MAGNETIC RESONANCE
BIOEFFECTS,
SAFETY, AND
PATIENT MANAGEMENT

SECOND EDITION

1

Bioeffects of Static Magnetic Fields

There are numerous areas of consideration for safety issues concerning the magnetic resonance (MR) environment, but none seems to be as prevalent and disconcerting as that related to the effects of the powerful static magnetic fields used for MR procedures. For more than 2,000 years, the effects of magnets on biologic processes have been investigated and debated. Static magnetic fields are measured in gauss (G) or tesla (T), with 10,000 G being equal to 1 T. For comparison's sake, the earth's magnetic field varies from approximately 0.3 to 0.7 G between the equator and the poles, respectively, whereas a small refrigerator door magnet may be used as strong as 150 G to 250 G. The strengths of the static magnetic fields used in clinical and research MR systems for imaging and/or spectroscopy range from 0.012 T to more than 10 T (100,000 G). According to the most current recommendations and guidelines provided by the United States Food and Drug Administration (FDA), clinical MR systems are permitted to function on a routine clinical basis at static magnetic field strengths of up to 2.0 T (1). However, should the static magnetic field strength exceed 2.0 T, evidence of safety must be provided by the sponsor or device manufacturer before routine clinical use (1).

There are two major areas of safety issues regarding the static magnetic fields used for MR procedures. The first deals with the bioeffects associated with exposure to the static magnetic fields. The second deals with the effects of the forces exerted by the magnetic fields of the MR systems on certain metallic objects. This chapter discusses the former, with the latter issues addressed in Chapters 10 and 11.

GENERAL CONSIDERATIONS

The available information regarding the possible adverse effects of static magnetic fields on biologic tissues is extensive. Most of these studies have concluded that static magnetic fields of up to 2 T produce no substantial harmful bioeffects, including no alterations in cell growth and morphology, DNA structure and gene expression, pre- and postnatal reproduction and development, visual functions, nerve bioelectric activity, animal behavior, visual response to photic stimulation, cardiovascular dynamics, hematologic indices, physiological regulation and circadian rhythms, or immune responsiveness (2–8).

However, the available data are contradictory and often confusing. Some experiments have demonstrated positive, significant static magnetic field–induced bioeffects. The findings of these studies were subsequently contraindicated, either because of the inability of investigations to replicate the findings or because methodologic inaccuracies were identified (3). Budinger (4) states: "From the vast literature on experiments with cell cultures, animals, and man, no experimental protocol has been found that, when repeated by other investigators, gives similar positive results."

There have been numerous general articles regarding potential bioeffects of static magnetic fields, particularly with respect to those exposure levels that are found in association with MR systems (2–49). Most of the data are based on animal experimental findings that cannot be readily extrapolated to human subjects. Furthermore, in several instances the investigators have not given appropriate consideration to certain variables such as the duration of exposure, field strength, and direction of the static magnetic field.

One of the first comprehensive studies examining static magnetic field bioeffects was conducted by Vyalov (16) at the Moscow Scientific Research Institute, where he studied workers chronically exposed to static magnetic fields of up to 0.35 T. Headaches, fatigue, chest pain, loss of appetite, vertigo, insomnia, and other nonspecific complaints were reportedly associated with exposure to the static magnetic fields (16). The inherent problems related to this study include the absence of strict control populations, results that were qualitative, no statistical analysis of the data, and the lack of an attempt to evaluate potential contributions from other confounding factors such as chemical agents in the environment; also, the data have not been replicated by other investigators (12).

CELL REPRODUCTION AND TERATOGENICITY

The available data on pregnancy-related issues and possible interactions with the static and other electromagnetic fields used for MR procedures is somewhat reassuring but, at the same time, remains controversial (14,16,18–49). This is primarily because there have not been enough investigations to demonstrate definitively the absolute safety of the electromagnetic fields used for MR with respect to cell reproduction and teratogenicity. The reader is referred to Chapter 4 for a more in-depth discussion of these issues.

ANIMAL HOMING CAPABILITIES

Certain animals, such as pigeons and dolphins, are known to have "homing" capabilities. This is partially explained by specialized sensitivity to magnetic fields that is species specific. At least one study has suggested that human subjects are also sensitive to magnetic fields and may display homing capability (50), but this is a somewhat controversial idea. Investigators have refuted the data pertaining to human magnetoreception because they have been unable to reproduce the positive results that were previously observed (51,52).

CELL FUNCTIONS

Shivers et al. (53) found that 23 min of exposure to the electromagnetic fields used for an MR imaging procedure at 0.15 T temporarily modified the permeability of the rat's blood–brain barrier. Although this finding may not be specific to exposure to the static magnetic field component of the MR system, it is unclear as to what form of electromagnetic radiation to which it may be related. Preliminary work performed by Adzamli et al. (54) suggests that the effects of static magnetic fields on the blood–brain barrier may apply only to exposure to lower (i.e., <0.5 T) static magnetic field strengths of MR systems. These findings require additional evaluation and characterization of the mechanism(s) responsible for the effect of the static magnetic field on the blood–brain barrier.

There has also been much controversy regarding the effects of magnetic fields on growth and healing of bone. This field is replete with conflicting points of view, with no clear statements that can yet be made, except that more data are required before a reliable opinion can be reached (55,56).

Human malignant melanoma cells were studied by Short et al. (57) to determine if the presence of external magnetic fields would affect their cell number or viability. Although for these parameters, both malignant melanoma cells as well as the normal fibroblasts, were unaffected by the static magnetic fields, there was an impairment of the ability of the tumor cells to remain attached to the tissue culture surface (57).

THROMBOLYSIS

In rabbits, accelerated thrombolysis was reported to be associated with exposure to static magnetic fields of up to 0.3 T (58). Interestingly, these changes did not seem to be related to the intensity of the magnetic field over the range to which they were exposed. The same researchers also found that exposure of guinea pigs to magnetic fields of as low as 50 G (and up to 3,000 G) for 1 h daily for 6 weeks resulted in a decreased platelet count, increased platelet aggregation, increased prothrombin and partial thromboplastin times, decreased fibrinogen, and increased fibrinolysis (59). Each of these indices reversed within 2 months after cessation of exposure to the static magnetic fields (59). In a similar experiment, prostacyclin levels in rat aortas increased after exposure to static magnetic fields of either 80 G or 1,500 G for 1 h per day, daily, for 7 weeks (60). The implications of the above findings to human subjects exposed to static magnetic fields during MR procedures is unknown.

NERVE FUNCTION

Several studies have been conducted to assess the effect of exposure to static magnetic fields on various aspects of nerve function (61–75). An experiment was performed on rats placed in a T-maze with a strong static magnetic field (up to 4.0 T) located at one portion of the maze (the gradient was up to 13 T/m) and a mock magnet bore located at the other (61). A very strong avoidance or aversion behavior pattern to the side of the T-maze with the static magnetic field was displayed. More than 90% of the time, the rats showed this reaction. Even with the sides of the T-maze reversed, more than 90% of the time the rats refused to enter the area with the exposure to the magnetic field (61).

Hong et al. (62) found that exposing the nerve from a rat tail to static magnetic fields of more than 0.5 T for more than 30 s significantly increased its excitability. This interesting finding was not found in human subjects exposed to a static magnetic field of 1.5 T (68).

Prato et al. (63) concluded that the static magnetic field component of MR exposure seemed to have no effect on morphine-induced analgesia, while the time-varying magnetic field abolished and the presence of the RF field markedly diminished analgesic effects. Interestingly, several other investigators also demonstrated that exposure to MR procedures appeared to have an attenuating effect on morphine-induced analgesia (64,65).

Von Klitzing et al. (66) reported alterations in brainstem auditory and somatosensory–evoked potentials and changes in electroencephalogram (EEG) tracings related to exposure to 0.35 T static magnetic fields used for MR procedures. However, studies by others (67–69) failed to support these findings. Furthermore, there was no observable effect on nerve conduction velocities or somatosensory, visual, and auditory–evoked potentials associated with exposure to a 1.0 T static magnetic field (70).

Yuh et al. (71) investigated an amputee patient who suffered from increased phantom limb pain during exposure to static magnetic fields of 0.5 and 1.5 T MR systems. Electrical stimulation studies revealed that the residual limb was unusually sensitive to subthreshold levels of current; however, the precise explanation for the symptomology that was present was unclear (71).

There have been several studies performed to assess neuropsychiatric and cognitive function alterations related to exposure to MR procedures (9,72–75). These investigations did not identify any effects associated with exposure to the static magnetic fields of the MR systems, either with respect to cognition, acute or chronic behavioral changes, or memory alterations.

Based on the above information, exposure to static magnetic fields of MR systems of up to 2.0 T do not appear to substantially influence nerve function in human subjects. Interestingly, normal subjects exposed to the static magnetic field of a 4.0-T MR system have reported unusual sensations including nausea, vertigo, and a metallic taste (76,77). These findings were suggested to be associated with alteration in nerve function as a result of interaction with direct exposure to or movement through the high-intensity static magnetic field (e.g., stimulation of the vestibulo-labyrinthine complex may explain the presence of vertigo) (76,77). Additional research is ongoing to study these phenomena.

CARDIOVASCULAR

A number of studies have reported small increases in blood pressure during or after exposure to static magnetic fields (12,16,17). Marsh et al. (12) also observed a reproducible slight leukopenia that was related to exposure to intense magnetic fields. The absolute white cell count, however, remained within the normal range (12).

A study on isolated, perfused rabbit hearts exposed to a static magnetic field of 4.7 T in conjunction with 5 G RF pulsing techniques did not produce any increased ventricular vulnerability or alteration in the threshold for ventricular fibrillation (78). Static magnetic fields of 2.11 T were also found to produce no acute physiologic changes either in the normoxic or hypoxic rat myocardium (79). There are also data that suggest that there is no significant alteration in cardiovascular parameters related to exposure to static magnetic fields of the MR systems, despite the presence of this cardiac effect (80) (see below).

A direct cardiac effect may be observed as a result of blood, a conductive fluid, flowing through the static magnetic field and generating a biopotential (80–82). This induced biopotential is typically exhibited by an augmentation of T-wave amplitude as well as other nonspecific waveform changes that are apparent on the electrocardiogram. This cardiac effect may be seen at static magnetic field strengths of as low as 0.1 T (80–82). The increase in T-wave amplitude is directly proportional to the intensity of the static magnetic field such that, at low static magnetic field strengths, the effects are not as predominant compared with the higher ones. Alternative lead positions can be used to attenuate the static magnetic field–induced electrocardiogram (EKG) changes in order to facilitate cardiac gated studies (83) (also see information in Chapter 7).

Because there are no other circulatory alterations that coincide with the EKG changes, no short-term biologic risks are believed to be associated with the cardiac effect that occurs in conjunction with exposure to static magnetic field strengths up to 2.0 T (80–82). However, because an elevation in T-wave amplitude is indicative of myocardial infarction, ischemia, or potassium toxicity, it is necessary to monitor the electrocardiogram immediately before and after MR procedures (especially if performed with high field–strength MR systems) without the influence of the static magnetic field to assess these conditions in high-risk cardiac patients. Of note is that changes in cardiac rhythm manifested as a slight decrease in heart rate have been induced by exposure to a static magnetic field of 2.0 T (84).

TEMPERATURE

There are conflicting statements in the literature regarding the effect of static magnetic fields on body and skin temperatures of mammals. Reports have indicated that static magnetic fields either increase or both increase and decrease temperature depending on the orientation of the organism in reference to the static magnetic fields (85). Other articles state that static magnetic fields have no effect on skin and body temperatures of mammals (86–88).

None of the investigators that identified a static magnetic field effect on temperatures proposed a plausible mechanism for this response. In addition, studies that reported static magnetic field–induced skin and/or body temperature changes used laboratory animals that are known to have labile temperatures or used instrumentation that may have been perturbed by the static magnetic fields.

Investigations conducted in laboratory animals and human subjects indicated that exposure to intense static magnetic fields and/or gradient magnetic fields do not alter skin and body temperatures (86–88). The studies performed in human subjects used a special fluoroptic thermometry system known to be unperturbed by high intensity static magnetic fields (86,87).

MAGNETOPHOSHENES

In 1892, d'Arsonval (89) first reported that movement in a static magnetic field of sufficient strength was able to elicit visual sensations described as flashes of light. These visual sensations are referred to as "magnetophosphenes."

Although their precise etiology is still unclear, magnetophosphenes are believed to result from direct excitation of the optic nerve and/or retina by currents that are induced by rapid gradient magnetic fields or, alternatively, rapid eye or head movements within a static magnetic field (75,76,89–91). Although there have been no instances of magnetophosphene induction related to the exposure to static magnetic fields up to 2.0 T, volunteer subjects exposed to a static magnetic field of 4.0 T have reported the presence of magnetophosphenes (76,77) (see Chapter 2 for additional information).

CELL ALIGNMENT

Researchers have shown that deoxygenated sickled red blood cells in vitro will align against or perpendicular to a static magnetic field (92,93). This phenomenon is attributed to paramagnetic anisotropy retained by the heme of hemoglobin S that is polymerized by deoxygenation. Further investigation, however, concluded that there did not seem to be any clinical significance for human subjects exposed to static magnetic fields with respect to this finding (94).

Normal erythrocytes do not deform in the presence of a strong magnetic field, although echinocytes do have such a preferential behavior pattern (95). Similarly, in vitro alignment of fibrin (96), and fibrogen (97) in the presence of strong magnetic fields, has been reported. However, clinical experience suggests that the aligning forces do not have an effect that is considered clinically significant, in vivo (98). There is a known effect in vitro of alignment of photoreceptor cells of the globe in the presence of magnetic fields of the strengths used for clinical MR procedures. Such an effect is not apparently seen in vivo, and this does not have any clinically significant or harmful effect(s).

CONCLUSIONS

There is no conclusive evidence for irreversible or hazardous bioeffects related to acute, short-term exposures of humans to static magnetic fields up to field strengths of 2.0 T. However, as of 1996, there are several 3.0 and 4.0 T MR systems operating at various research and clinical facilities around the world. Studies have indicated that volunteer subjects exposed to the 4.0-T MR system have experienced various forms of unwanted side effects (76,77). Obviously, the intense static magnetic fields of these MR systems can produce significant undesirable physiologic changes in human subjects and, therefore, considerable research is required to study the mechanisms responsible for these bioeffects and to determine possible means to counter-balance them.

REFERENCES

1. Food and Drug Administration. Magnetic resonance diagnostic device: panel recommendation and report on petitions for MR reclassification. *Fed Reg* 1988;53:7575–7579.
2. Tenforde T. Biological effects of dosimetry of stationary magnetic fields. In: Grandolfo M, Michaelson S, Rindi A, eds. *Biological effects and dosimetry of static and ELF electromagnetic fields.* New York: Plenum; 1985:93–127.
3. Tenforde T, Budinger T. Biological effects and physical safety aspects of NMR imaging and in vivo spectroscopy. In: Thomas S, Dixon R, eds. *NMR in medicine: instrumentation and clinical applications.* New York: American Association of Physicists in Medicine, Medical Monograph No. 14; 1986:493–548.
4. Budinger T. Nuclear magnetic resonance (NMR) in vivo studies: Known thresholds for health effects. *J Comput Assist Tomogr* 1981;5:800–811.
5. Budinger T. Thresholds for physiological effects due to RF and magnetic fields used in NMR imaging. *IEEE Trans Nucl Sci* 1979;NS-26:2821–2825.
6. Budinger T, Cullander C. Chapter 19. Biophysical phenomena and health hazards of in vivo magnetic resonance. In: Margulis A, Higgins C, Kaufman L, Crooks L, eds. *Clinical magnetic resonance imaging.* San Francisco: Radiology Research and Education Foundation; 1983:303–320.

7. Stuchly MA. Human exposure to static and time-varying magnetic fields. *Health Physics* 1986;51:215–241.
8. Becker R. The biological effects of magnetic fields: a survey. *Med Electron Biol Eng* 1963;1: 293–303.
9. Bartels V, Mann K, Matejcek M, Puttkammer M, Schroth G. Magnetresonanztomographie und sicherheit. *Fortschr Rontgenstr* 1986;145:383–385.
10. Gonet B. Influence of constant magnetic fields on certain physiochemical properties of water. *Bioelectromagnetics* 1985;6:169–175.
11. Kanal E, Shellock F, Talagala L. Safety considerations in MR imaging. *Radiology* 1990;176: 593–606.
12. Marsh J, Armstrong T, Jacobson A, Smith R. Health effects of occupational exposure to steady magnetic fields. *Am Ind Hyg Assoc J* 1982;43:387–394.
13. Papatheofanis F. A review on the interaction of biological systems with magnetic fields. *Physiol Chemistry Physics Med NMR* 1984;16:251–255.
14. Persson B, Stahlberg F. *Health and safety of clinical NMR examinations.* Boca Raton: CRC Press; 1989.
15. Shellock FG, Kanal E. Policies, guidelines, and recommendations for MR imaging safety and patient management. *J Magn Reson Imag* 1991;1:97–101.
16. Villa M, Mustarelli P, Caprotti M. Mini-review: biological effects of magnetic fields. *Life Sci* 1991;49:85–92.
17. Vyalov A. Clinico-hygienic and experimental data of the effects of magnetic fields under industrial conditions. In: Kholodov Y, ed. *Influence of magnetic fields on biological objects.* Moscow: Translated by the Joint Publications Research Service, 1974:163–174. vol JJPRS–63038.
18. Kanal E, Gillen J, Evans J, Savitz D, Shellock F. Survey of reproductive health among female MR workers. *Radiology* 1993;187:395–399.
19. LaForge H, Sadeghi M, Seguin M. Magnetostatic field effect: stress syndrome pattern and functional relation with intensity. *J Psychol* 1986;120:299–304.
20. Ngo F, Blue J, Roberts W. The effect of a static magnetic field on DNA synthesis and survival of mammalian cells irradiated with fast neurons. *Magn Reson Med* 1987;5:307–317.
21. Barnothy J. Growth rate of mice in static magnetic fields. *Nature* 1963;200:86–87.
22. Asashima M, Shimada K, Pfeiffer C. Magnetic shielding induces early developmental abnormalities in the newt, Cynops pyrrhogaster. *Bioelectromagnetics* 1991;12:215–224.
23. Ramirez E, Monteagudo J, Garcia-Gracia M, Delgado J. Oviposition and development of Drosophila modified by magnetic fields. *Bioelectromagnetics* 1983;4:315–326.
24. Sutherland R, Marton J, MacDonald J, Howell R. Effect of weak magnetic fields on growth of cells in tissue culture. *Physiol Chemistry Physics* 1978;10:125–131.
25. Strand J, Abernathy C, Sakalski J, Genoway R. Effects of magnetic field exposure on fertilization success in rainbow trout, Salmo gairdneri. *Bioelectromagnetics* 1983;4:295–301.
26. Joshi M, Kahn M, Damle P. Effect of magnetic field on chick morphogenesis. *Differentiation* 1978;10:39–43.
27. Neurath P. The effect of high gradient, high strength magnetic fields on the early embryonic development of frogs. In: Barnothy M, ed. *Biological effects of magnetic fields.* New York: Plenum Press; 1969;1, pp 146.
28. Liboff A, Williams T, Strong D, Wistar R. Time-varying magnetic fields: effect on DNA synthesis. *Science* 1984;223:818–820.
29. Tofani S, Agnesod G, Ossola P. Effects of continuous low-level exposure to radiofrequency radiation on intrauterine development in rats. *Health Physics* 1986;51:489–499.
30. Peeling J, Lewis J, Samoiloff M, Bock E, Tomchuk E. Biological effects of magnetic fields: chronic exposure of the nematode Panagrellus Redivivus. *Magn Reson Imag* 1988;6:655–660.
31. Ueno S, Harada K, Shiokawa K. The embryonic development of frogs under strong DC magnetic fields. *IEEE Trans Magnet* 1984;MAG-20:1663–1665.
32. Kay H, Herfkens R, Kay B. Effect on magnetic resonance imaging on Xenopus Laevis embryogenesis. *Magn Reson Imag* 1988;6:501–506.
33. Prasad N, Wright D, Ford J, Thornby J. Safety of 4-T MR imaging: study of effects on developing frog embryos. *Radiology* 1990;174:251–253.
34. Prasad N, Bushong S, Thronby J, Bryan R, Hazelwood C, Harrell J. Effect of nuclear magnetic resonance on chromosomes of mouse bone marrow cells. *Magn Reson Imag* 1984;2:37–39.

35. Malinin G, Gregory W, Morelli L, Sharma V, Houch J. Evidence of morphological and physiological transformation on mammalian cells by strong magnetic fields. *Science* 1976;194:844.
36. Geard C, Osmak R, Hall E, Simon H, Maudsley A, Hilal S. Magnetic resonance and ionizing radiation: a comparative evaluation in vitro of oncogenic and genotoxic potential. *Radiology* 1984;152:199–202.
37. Cooke P, Morris P. The effects of NMR exposure of living organism. II. A genetic study of human lymphocytes. *Br J Radiol* 1981;54:622–625.
38. Wolff S, Crooks L, Brown P, Howard R, Painter R. Test for DNA and chromosomal damage induced by nuclear magnetic resonance imaging. *Radiology* 1980;136:707–710.
39. Wolff S, James T, Young G, Margulis A, Bodycote J, Afzal V. Magnetic resonance imaging: absence of in vitro cytogenetic damage. *Radiology* 1985;155:163–165.
40. Schwartz J, Crooks L. NMR imaging produces no observable mutations or cytotoxicity in mammalian cells. *AJR Am J Roentgenol* 1982;139:583–585.
41. Ardito G. Lamberti L, Bigatti P, Prono G. Influence of a constant magnetic field on human lymphocyte cultures. *Boll Soc It Biol Spec* 1984;60:1341–1346.
42. Sikov M, Mahlum D, Montgomery L, Decker J. Development of mice after intrauterine exposure to direct current magnetic fields. Proceedings of the 18th Hanford Life Sciences Symposium. Richland, WA. Technical Information Center, US Department of Energy, 1979:462–473.
43. Mahlum D, Sikov M, Decker J. Dominant lethal studies in mice exposed to direct current magnetic fields. Proceedings of the 18th Hanford Life Sciences Symposium. Richland, WA. Technical Information Center, US Department of Energy, 1979:474–484.
44. Tyndall D, Sulik K. Effects of magnetic resonance imaging on eye development in the C57BL/6J mouse. *Teratology* 1991;43:263–275.
45. Kale P, Baum J. Genetic effects of strong magnetic fields in Drosophilia melanogaster. *Mutation Res* 1982;105:79–83.
46. Heinrichs W, Fong P, Flannery M, et al. Midgestational exposure of pregnant balb/c mice to magnetic resonance imaging. *Magn Reson Imag* 1988;6:305–313.
47. McRobbie D, Foster M. Pulsed magnetic field exposure during pregnancy and implications for NMR foetal imaging: a study with mice. *Magn Reson Imag* 1985;3:231–234.
48. Adey W. Tissue interactions with nonionizing electromagnetic fields. *Physiol Rev* 1981;61:435–514.
49. Beers J. Biological effects of weak electromagnetic fields from 0 Hz to 200 MHz: a survey of the literature with special emphasis on possible magnetic resonance effects. *Magn Reson Imag* 1989;7:309–331.
50. Baker R. Goal orientation by blindfolded humans after long-distance displacement: possible involvement of a magnetic sense. *Science* 1980;210:555–557.
51. Fildes B, O'Loughlin B, Bradshaw J. Human orientation with restricted sensory information: no evidence for magnetic sensitivity. *Perception* 1984;13:229–236.
52. Gould J, Able K. Human homing: an elusive phenomenon. *Science* 1981;212:1061–1063.
53. Shivers R, Kavaliers M, Teskey G, Prato F, Pelletier RM. Magnetic resonance imaging temporarily alters blood–brain barrier permeability in the rat. *Neurosci Lett* 1987;76:25–31.
54. Adzamli IK, Jolesz FA, Blau M. An assessment of blood–brain barrier integrity under MRI conditions: brain uptake of radiolabeled Gd-DTPA and In-DTPA-IgG. *J Nucl Med* 1989:30:839.
55. Linder-Aronson S, Lindskog S. A morphometric study of bone surfaces and skin reactions after stimulation with static magnetic fields in rats. *Am J Orthod Dentofac Orthop* 1991;99:44–48.
56. Bruce G, Howlett C, Huckstep R. Effect of a static magnetic field on fracture healing in rabbit radius. *Clin Orthop* 1987;222:300–306.
57. Short W, Goodwill L, Taylor C, Job C, Arthur M, Cress A. Alteration of human tumor cell adhesion by high-strength static magnetic fields. *Invest Radiol* 1991;27:836–840.
58. Gorczynska E. Dynamics of the thrombolytic process under conditions of a constant magnetic field. *Clin Phys Physiol Meas* 1986;7:225–235.
59. Gorczynska E, Wegrzynowicz R. The effect of magnetic fields on platelets, blood coagulation, and fibrinolysis in guinea pigs. *Physiol Chem Phys Med NMR* 1983;15:459–468.
60. Gorczynska E, Wegrzynowicz R. Magnetic field provokes the increases of prostacyclin in aorta of rats. *Naturwissenschaftern* 1986;73:675–677.

61. Weiss M, Herrick R, Tabor K, Contant C, Plishker G. Bioeffects of high magnetic fields: a study using a simple animal model. *Magn Reson Imag* 1992;10:689–694.
62. Hong CZ, Harmon D, Yu J. Static magnetic field influence on rat tail nerve function. *Arch Phys Med Rehabil* 1986;67:746–749.
63. Prato F, Ossenkeopp KP, Kavaliers M, Sestini E, Teskey G. Attenuation of morphine-induced analgesia in mice by exposure to MRI: separate effects of the static, radiofrequency and time-varying magnetic fields. *Magn Reson Imag* 1987;5:9–14.
64. Ossenkopp KP, Kavaliers M, Prato F, Teskey G, Sestini E, Hirst M. Exposure to nuclear magnetic resonance imaging procedure attenuates morphine-induced analgesia in mice. *Life Sci* 1985;37:1507–1514.
65. Kavaliers M, Ossenkopp KP. Tolerance to morphine-induced analgesia in mice: magnetic fields function as environmental specific cues and reduce tolerance development. *Life Sci* 1985;37:1125–1135.
66. Klitzing LV. Do static magnetic fields of NMR influence biological signals? *Clin Phys Physiol Meas* 1986;7:157–160.
67. Buettner U. Human interactions with ultra-high fields. *Ann NY Acad Sci* 1992:59–66.
68. Hong CZ, Shellock F. Short-term exposure to a 1.5 Tesla static magnetic field does not affect somato-sensory-evoked potentials in man. *Magn Reson Imag* 1990;8:65–69.
69. Muller S, Hotz M. Human brainstem auditory evoked potentials (BAEP) before and after MR examinations. *Magn Reson Med* 1990;16:476–480.
70. Vogl T, Pasulus W, Fuchs A, Krafczyk S, Lissner J. Influence of magnetic resonance imaging on evoked potentials and nerve conduction velocities in humans. *Invest Radiol* 1991;26:432–437.
71. Yuh W, Fisher D, Shields R, Ehrhardt J, Shellock, F. Phantom limb pain induced in amputees by strong magnetic fields. *J Magn Reson Imag* 1992;2:221–223.
72. Brockway J, Bream P. Does memory loss occur after MR imaging? *J Magn Reson Imag* 1992;2: 721–728.
73. Besson J, Foreman E, Eastwood L, Smith F, Ashcroft G. Cognitive evaluation following NMR imaging of the brain. *J Neurol Neurosurg Psychiatry* 1984;47:314–316.
74. Ossenkopp KP, Innis N, Prato F, Sestini E. Behavioral effects of exposure to nuclear magnetic resonance imaging: I. Open-field avoidance behavior and passive avoidance learning in rats. *Magn Reson Imag* 1986;4:275–280.
75. Innis N, Ossenkopp KP, Prato F, Sestini E. Behavioral effects of exposure to nuclear magnetic resonance imaging: II. Spatial memory tests. *Magn Reson Imag* 1986;4:281–284.
76. Redington R, Dumoulin C, Schenck J, et al. MR imaging and bioeffects on a whole body 4.0 Tesla imaging system. In: *Book of Abstracts, Society of Magnetic Resonance in Medicine.* Berkeley, CA: Society of Magnetic Resonance in Medicine; 1988; 1:4.
77. Schenck J. Health and physiological effects of human exposure to whole body 4 Tesla magnetic fields during MRI. In: Magin R, Liburdy R, Persson B, eds. *Biological effects and safety aspects of nuclear magnetic resonance imaging and spectroscopy.* New York Academy of Sciences; 1991;285–301.
78. Doherty J, Whitman G, Robinson M, et al. Changes in cardiac excitability and vulnerability in NMR fields. *Radiology* 1985;20:129–135.
79. Gulch R, Lutz O. Influence of strong static magnetic fields on heart muscle contraction. *Phys Med Biol* 1986;31:763–769.
80. Keltner J, Roos M, Brakeman P, Budinger T. Magnetohydrodynamics of blood flow. *Magn Reson Med* 1990;16:139–149.
81. Beischer D, Knepton J. The electroencephalogram of the Squirrel monkey (Saimiri sciureus) in a very high magnetic field. In: Naval Aerospace Medical Institute, Pensacola, FL, 1964.
82. Mezrich R, Reichek N, Kressel H. ECG effects in high-field MR imaging. *Radiology* 1985;157(P):219.
83. Dimick RN, Hedlund LW, Herfkens RJ, Fram EK, Utz J. Optimizing electrocardiographic electrode placement for cardiac-gated magnetic resonance imaging. *Invest Radiol* 1987;22:17–22.
84. Jehenson P, Duboc D, Lavergne T, et al. Change in human cardiac rhythm induced by a 2-T static magnetic field. *Radiology* 1988;166:227–230.
85. Gemmel H, Wendhausen H, Wunsch F. Biologische effekte statischer magnetfelder bei NMR-tomographie am menschen. *Radiologische Klinik* 1983; Wiss. Mitt. Univ. Kiel.

86. Shellock F, Schaefer D, Gordon C. Effect of a 1.5 T static magnetic field on body temperature of man. *Magn Reson Med* 1986;3:644–647.
87. Shellock F, Schaefer D, Crues J. Exposure to a 1.5 T static magnetic fields does not alter body and skin temperatures in man. *Magn Reson Med* 1989;11:371–375.
88. Tenforde T, Levy L. Thermoregulation in rodents exposed to homogeneous (7.55 Tesla and gradient (60 Tesla/per second) DC magnetic fields. The Bioelectromagnetics Society 7th Annual Meeting Abstracts. 1985: pp 7.
89. d'Arsonval M. Action physiologique des courants alternatifs a grande frequence. *Arch Physiol* 1893;5:401.
90. Barlow H, Kohn H, Walsh E. Visual sensations aroused by magnetic fields. *Am J Physiol* 1947;148:372–375.
91. Lovsund P, Nillson S, Reuter T, Oberg P. Magnetophosphenes: a quantitative analysis of thresholds. *Med Biol Eng Comp* 1980;18:326–334.
92. Brody A, Sorette M, Gooding C, et al. Induced alignment of flowing sickle erythrocytes in a magnetic field: a preliminary report. *Invest Radiol* 1985;20:560–566.
93. Murayama M. Orientation of sickled erythrocytes in a magnetic field. *Nature* 1965;206:420–422.
94. Leitmannova A, Stosser R, Glaser R. Changes in the shape of human erythrocytes under the influence of a static homogeneous magnetic field. *Acta Biolog Med Germ* 1977;36:931–944.
95. Brody A, Embury S, Mentzer W, Winkler M, Gooding C. Preservation of sickle cell blood flow patterns during MR imaging: an in vivo study. *AJR Am J Roentgenol* 1988;151:139–141.
96. Hurdy-Clergeion G, Freyssinet J, Talbot J, Marx J. Orientation of fibrin in strong magnetic fields. *Ann NY Acad Sci* 1983:380–387.
97. Freyssinet JM, Torbet J, Hurdy-Clergeon G. Fibrinogen and fibrin in strong magnetic fields: complementary results and discussion. *Biochemie* 1984;66:81–85.
98. Certaines JD. Molecular and cellular responses to orientation effects in static and homogeneous ultra high magnetic fields. *Ann NY Acad Sci* 1992:35–43.

2

Bioeffects of Gradient Magnetic Fields

During magnetic resonance (MR) imaging there are numerous gradient magnetic fields that are turned on and off at rapid rates, at varying frequencies, for varying durations, and to varied peak gradient amplitudes. All spatial localization is accomplished in MR imaging with the use of these gradient magnetic fields. According to Faraday's Law of Induction, exposure of any conductor to time-varying magnetic fields will induce a voltage in the conductor that is oriented perpendicular to the time rate of change of the magnetic field. Thus, by placing the body within the MR system and rapidly switching on and off the current within the gradient magnetic field coils, two results are simultaneously achieved. Not only is there the creation of a gradient magnetic field, but there is also the potential of inducing voltages within the tissues of (and/or other electrical conductors on or in) the patient in the bore of the MR system and its three orthogonally oriented sets of gradient coils.

Thus, the nature of MR procedures is likely to induce electrical voltages and/or currents within the patient. The magnitude of these voltages and/or currents will be determined by several factors, including the electrical resistance in the induced circuit in the tissue(s), the cross-sectional area of the induced current flow, and the rate of change (i.e., changing magnitude versus time) of the gradient magnetic field itself. Consequently, all induced voltages or currents will occur during the times that the gradient magnetic field strengths are changing, namely, the rise and fall times of the gradients. Furthermore, the greater the magnitude of the rise and fall times, the greater the induced voltage and current.

To approximate the values that might be achieved during a typical MR imaging procedure, let us assume a maximum, peak gradient amplitude of 1.0 G per centimeter achieved at a rise time of 500 microseconds (0.5 μs). Many of today's state-of-the-art gradient subsystems can achieve twice or more this rise time or gradient amplitude. At approximately 30 cm from the center of the gradient coils (i.e., the center of the MR magnet), this would correspond to 2,000 G/s times 30 cm, or 60,000 G/s, or 6 T/s. Note that there is a greater changing magnetic field over time, or dB/dt, as one proceeds farther away from the center and toward the ends of the gradient coils, where the time rate of change of the gradient magnetic fields (dB/dt) is the greatest.

These induced voltages will recur for every gradient that is switched on. Although this frequency is determined by factors such as the type of MR imaging sequence performed, the timing parameters of the pulse sequence, and the number of section locations being imaged, a typical MR imaging pulse sequence might re-excite the same set of gradient coils at a rate of tens of times per second.

Theoretically, there are at least two possible bioeffects related to gradient magnetic fields from induced currents or voltages in the human body. One is associated with induced currents and voltages that may result in power deposition and subsequent tissue heating while the patient is exposed to the gradient magnetic fields during the MR procedure. However, it is well accepted that the thermal effects that result from the gradient switching during MR imaging are essentially negligible and, therefore, they are considered clinically insignificant (1–3).

The same conclusion, however, is not applicable to the possibility of direct neuromuscular stimulation or excitation caused by the induced currents or voltages. Both theory and practice have demonstrated that, with sufficient gradient magnetic field switching of appropriate gradient magnitudes, neuromuscular stimulation may occur. This may partially result from direct stimulation or from induced voltages exceeding the threshold necessary for achieving neural action potential discharge.

Thus, there is reasonable cause to investigate whether the magnitude of induced currents from clinically applied MR procedures might be sufficient to induce seizures, magnetophosphenes (electromagnetically induced visual flashes of light), alterations of nerve conduction velocity, peripheral nerve stimulation, skeletal muscular contractions, or even cardiac arrhythmias.

To determine if tissues will be affected, adversely or otherwise, by induced currents and voltages, it is necessary to determine the amplitude of such induced voltages. Furthermore, to calculate induced current densities, it is important to know the electrical conductivity or resistivity of the induced current loop. This is determined by the tissues through which the induced voltage will attempt to induce a current flow. Even with this information, the answers to the questions posed above are not necessarily defined clearly.

It is well known that there are several factors that are responsible for inducing a physiologic response to an induced voltage, including the strength of the static magnetic field, the orientation of the gradient magnetic fields being switched relative to the patient's tissues, the size of the greatest diameter of the patient's body, the frequency of the stimulus, the duration of the induced voltage, the shape of the waveform, the width of the pulse, the sensitivity of the tissue, and other factors that can all affect the threshold at which a response or measurable effect is observed (4–10). In consideration of the above, it becomes readily apparent why there may be different thresholds for eliciting excitation for different tissues.

The United States Food and Drug Administration (FDA) has issued safety guidelines and suggested operating limitations for MR imaging devices regarding the gradient magnetic fields associated with MR imaging procedures. The specific wording of the guidelines issued in 1988 is as follows (11):

"Rate of change of magnetic field:

Limit patient exposure to time-varying magnetic fields with strengths significantly less than those required to produce peripheral nerve stimulation.

There are three alternatives:

1. Demonstrate that the maximum dB/dt of the system is 6 T/s or less; or
2. Demonstrate that for axial gradients:
   dB/dt<20 T/s for $T > 120$ μs; or
   dB/dt $<$ 2,400/t (μs) T/s for 12 μs $< T <$ 120 μs; or
   dB/dt $<$ 200 T/s for $T <$ 12 μs

   For transverse gradients: dB/dt is considered to be below the level of concern when less than three times the above limits for axial gradients; or
3. Demonstrate with valid scientific evidence that the rate of change of magnetic field for the system is not sufficient to cause peripheral nerve stimulation by an adequate margin of safety (at least a factor of three):

   The parameter of dB/dt cited above must be shown to fall below either of the two levels of concern by presentation of valid scientific measurement of calculated evidence sufficient to demonstrate that the time rate of magnetic filed change (dB/dt) is of no concern."

On April 21, 1995, the Center for Devices and Radiological Health released a document for public comment that contained draft revisions to the August 2, 1988 "Guidance for the Content and Review of a Magnetic Resonance Diagnostic Device 510(k) Application" document. The revisions in that draft related to operating at gradient magnetic field rates of change (dB/dt levels) exceeding those levels of concern as they had been listed in the original guidance document. Comments were solicited regarding this draft from MR system manufacturers, MR user groups, and technical experts. Feedback was also obtained at a public hearing regarding this draft guidance document that was held on September 21, 1995.

As a result of the feedback from the above-named sources, a draft MRI Guidance Update for dB/dt was issued by the Office of Device Evaluation, Center for Devices and Radiological Health, on October 11, 1995. This document outlines several modifications to the prior levels of concern. For example, it was decided that painful peripheral nerve stimulation be the target threshold to avoid (as opposed to simple twitching or simple biologic detectability of this low level of stimulation), and that an exam be terminated if the patient complains of severe discomfort or pain.

The actual wording is as follows: "Equipment intended for routine clinical MRI use should be limited so that painful stimulation is not induced."

Indeed, it was specifically noted in the comments to the draft document that mild stimulation is not considered hazardous, and that an examination need not be terminated if the patient experiences mild peripheral nerve stimulation.

The draft guidance update document also states that for equipment that can exceed certain dB/dt thresholds, the manufacturers of these MR systems are required to study at least 20 volunteers using maximal dB/dt attainable values that can be produced by the MR systems (12). The number of volunteer subjects who experience stimulation and the level (mild, moderate, or painful) of the stimulation must be reported.

This document also contains a "Warnings" section, stating that special patient populations should be studied only in controlled clinical settings under supervision by the Institutional Review Board (12). The indicated special patient populations include children, pregnant women, epileptics, patients with metallic implants, cardiac arrhythmias, peripheral neuropathy, comatose patients, or patients who are unable to communicate (12).

Operators of the MR systems are to be warned by the MR system manufacturers regarding the types of imaging techniques available on the specific MR system that may produce peripheral nerve stimulation (12). They also need to be provided with a description of the types of sensations of peripheral nerve stimulation that are capable of being produced. Whenever these techniques are used, operators are to be instructed to inform the patient that peripheral nerve stimulation may occur, describing the nature of such sensations to the patient.

The MR operator is to maintain constant contact with the patient during the procedures in which peripheral nerve stimulation may be induced. The patient is to be instructed not to clasp their hands (to avoid creating a conductive loop, thus increasing the likelihood of neural stimulation) and to inform the operator if they experience severe discomfort or pain. In these instances, the MR procedure must be terminated and a report regarding the incident should be completed and immediately submitted to the manufacturer of the MR system, as well as to the FDA (12).

NEURAL, SKELETAL MUSCLE, AND CARDIAC MUSCLE STIMULATION

As noted above and for the purpose of discussion and comparison, we can use the approximation of 1 $\mu A/cm^2$ for a dB/dt of 1.0 T/s as a reasonably expectable current density that will be experienced because of gradient magnetic fields typically used in clinical MR imaging procedures (13). The MR systems used to date can be expected routinely to produce current densities of approximately 3 $\mu A/cm^2$ for a dB/dt of 3.0 T/s, which is below the level where biologic effects can be expected (14,15). By comparison, roughly 15 to 100 $\mu A/cm^2$ are needed to produce tetanic contractions of the skeletal muscles involved in breathing, whereas 0.2 to 1.0 $\mu A/cm^2$ appears to be the threshold current density required to produce ventricular fibrillation in the human heart (at frequency ranges of 20–200 Hz for sinusoidal voltages) (13,16). The shorter the stimulus duration, the greater the threshold required to produce cardiac fibrillation. This can be approximated by an inverse square root ratio between the amplitude of the stimulus and the shock duration necessary to elicit cardiac fibrillation (17). The current densities required to elicit extra systoles in guinea pig hearts have been reported to be three to five times less than that required to produce fibrillation (16). In addition, cardiac thresholds are significantly greater than those necessary to elicit neuromuscular excitations (18–20).

Seizure induction thresholds seem to be even higher; that is, to elicit a convulsive seizure current densities of roughly 3 $\mu A/cm^2$ (and sustained for 300 ms) would be required (21). Animal data suggest that current densities of approximately 1 $\mu A/cm^2$ would be needed to induce reversible nerve damage (13). This is roughly a million-fold lower than those induced by routine MR imaging studies today.

Mathematical calculations (13) suggest that the threshold currents required to induce ventricular fibrillation in a healthy heart are significantly greater than those that will be achieved during routine MR procedures today. Similar statements can be made concerning present-day (non-echo planar) MR imaging techniques and hardware capabilities and peripheral nerve stimulation, muscular contraction, or seizures (14,15).

One should recognize that the MR industry has been steadily moving toward developing and using more capable (i.e., both stronger maximum amplitudes and faster dB/dt, or rise/fall times) gradient subsystems. These will be accompanied by proportionately higher induced voltages and current densities in the patients who are exposed to these MR systems.

It is also important to realize that the preceding statements are based on calculations and observations using normal human tissue. If the electrical resistance of the circuit decreases, such as by the incorporation of a highly conductive metallic structure or wire into the conductive loop, total circuit resistance may decrease, and current may increase.

As an example, epicardial pacer wires may be found in a patient referred for an MR procedure. This occurs often because, after a successful postoperative surgical recovery, epicardial pacing wires that have been placed intraoperatively are typically pulled from the chest and epicardium percutaneously. The pacing wires may get "stuck" and cannot be removed easily. If this occurs, the clinician depresses the skin and cuts the leads at the skin entry site. These retained electrical conductors have one end in the epicardial tissue and the other in the subcutaneous tissue of the chest. Similar concerns may be raised regarding the pacing wires that have been left in place within the heart after removal of a pacemaker. The concern in each of these cases is that the increased electrical conductivity of the part of the wires may sufficiently decrease the overall resistivity of the circuit to yield enough current to induce neuromuscular excitation during certain types of MR imaging procedures, in what may be already excitable myocardial tissue.

There has been at least one report of pacing the cardiac rate at the frequency of the applied MR imaging pulse in dogs with implanted cardiac pacemakers undergoing an MR procedure using a 1.5-T MR system (22). Although it should be stressed that there are no data available to demonstrate arrhythmias or other harmful effects to patients as a result of induced currents from MR imaging, one should at least be aware of the theoretical concern noted above. In addition, there have been several fatalities involving patients with cardiac pacemakers who had been inadvertently permitted into the MR imaging environment (23). Even though the cause of death in these patients is unknown, the possibility of an arrhythmia-induced injury has not been excluded.

If the tissue is inherently abnormal, there is the possibility that the current densities necessary to induce neural activation may decrease significantly. There has been one case report of phantom limb pain in an amputee patient that was apparently induced by strong changing magnetic fields (24), the precise etiology of which is still unknown. Several patients with seizure disorders have also experienced seizures during MR imaging procedures (25). It is entirely unclear if there was any causal relationship between the MR procedures and the development of the seizures. Even if there is an association between seizures and MR procedures, it is unknown whether there is any association with the gradient magnetic fields used for MR imaging or whether the association is with, for example, auditory or stress-related stimuli. Nevertheless, the potential interactions are present with virtually no data to support or refute these possible relationships.

The factors and thresholds necessary for neural stimulation are controversial (6,26,27). Obviously, as our understanding of the processes of neural stimulation are still evolving, we may not be able to state definitively whether stimulation can or should result for any given situation. Therefore, it may be appropriate to leave a larger than usual safety factor for these issues until more is known about the science of neural stimulation itself, as well as the inductive effects of MR imaging techniques.

MAGNETOPHOSPHENES

D'Arsonval first reported in 1893 that motion in a sufficiently strong magnetic field could elicit what was subjectively reported as visual sensations, often described as flashes of light (28). These visual sensations are referred to as "magnetophosphenes," and result from direct excitation of the optic nerve and/or retina by currents that are induced by rapid gradient magnetic fields or, alternatively, by rapid eye motion within a static magnetic field. There has been extensive work in this area with such experiences noted even in blind individuals (29–31).

Magnetophosphenes have been elicited by current densities of as low as roughly 17 μA/cm^2 (13). Although there have been no cases of magnetophosphenes reported for fields of up to and including 1.95 T, magnetophosphenes, metallic taste, headache, and symptoms of vertigo seem also to be relatively reproducible symptoms associated with rapid motion within the static magnetic field of 4-T MR systems (32). Although these symptoms have been reported to be related to the high static magnetic field of those MR systems, it is apparent that they seem to result from the gradient magnetic field effects of induced voltages and currents that are produced from motion in the environment of the static magnetic fields (i.e., changing magnetic fields inducing electrical voltages). It is for this reason that these bioeffects were also discussed in Chapter 1, Bioeffects of Static Magnetic Fields. Although these physiologic changes are at the level of biologic detectability, they are not necessarily harmful responses.

AUDITORY CONSIDERATIONS

The generation of a gradient magnetic field in the presence of the background of a powerful static magnetic field results in a torque, or rotational force, on the gradient coils themselves, as the induced magnetic field opposes or aligns with the static magnetic field. Because these gradient coil currents will be alternated between on and off states dozens of times per second (if not more), these forces will be rapidly alternated between on and off states, and will result in a vibrational motion of the gradient coils. This produces what can be loosely described as an auditory, "banging" or "knocking" noise. The reader is referred to Chapter 5 for further discussion regarding the auditory effects associated with gradient magnetic fields during MR procedures.

NEURAL STIMULATION AND ECHO PLANAR IMAGING MR SYSTEMS

Any discussion of the gradient magnetic fields used for MR imaging and their secondary induced voltages is incomplete without bringing up the gradient strengths and rise time capabilities of the MR imagers used for echo planar techniques. As previously discussed, the direction in which the MR industry is heading currently is one wherein there is a marked advance in the peak gradient amplitudes and decreased rise times to maximum amplitude capabilities of the gradient magnetic field subsystems of the MR imagers. Whereas only a few years ago many MR systems would have had 1 G/cm maximum gradient amplitudes with 600 or 700 μs rise times, today it is not uncommon to find clinical MR systems with 15 or more G/cm maximum gradient magnetic field strengths and 300 to 500 μs rise times.

Additionally, with the development and introduction of echo planar imaging technology and hardware into the clinical MR setting, 2.5 G/cm maximum amplitudes and <300 μs rise times are now the range of the hardware specifications for MR systems to be imminently delivered to clinical MR sites. Therefore, the potential for exposing numerous patients (not just volunteer subjects) to considerably increased levels of induced voltages will soon be created.

Several investigators using MR systems from various manufacturers have already reported what is believed to represent direct peripheral muscle stimulation in the form of uncontrolled, involuntary skeletal muscular contractions and/or twitching in human subjects induced from echo planar imaging sequences (10,33–36). The threshold for these gradient magnetic field–induced bioeffects have been observed at and beyond 60 T/s. These have included sensory stimulation in the form of creeping sensations along the back or twitching along the bridge of the nose or feelings like electric shocks, and have ranged from imperceptible to painful sensations. The positioning of the subject or patient also seems to play a role in the severity of the response to stimulation (33). Of additional note is that cardiac and respiratory functions at gradient magnetic field values of up to 60 T/s have been found to be unaffected in anesthetized rabbits (37).

OTHER BIOEFFECTS

Several studies have reported positive results during experiments with respect to exposure to gradient magnetic fields used for MR procedures. For example, Teskey et al. (38) found a decrease in the fentanyl-induced analgesia experienced by mice when exposed to the gradient magnetic fields at levels used in MR imaging. Morphine-induced analgesia was also found to be inhibited or reduced when mice were exposed to gradient magnetic fields (39). Garber et al. (40) found an increase in the brain mannitol space that seemed to be directly related to exposure to gradient magnetic fields. Peeling et al. (41) found a slight decrease in the overall survival, growth, and maturity of nematode populations exposed to gradient magnetic fields in the presence of static magnetic fields of various strengths. Interestingly, there was no observed effect of the gradient magnetic fields alone in this study, whereas Weiss et al. (42) found a reproducible avoidance behavior pattern in rats exposed to a strong magnetic field gradient, as they were presumably able to detect and avoid exposure to the changing field under the experimental conditions.

Conversely, there have been experiments that failed to reveal any association with bioeffects related to exposure to gradient magnetic fields, including no effect on normal amphibian embryogenesis (43) or effects on murine natural killer cell cytotoxicity (44), either with or without interleukin-2 (45). Studies were also performed on pregnant mice that failed to demonstrate any associated changes in litter number or growth rates of exposed versus control groups (46). These studies included exposure not only to gradient magnetic fields, but also to radiofrequency radiation and static fields of 0.15, 2.35, or 4.5 T, yet they still failed to reveal any adverse bioeffect.

CONCLUSIONS

There has been increased public awareness and concern regarding bioeffects of gradient magnetic fields (47), which should be met with a review of the known data and maintenance of reasonable limits and standards of application of this technology. Certainly this issue must be revisited again as the maximum strengths and the rise time capabilities (dB/dt) of the newer and faster MR systems continue to improve. Similarly, these considerations should be foremost in the mind for those patients in whom there are electrical conductors in anatomically sensitive locations, such as epicardial or retained intracardiac pacer wires, because the generated current densities may be sufficiently high in these anatomic areas and in these patients to exceed thresholds for biologic detectability for some functions. Although there have been numerous studies that have failed to reveal any adverse bioeffects related to exposure to gradient magnetic fields, there have been a few whose outcomes have raised questions regarding potential interactions between some biologic functions and the gradient magnetic field component of an MR imaging examination. Thus, as the years pass and as the field of MR continues to progress, the potential safety issues related to gradient magnetic fields promises to be of greater concern and will bear watching with even further scrutiny.

REFERENCES

1. Bottomley P, Edelstein W. Power deposition in whole body NMR imaging. *Med Physics* 1981;8:510–512.
2. Schaefer D. Safety aspects of magnetic resonance imaging. In: Wehrli F, Shaw D, Kneeland B, eds. *Biomedical magnetic resonance imaging: principles, methodology, and applications.* New York: VCH Publishers; 1988:553–578.
3. Persson B, Stahlberg F. Extremely low frequency (ELF) magnetic fields. In: Persson B, Stahlberg F, eds. *Health and safety of clinical NMR examination.* Boca Raton, Fla: CRC Press; 1989:49.
4. Schaefer D. Dosimetry and effects of MR exposure to RF and switched magnetic fields. In: Liburdy R, Persson B, eds. *Biological effects and safety aspects of nuclear magnetic resonance imaging and spectroscopy.* New York: The New York Academy of Sciences; 1992;649: 225–236.
5. Reilly J. Peripheral nerve stimulation by induced electrical currents: exposure to time-varying magnetic fields. *Med Biol Eng Comput* 1989;27:101–110.
6. Reilly J. Principles of nerve and heart excitation by time varying magnetic fields. In: Magin R, Liburdy R, Persson B, eds. *Biological effects and safety aspects of nuclear magnetic resonance imaging and spectroscopy.* New York: The New York Academy of Sciences; 1992;649:96–117.
7. Reilly J. Excitation models. In: Reilly J, ed. *Electrical stimulation and electropathology.* Cambridge: Cambridge University Press; 1992:95–132.
8. McRobbie D, Foster M. Thresholds for biological effects of time-varying magnetic fields. *Clin Phys Physiol Meas* 1984;5:67–78.
9. Yamagata H, Kuhara S, Seo Y, Sato K, Hiwaki O, Ueno S. Evaluation of dB/dt thresholds for nerve stimulation elicited by trapezoidal and sinusoidal gradient fields in echo-planar imaging. In: *Book of Abstracts, Society of Magnetic Resonance in Medicine.* Berkeley, CA: Society of Magnetic Resonance in Medicine; 1991:1277.
10. Budinger T, Fischer H, Hentschel D, Reinfelder HE, Schmitt F. Physiologic effects of fast oscillating magnetic field gradients. *J Comput Assist Tomogr* 1991;15:909–914.

11. FDA. Federal Register: guidance for content and review of a magnetic resonance diagnostic device 510(k) application. 1988.
12. Guidance update for dB/dt for the "Guidance for content and review of a magnetic resonance diagnostic device 510(k) application" document. Office of Device Evaluation/Center for Devices and Radiological Health. Robert A. Phillips, Computed Imaging Devices Branch. Rockville, MD, Oct. 11, 1995.
13. Budinger T. Nuclear magnetic resonance (NMR) in vivo studies: known thresholds for health effects. *J Comput Assist Tomogr* 1981;5:800–811.
14. Budinger T, Cullander C. Biophysical phenomena and health hazards of in vivo magnetic resonance. In: Margulis A, Higgins C, Kaufman L, Crooks L, eds. *Clinical magnetic resonance imaging.* San Francisco: Radiology Research and Education Foundation; 1983:303–320.
15. Budinger T. Thresholds for physiological effects due to RF and magnetic fields used in NMR imaging. *IEEE Trans Nucl Sci* 1979;NS-26:2821–2825.
16. Tenforde T, Budinger T. Biological effects and physical safety aspects of NMR imaging and in vivo spectroscopy. In: Thomas S, Dixon R, eds. *NMR in medicine: instrumentation and clinical applications.* New York: American Association of Physicists in Medicine; 1986:493–548. (Medical Monograph No. 14)
17. Dalziel C. *Trans AIEEE* 1960;79:667.
18. McRobbie D, Foster M. Cardiac response to pulsed magnetic fields with regard to safety in NMR imaging. *Phys Med Biol* 1985;30:695–702.
19. Reilly J. Stimulation via electrical and magnetic fields. In: Reilly J, ed. *Electrical stimulation and electropathology.* Cambridge: Cambridge University Press; 1992:328–382.
20. Smith M, Tassone R, Mosher T. Potential health risk due to cardiac applications of echo planar imaging. In: Magin R, Liburdy R, Persson B, eds. *Biological effects and safety aspects of nuclear magnetic resonance imaging and spectroscopy.* New York: The New York Academy of Sciences; 1992:359–362.
21. Fink M. *Convulsive therapy: theory and practice.* New York: Raven Press; 1979.
22. Hayes D, Holmes D, Gray J, et al. Effect of a 1.5 T nuclear magnetic resonance imaging on implanted permanent pacemakers. *J Am Coll Cardiol* 1987;10:782–786.
23. Kanal E, Shellock FG, Talagala L. Safety considerations in MR imaging. *Radiology* 1990;176: 593–606.
24. Yuh W, Fisher D, Shields R, Ehrhardt J, Shellock FG. Phantom limb pain induced in amputees by strong magnetic fields. *J Magn Reson Imag* 1992;2:221–223.
25. Kanal E, Shellock FG, Sonnenblick D. MRI clinical site safety survey: Phase I results and preliminary data. *Magn Reson Imag* 1988;7(S1):106.
26. Mansfield P, Harvey P. Limits to neural stimulation in echo planar imaging. *Magn Reson Med* 1993;29:746–758.
27. Irnich W. Magnetostimulation in MRI. In: *Book of Abstracts, Society of Magnetic Resonance in Medicine.* Berkeley, CA: Society of Magnetic Resonance in Medicine; 1993;3:1372.
28. d'Arsonval M. Action physiologique des courants alternatifs a grande frequence. *Arch Physiol* 1983;5:401.
29. Magnusson C, Stevens H. Visual sensations caused by changes in the strength of a magnetic field. *Am J Physiol* 1911;29:124–136.
30. Lovsund P, Nillson S, Reuter T, Oberg P. Magnetophosphenes: a quantitative analysis of thresholds. *Med Biol Eng Comp* 1980;18:326–334.
31. Barlow H, Kohn H, Walsh E. Visual sensations aroused by magnetic fields. *Am J Physiol* 1947;148:372–375.
32. Redington R, Dumoulin C, Schenck J, et al. MR imaging and bioeffects on a whole body 4.0 Tesla imaging system. In: *Book of Abstracts, Society of Magnetic Resonance in Medicine.* Berkeley, CA: Society of Magnetic Resonance in Medicine; 1988;1:4.
33. Ehrhardt J, Lin CS, Magnotta V, Fisher D, Yuh W. Neural stimulation in a whole body echo-planar imaging system. In: *Book of Abstracts, Society of Magnetic Resonance in Medicine;* Berkeley, CA: Society of Magnetic Resonance in Medicine; 1993;3:1372.
34. Cohen M, Weisskoff R, Redzian R, Kantor H. Sensory stimulation by time-varying magnetic fields. *Magn Reson Med* 1990;14:409–414.
35. Fischer H. Physiologic effects by fast oscillating magnetic field gradients. *Radiology* 1989;173(P):382.
36. Budinger T, Fischer H, Hentschel T, Reinfelder HE, Schmitt F. Neural stimulation dB/dt

thresholds for frequency and number of oscillations using sinusoidal magnetic gradient fields. In: *Book of Abstracts, Society of Magnetic Resonance in Medicine.* Berkeley, CA: Society of Magnetic Resonance in Medicine; 1990; 1:276.

37. Gore J, McDonnell M, Pennock J, Stanbrook H. An assessment of the safety of rapidly changing magnetic fields in the rabbit: implications for NMR imaging. *Magn Reson Imag* 1982; 1: 191–195.
38. Teskey G, Prato F, Ossenkopp KP, Kavaliers M. Exposure to time varying magnetic fields associated with magnetic resonance imaging reduces fentanyl-induced analgesia in mice. *Bioelectromagnetics* 1988; 9:167–174.
39. Prato F, Ossenkopp KP, Kavaliers M, Sestini E, Teskey G. Attenuation of morphine-induced analgesia in mice by exposure to MRI: differential effects of static radiofrequency and time-varying magnetic fields components. *Magn Reson Imag* 1987; 5:9–14.
40. Garber H, Oldendorf W, Braun L, Lufkin R. MRI gradient fields increase in brain mannitol space. *Magn Reson Imag* 1989; 7:605–610.
41. Peeling J, Lewis J, Samoiloff M, Bock E, Tomchuk E. Biological effects of magnetic fields: chronic exposure of the nematode *Panagrellus Redivivus. Magn Reson Imag* 1988; 6:655–660.
42. Weiss J, Herrick RC, Taber KH, Contant C, Plisker GA. Bio-effects of high magnetic fields: a study using a simple animal model. *Magn Reson Imag* 1992; 10:689–694.
43. Prasad N, Wright D, Ford J, Thornby J. Safety of 4 T MR imaging: study of effects on developing frog embryos. *Radiology* 1990; 174:251–253.
44. Prasad N, Lotzova E, Thornby J, Madewell J, Ford J, Bushong S. Effects of MR imaging on murine natural killer cell cytotoxicity. *AJR Am J Roentgenol* 1987; 148:415–417.
45. Prasad N, Lotzova E, Thornby J, Tabor K. The effects of 2.35-T MR imaging on natural killer cell cytotoxicity with and without interleukin-2. *Radiology* 1990; 175:261–263.
46. McRobbie D, Foster M. Pulsed magnetic field exposure during pregnancy and implications for NMR foetal imaging: a study with mice. *Magn Reson Imag* 1985; 3:231–234.
47. Egerter D. MR nerve stimulation: new safety concern? *Diagn Imag* 1990;August:127–131.

3

Bioeffects of Radiofrequency Electromagnetic Fields

Radiofrequency (RF) radiation is defined as nonionizing electromagnetic radiation in the frequency range of 0 to 3,000 GHz, as distinguished from the very high photon energies and frequencies associated with ionizing electromagnetic radiation (e.g., gamma and x-rays) (1–4). The RF spectrum includes radar, ultra high frequency (UHF) and very high frequency (VHF) television, AM and FM radio, and microwave communication frequencies.

Research studies conducted over the past 30 years have reported that exposure to RF radiation may produce various physiologic effects including alterations in visual, auditory, endocrine, neural, cardiovascular, immune, reproductive, and developmental functions (1–4). These biologic changes are generally felt to occur because of RF radiation–induced heating of tissues (1–10).

During MR procedures, most of the RF power transmitted for imaging or spectroscopy (especially for carbon decoupling) is transformed into heat within the patient's tissue as a result of resistive losses (11–21). Not surprisingly, the primary bioeffects associated with the RF radiation used for MR procedures are directly related to the thermogenic qualities of this electromagnetic field (11–21).

Exposure to RF radiation may also cause athermal, field-specific alterations in biologic systems that are produced without a substantial elevation in temperature (1,4,5,22). The athermal bioeffects of RF radiation are somewhat controversial because of assertions concerning the role of electromagnetic fields in causing cancer as well as developmental abnormalities, along with the concomitant ramifications of such effects (1,4,5,8,22).

A report from the U.S. Environmental Protection Agency indicated that the existing evidence on this issue is sufficient to demonstrate a relationship between chronic exposures to low level, electromagnetic fields and cancer (8). Therefore, there is an ongoing effort to determine if there is any association between exposure to athermal levels of RF radiation and the abnormalities described above. To date, no research has been performed to investigate the potential athermal bioeffects of RF radiation associated with MR procedures. Those interested in thorough discussions of this topic are referred to extensive reviews written by Adey (5) and Beers (22).

Before 1985, there were no published reports concerning the thermal and other physiologic responses of human subjects exposed to RF radiation during MR procedures. In fact, there has been a general lack of quantitative data on thermal responses of human subjects exposed to RF radiation from any source. The previous investigations performed on this topic typically examined physiologic responses to therapeutic applications of diathermy or the thermal sensations related to exposure to RF radiation (1,3,4,23,24). These studies usually involved exposures to RF energy that were limited or localized to small regions of the body.

Although there have been many investigations performed using laboratory animals to determine thermoregulatory reactions to tissue heating associated with exposure to RF radiation, these experiments do not directly apply to the conditions that occur during MR procedures, nor can they be extrapolated to provide useful information for various reasons (2,3). For example, the pattern of RF absorption or the coupling of radiation to biologic tissues primarily depends on the organism's size, anatomic features, the duration of exposure, the sensitivity of the involved tissues (e.g., some tissues are more "thermal sensitive" than others), and a myriad of other variables (1,3,4,17,25). Furthermore, there is no laboratory animal that sufficiently mimics or simulates the thermoregulatory responses of an organism with the dimensions and specific responses to that of a human subject. Therefore, experimental results obtained in laboratory animals cannot be simply "scaled" or extrapolated to predict thermoregulatory or other physiologic changes in human subjects exposed to RF radiation–induced heating during MR procedures (17,18,25).

Elaborate mathematic models have been devised to predict "worst-case" scenarios of how human subjects may respond to the RF energy that is absorbed during MR procedures (26–28). A recognized major limitation of modeling is that it is difficult to account for the numerous critical variables (i.e., the subject's age, the amount of subcutaneous fat, the physical condition of the individual) that can affect the thermoregulatory responses of human subjects. Many individuals that are exposed to RF radiation during MR procedures have some underlying health condition (e.g., hypertension, diabetes, cardiovascular disease, etc.) or are taking medication(s) (e.g., β-blockers, calcium blockers, vasodilators, vasoconstrictors, tranquilizers, sedatives, etc.) that can alter or seriously impair their ability to dissipate a heat load. More importantly, none of the mathematic models developed to predict thermal responses to RF radiation have ever been validated by experiments performed in human subjects or, more importantly, in a patient population.

Several investigations have been performed directly in human subjects in recent years that have yielded extremely useful and important data about the thermoregulatory responses and other physiologic reactions to the tissue heating produced by RF radiation during MR procedures (14,18,21). This chapter will review and discuss these studies.

CHARACTERISTICS OF RF RADIATION–INDUCED HEATING DURING MR PROCEDURES

The physical dimensions and configuration of the tissue in relation to the incident wavelength are important factors that determine the relative amount and pattern of energy that is absorbed during exposure to RF radiation (1–4). If the tissue size is large in relation to the incident wavelength, energy is predominantly absorbed on the surface (1–4). If it is small relative to the wavelength, there is little absorption of RF power (1–4).

The most efficient absorption of RF energy occurs when the tissue is approximately 50% the size of the incident wavelength; this frequency of maximum absorption is known as the "resonant frequency." Exposure to a resonant frequency of RF power is the most hazardous from a bioeffects standpoint because of deep and often uneven absorption patterns (1–4). Because of the aforementioned factors, RF radiation–induced heating is considered to be a unique means of elevating the tissue temperature because of its ability to penetrate superficial tissues and directly heat internal sites of the body at certain wavelengths (2–3).

Tissue heating that results from the RF radiation used for MR procedures is primarily caused by magnetic induction, with a negligible contribution from the electric fields (11–20). Therefore, the "ohmic heating" of tissue during MR procedures is greatest at the surface or periphery and minimal at the center of the body of human subjects (Fig. 3-1). Predictive calculations and measurements obtained in phantoms and in human subjects exposed to MR imaging support this pattern of temperature distribution (11–20).

The actual increase in tissue temperature caused by exposure to RF radiation depends on a variety of factors associated with the thermoregulatory system of the individual and the surrounding environment (2,3,14–18). With regard to the thermoregulatory system, when subjected to a thermal challenge the human body loses heat by means of convection, conduction, radiation, and evaporation. Each of these mechanisms is responsible to a varying degree for heat dissipation as the body attempts to maintain thermal homeostasis (2,3). If the thermoregulatory effectors are not capable of totally dissipating the heat load, then an accumulation or storage of heat occurs, along with an elevation in local and/or overall tissue temperatures (2,3).

As previously mentioned, there are various underlying health conditions that may affect an individual's ability to tolerate a thermal challenge. These conditions include cardiovascular disease, hypertension, diabetes, fever, old age, and obesity (29–35). Various medications (diuretics, β-blockers, calcium blockers, amphetamines, muscle relaxers, sedatives) can also alter the thermoregulatory

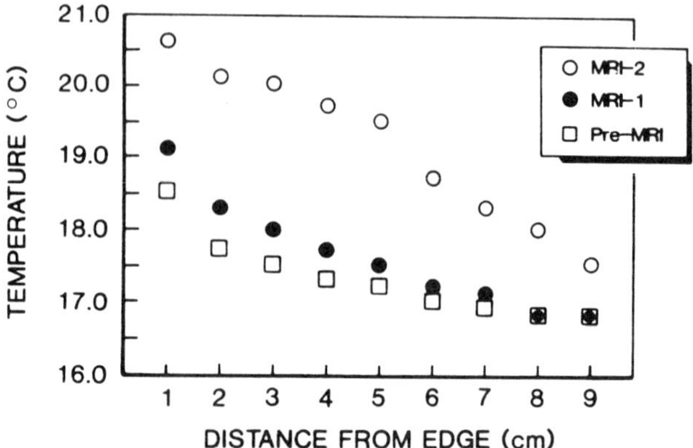

FIG. 3-1. MR imaging was performed on a spherical, seedless watermelon (diameter, 24 cm) to study the depth of temperature changes related to RF radiation–induced heating. Thermistor needles were inserted into the watermelon immediately before (*opened square*) and after MR imaging performed with a 1.5 T/64 MHz MR system using a quadrature transmit/receive body coil at whole-body–averaged SARs of 1.0 W/kg (*closed circle*) and 2.5 W/kg (*opened circle*) for 30 min. Room temperature was 20.5°C and relative humidity was 45%. The temperature plots show that there is predominantly surface or peripheral heating that occurs under these experimental conditions.

responses to a heat load. Of note is that certain medications have a synergistic effect with respect to tissue heating if the heating is caused by exposure to RF radiation (36,37). In consideration of the above, investigations designed to evaluate thermal responses in human subjects exposed to RF electromagnetic fields during clinical MR procedures must include data derived from patient subjects with health conditions in order to assess their specific responses, in addition to those reactions of patients with normal thermoregulatory function.

The environmental conditions that exist in and around the MR system will also affect the tissue temperature changes that occur during RF radiation–induced heating. During an MR procedure, the amount of tissue heating that occurs and concomitant exposure to RF energy that is tolerable depend on environmental factors that include the ambient temperature, relative humidity, and air flow.

With respect to the environmental conditions of the MR setting, it has been proposed that, in order to counterbalance any excessive tissue heating that may occur during exposure to high levels of RF energy, patients should be "pre-cooled" before performance of certain MR procedures (unpublished communication, 1994). However, it should be noted that the subjective perception of human subjects to the environmental temperature depends on the gradient of temperature that is sensed by the peripheral thermoreceptors. Therefore, patients going from a cooler (i.e., the "pre-cooling" room) to a warmer environment (i.e., the MR system) would likely be more uncomfortable. Preliminary data obtained during recently performed experiments supports this contention (unpublished observations, 1994).

MR PROCEDURES AND THE SPECIFIC ABSORPTION RATE (SAR) OF RF RADIATION

The thermoregulatory and other physiologic changes that a human subject displays in response to exposure to RF radiation depend on the amount of energy that is absorbed. The dosimetric term used to describe the absorption of RF radiation is the "specific absorption rate," or SAR (1–4). The SAR is the mass normalized rate at which RF power is coupled to biologic tissue and is typically indicated in units of watts per kilogram (W/kg) (1–4). The relative amount of RF radiation that an individual encounters during an MR procedure is usually characterized with respect to the whole-body–averaged and peak SAR levels (i.e., the SAR averaged in 1 g of tissue) of the exposure.

Measurements or estimates of SAR are not trivial, particularly in human subjects, and there are several methods of determining this parameter for the purpose of RF energy dosimetry associated with MR procedures (11–21). The SAR that is produced during an MR procedure is a complex function of numerous variables including the frequency (which, in turn, is determined by the static magnetic field strength), the type of RF pulse used (i.e., 90° or 180°), the repetition time, the pulse width, the type of RF coil used (i.e., transmit/receive body coil or send/receive surface coil), the volume of tissue contained within the coil, the resistivity of the tissue, the configuration of the anatomical region exposed, the orientation of the body to the field vectors, as well as other factors (11–21).

RECOMMENDED SAFE LEVELS OF EXPOSURE TO RF RADIATION DURING AN MR PROCEDURE

The United States Food and Drug Administration (FDA) is responsible for providing guidelines and recommendations for the safe use of MR systems. In 1988, MR systems were reclassified from class III, in which premarket approval is required, to class II, which is regulated by performance standards, as long as the MR system is within the "umbrella" of certain defined limits (38). Subsequent to this reclassification, new MR systems had only to demonstrate that they were "substantially equivalent" to any class II device that was brought to market using the premarket notification process (510[k]) or, alternatively, to any of the devices described by the various MR system manufacturers that had petitioned the FDA for such a reclassification.

Currently, the FDA provides recommendations for two alternative safe levels of exposure to RF radiation during MR procedures, primarily in an effort to control the risk of systemic thermal overload and local thermal injury. Either the following specific SAR levels or temperature criteria may be adhered to by MR health care practitioners performing MR procedures, as follows (38):

1. The exposure to RF energy below the level of concern is an SAR of 0.4 W/kg or less averaged over the body, and 8.0 W/kg or less spatial peak in any 1 g of tissue, and 3.2 W/kg or less averaged over the head; or
2. the exposure to RF energy that is insufficient to produce a core temperature increase of 1°C and localized heating to no greater than 38°C in the head, 39°C in the trunk, and 40°C in the extremities, except for patients with impaired systemic blood flow and/or perspiration (i.e., patients with compromised thermoregulatory systems).

The above exposure levels apply to normal clinical environments where the individual is resting and lightly dressed. For clinical MR systems, the exposures to RF radiation during MR procedures must be below either of the above two levels of concern by presentation of valid scientific measurement or calculational evidence sufficient to demonstrate that RF heating effects are of no concern (38).

ASSESSMENT OF THERMAL AND OTHER PHYSIOLOGIC RESPONSES TO RF RADIATION-INDUCED HEATING DURING AN MR PROCEDURE

Obtaining thermal and other physiologic measurements in human subjects within the harsh electromagnetic environment associated with the MR system is not a simple task. The strong static magnetic fields of the MR systems can easily create missiles out of monitoring devices because they usually contain ferromagnetic components (39–42). In addition, the static, gradient, and RF electromagnetic fields may adversely interfere with the proper operation of the monitor (39–42). In turn, the monitors themselves may produce subtle or significant imaging artifacts during operation by generating "RF noise" that can significantly distort the quality of the MR images (39–42). In consideration of the above, monitors must be specially adapted or modified and then rigorously tested before use in the MR environment (see Chapter 7 for additional information). Otherwise, the data pertaining to thermal and other physiologic responses may be erroneous.

Currently, there are a variety of MR-compatible monitors as well as other patient support devices that are commercially available for use in the MR environment (39–42). Every physiologic parameter that is obtainable under normal circumstances in the critical care area or operating room may be recorded during an MR procedure, including heart rate, oxygen saturation, end-tidal carbon dioxide, respiratory rate, blood pressure, cutaneous blood flow and, most importantly, body and skin temperatures (39–42).

For assessment of thermal responses during an MR procedure, volunteer subjects or patients have been continuously or semicontinuously monitored throughout the experimental procedures using several types of devices. For example, in various research studies, sublingual pocket or tympanic membrane temperature (note that there is a good relationship between temperatures measured in the sublingual pocket or tympanic membrane and esophageal temperatures—an indicator of "deep" body or "core" temperature) were typically obtained immediately before and after MR procedures using sensitive electronic thermometry or infrared devices (43–53). Skin temperatures were measured immediately before and after MR procedures using highly sensitive and accurate infrared thermometry or thermographic equipment (43–53). Body and skin temperatures measured at multiple sites were recorded before, during, and after MR procedures using a fluoroptic thermometry system that is unperturbed by electromagnetic radiation of all types, including static magnetic fields of up to 9.0 T (42). Heart rate, oxygen saturation, blood pressure, respiratory rate, and cutaneous blood flow, which are important physiologic variables that change in response to a thermal load, were typically monitored before, during, and after MR procedures to assess the reaction of the thermoregulatory system of human subjects exposed to RF radiation–induced heating. All these parameters were obtained with MR-compatible devices that have been extensively tested and demonstrated to provide sensitive and accurate data (43–53).

THERMAL AND OTHER PHYSIOLOGIC RESPONSES TO RF RADIATION–INDUCED HEATING DURING AN MR PROCEDURE

As previously mentioned, the increase in tissue temperature caused by exposure to RF energy during an MR procedure depends on multiple physiologic, physical, and environmental factors including the status of the patient's thermoregulatory system, underlying health conditions, duration of exposure, the rate at which energy is deposited, the ambient temperature, humidity, and airflow over and around the patient within the MR system. Although the primary cause of tissue heating during MR procedures is attributed solely to RF radiation, it should be noted that various reports have suggested that exposure to static magnetic fields used for MR procedures may also cause temperature changes (54,55).

The mechanism(s) responsible for such an effect remains unclear, but the results of these studies have warranted investigations in human subjects to determine if there is any contribution of the static magnetic field to the temperature changes that may be observed during an MR procedure. Therefore, studies have been conducted in human subjects exposed to a 1.5-T static magnetic field to determine if there was any effect on body and/or skin temperatures (56,57). The data revealed that there were no statistically significant alterations observed in any of the recorded temperature or other physiologic parameters (56,57). Tenforde (58) examined this phenomenon as well in laboratory animals exposed to static magnetic fields of as high as 7.55 T and also reported no effect. As far as the potential for production of heat by gradient magnetic fields is concerned, this is not believed to occur as a result of exposure to conventional pulse sequences used for clinical MR procedures (15).

The first study of human thermal responses to RF radiation–induced heating during an MR procedure was conducted by Schaefer et al. (59). Temperature changes and other physiologic alterations were assessed in volunteer subjects exposed to relatively high whole-body–averaged SARs (i.e., approximately 4.0 W/kg). The data indicated that there were no excessive temperature elevations or other deleterious physiologic consequences related to this exposure to RF radiation (59).

Several studies were subsequently conducted involving volunteer subjects and patients undergoing clinical MR procedures with the intent of obtaining information that would be applicable to the patient population typically encountered in the MR setting (43–45,47,50,52,59–62). The whole-body–averaged SARs ranged from approximately 0.05 W/kg (i.e., for MR procedures involving imaging with a transmit/receive head coil) to 4.0 W/kg (i.e., for MR procedures involving the imaging of the spine or abdomen with a transmit/receive body coil) (43–52). These studies demonstrated that changes in body temperatures were relatively minor (i.e., <0.6°C) (Figs. 3-2–3-6). There tended to be statistically significant increases in skin temperatures that were also of no serious physiologic consequence. Furthermore, there were no associated deleterious alterations in any of the hemodynamic parameters that were assessed during these investigations (i.e., heart rate, blood pressure, and cutaneous blood flow).

Of further note is that there was a poor correlation between body or skin temperature changes versus whole-body–averaged SARs during clinical MR imaging (Fig. 3-2). This is not unusual considering all the variables that may alter thermal responses in a patient population. Therefore, the thermal reactions to a given SAR may be quite variable depending on the individual's own thermoregulatory system and the presence of one or more underlying condition(s) that may alter or impair the ability to dissipate heat. In consideration of the above, it would appear that the safety criteria for exposure to RF radiation indicated by the FDA that relies on temperature changes is the more appropriate and meaningful parameter to adhere to as opposed to whole-body–averaged or peak SAR levels.

An extensive thermophysiology investigation using multiple fluoroptic thermometry probes that are unperturbed by electromagnetic fields demonstrated that human subjects with normal thermoregulatory systems exposed to MR imaging at whole-body–averaged SAR levels up to 4.0 W/kg [i.e., 10 times higher than the level currently recommended by the United States Food and Drug Administration (38)] had no statistically significant increases in body temperatures and have statistically significant elevations in skin temperatures that were not excessive (50) (Fig. 3-7). The results of this study indicated that the

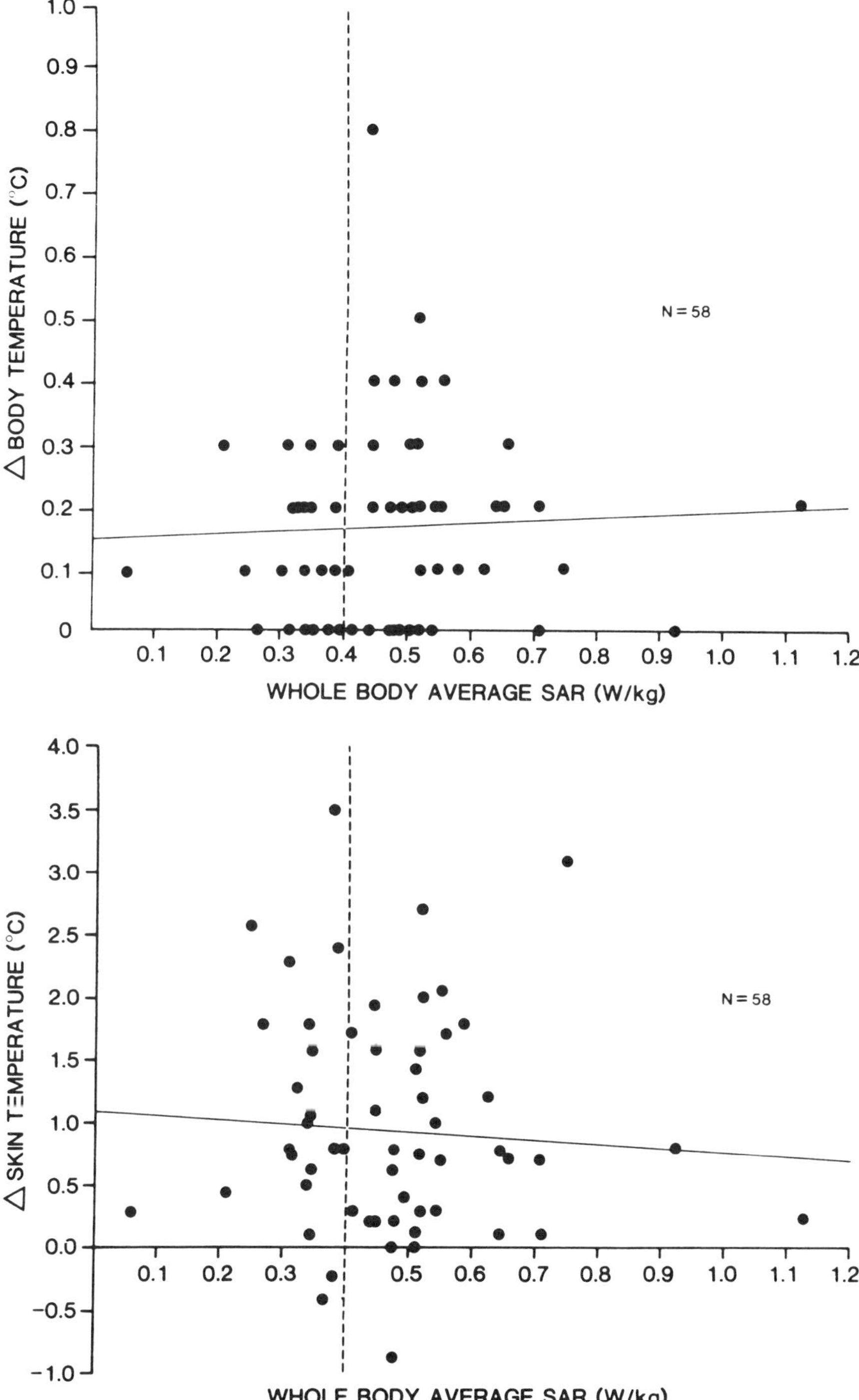

FIG. 3-2. Top: Changes in body temperature versus whole-body–averaged SARs during clinical MR imaging procedures. Note that there is a poor correlation between these two variables. **Bottom:** Changes in skin temperature versus whole-body–averaged SARs during clinical MR imaging procedures. Note that there is a poor correlation between these two variables.

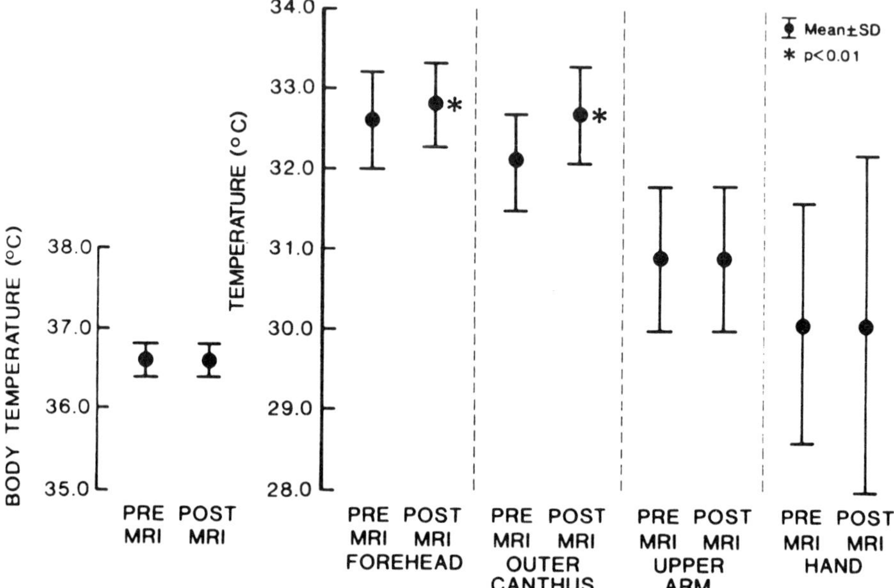

FIG. 3-3. Average body (sublingual pocket) temperature, forehead skin temperature, outer canthus skin temperature, upper arm skin temperature, and hand skin temperature measured immediately before and after clinical MR imaging of the brain at 1.5 T/64 MHz using a head coil. There were statistically significant increases ($p < 0.01$) in body, forehead skin, and outer canthus skin temperatures (see ref. 47).

SAR recommendations issued by the FDA for exposure to RF radiation for patients with normal thermoregulatory function may be too conservative (50).

An extensive research study was performed in volunteer subjects exposed to MR imaging performed at a whole-body–averaged SAR of 6.0 W/kg in cool (22°C) and warm (33°C) environments in order to characterize thermal and other physiologic responses to this high exposure to RF energy because some of the newly developed pulse sequences have very high SARs associated with their use (53). To date, this has been the highest level of RF power to which human subjects have ever been exposed.

Tympanic membrane temperature, six skin temperatures, heart rate, blood pressure, oxygen saturation, and skin blood flow were monitored before, during, and after exposure to the RF energy (Fig. 3-8). In the cool environment, there were statistically significant increases in tympanic membrane, abdomen, upper arm, hand, and thigh temperatures as well as heart rate and skin blood flow. In the warm environment, there were statistically significant increases in tympanic membrane, hand, and chest temperatures as well as systolic blood pressure and heart rate. Each of the temperature increases recorded were within FDA guidelines (38,53). These data indicate that MR imaging performed at 6.0

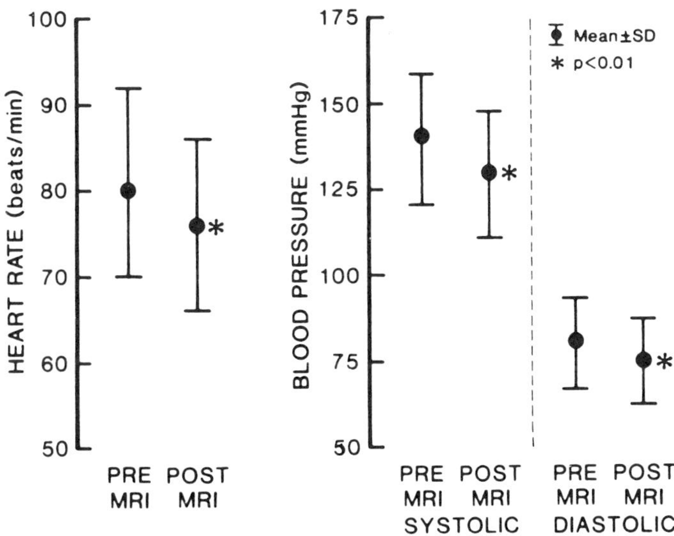

FIG. 3-4. Average heart rate, systolic and diastolic blood pressures obtained immediately before and after MR imaging of the brain at 1.5 T/64 MHz using a head coil. There were statistically significant decreases in each of these measured parameters (see ref. 47).

W/kg can be physiologically tolerated by individuals with normal thermoregulatory function (53).

Of additional note is that the subjective perception of tissue heating was greater when the subjects underwent MR imaging at an SAR of 6.0 W/kg in the cool environment compared with their experience in the warm environment. This indicates that it would not be useful to precool subjects that will subsequently undergo high SAR procedures to help them better tolerate these procedures, as has been suggested by some researchers and manufacturers of MR systems.

MR PROCEDURES AND TEMPERATURE-SENSITIVE ORGANS

Certain human organs that have reduced capabilities for heat dissipation, such as the testis and eye, are particularly sensitive to elevated temperatures. Therefore, these are primary sites of potentially harmful effects if RF radiation exposures during MR procedures are excessive (11–18,21).

Testis

Laboratory investigations have demonstrated detrimental effects on testicular function (i.e., a reduction or cessation of spermatogenesis, impaired sperm

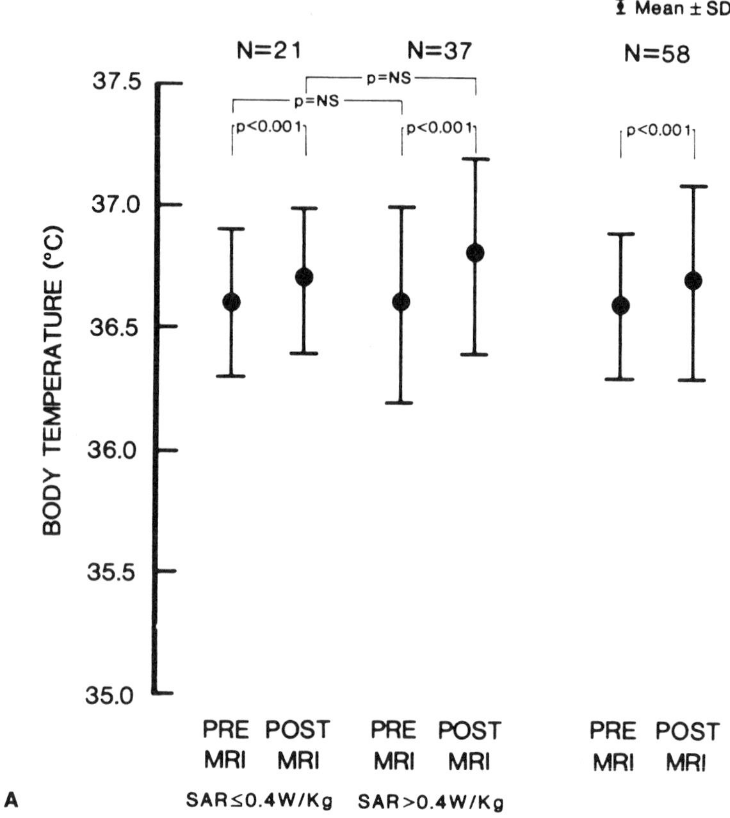

FIG. 3-5. Average body (sublingual pocket) temperature (**A**) and skin temperature (**B**) measured immediately before and after clinical MR imaging at 1.5 T/64 MHz. Data are displayed showing measured parameters during exposures to whole-body–averaged SARs above 0.4 W/kg, below 0.4 W/kg, and all the data combined (see ref. 43).

motility, degeneration of seminiferous tubules, etc.) caused by RF radiation–induced heating from exposures sufficient enough to raise scrotal and/or testicular tissue temperatures between 38 to 42°C (7). Scrotal skin temperatures (which are an index of intratesticular temperatures because a high correlation has been demonstrated between intratesticular and scrotal skin temperatures) (63) were measured in volunteer subjects undergoing MR imaging at a whole-body–averaged SAR of 1.1 W/kg (48). The largest change in scrotal skin temperature was 2.1°C and the highest scrotal skin temperature recorded was 34.2°C (48). These temperature changes were below the threshold known to impair testicular function (7,48). However, inordinately heating the scrotum during MR imaging could exacerbate certain pre-existing disorders associated with increased scrotal/testicular temperatures (e.g., acute febrile illnesses, vari-

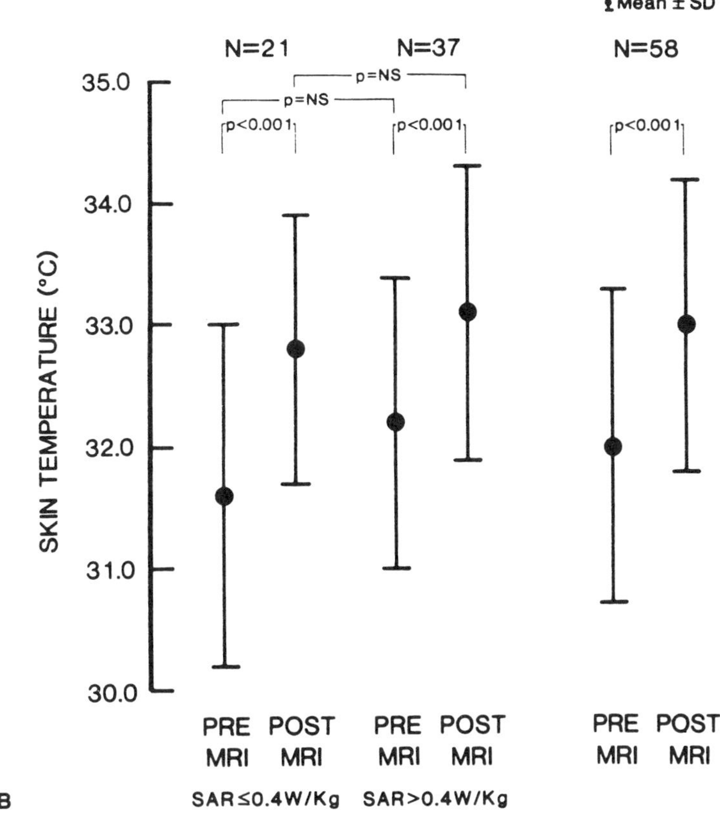

FIG. 3-5. *Continued.*

cocele, etc.) in patients who are already oligospermic and could lead to temporary or permanent sterility. Therefore, additional studies designed to investigate these issues are needed, particularly if patients are subjected to MR procedures that have associated SARs that are higher than those previously evaluated (which is entirely possible because there is a trend to use some of the newly developed pulse sequences to image the scrotum, such as fast spin echo or magnetization transfer contrast, which have associated high SARs).

Eye

Dissipation of heat from the eye is a slow and inefficient process because of its relative lack of vascularization (6). Acute near-field exposures of RF radiation to the eyes or heads of laboratory animals have been demonstrated to be

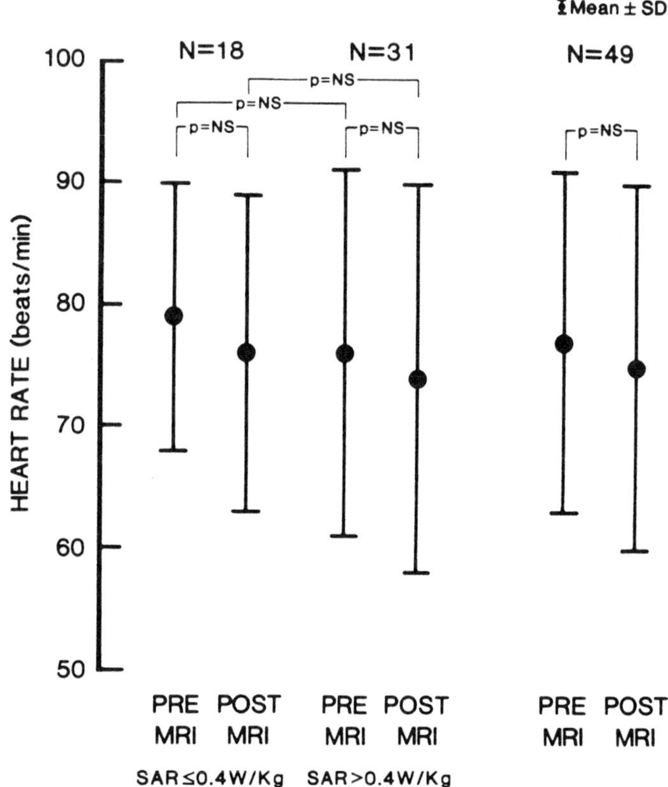

FIG. 3-6. Average heart rate (**A**) and mean blood pressure (**B**) obtained immediately before and after MR imaging at 1.5 T/64 MHz. Data are displayed showing measured parameters during exposures to whole-body–averaged SARs above 0.4 W/kg, below 0.4 W/kg, and all the data combined (see ref. 43).

cataractogenic as a result of the thermal disruption of ocular tissues if the exposure is of a sufficient intensity and duration (6). An investigation conducted by Sacks et al. (64) revealed that there were no discernible effects on the eyes of rats produced by MR procedures at exposures that far exceeded typical levels used in the clinical setting. However, as previously indicated, it may not be acceptable to extrapolate these data to human subjects considering the coupling of RF radiation to the anatomy and the tissue volume of laboratory rat eyes compared with those of human subjects.

Corneal temperatures (corneal temperature is a representative site of the average temperature of the human eye) (65) have been measured in patients undergoing MR imaging of the brain using a transmit/receive head coil at peak SARs of up to 3.1 W/kg (46). The largest corneal temperature change was 1.8°C and the highest temperature measured was 34.4°C. An additional study (49)

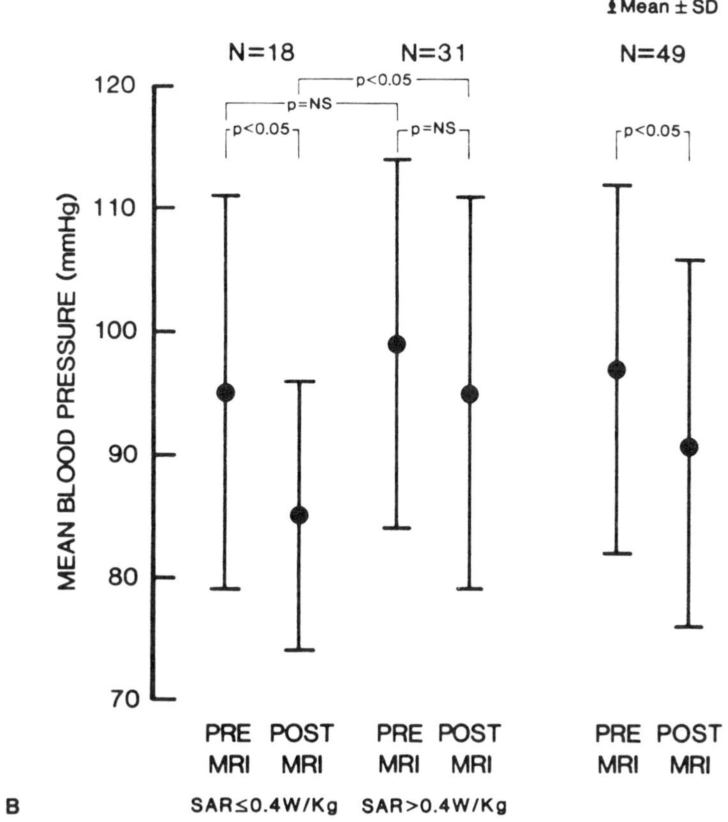

FIG. 3-5. *Continued.*

examined corneal temperatures in patients with suspected ocular pathology who underwent MR imaging using a special eye coil. Again, there were no excessive corneal temperature elevations. Because the temperature threshold for RF radiation–induced cataractogenesis in animal models has been demonstrated to be between 41 and 55°C for acute near-field exposures (6), it does not appear that clinical MR imaging using a head coil or an eye coil has the potential to cause thermal damage to ocular tissue. The effect of MR procedures performed using higher SARs on ocular tissue remains to be determined.

MR PROCEDURES AND "HOT SPOTS"

Theoretically, RF radiation "hot spots" caused by an uneven distribution of RF power may arise whenever current concentrations are produced in associa-

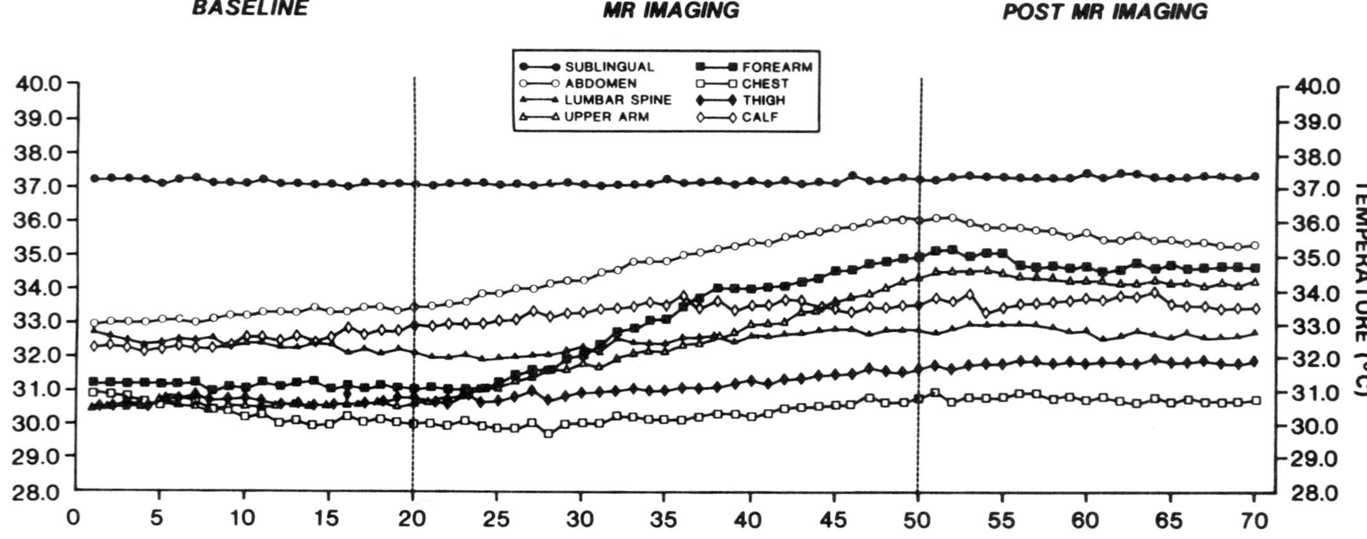

FIG. 3-7. Body (sublingual pocket) and multiple skin temperatures measured at 1-min intervals using a fluoroptic thermometry system (Luxtron) before (*baseline*), during (*MR imaging*), and after (*post-MR imaging*) MR imaging performed at whole-body–averaged SAR of 2.8 W/kg. Note that there was little or no change in sublingual or body temperature, whereas there were slight to moderate changes in skin temperatures (depending on the site of measurement) during MR imaging. After MRI, some skin temperatures returned to the baseline level, whereas others remained elevated during the 20-min post-MRI evaluation period (see ref. 50).

tion with restrictive conductive patterns (12–21). There has been the suggestion that RF radiation "hot spots" may occur during an MR procedure and generate thermal "hot spots" under certain conditions. Because RF radiation is mainly absorbed by peripheral tissues, thermography has been used to study the heating pattern associated with MR procedures performed at high whole-body–averaged SARs (44,60). This research demonstrated that there was no evidence of surface thermal "hot spots" related to performing MR imaging in human subjects. The thermoregulatory system apparently responds to the thermal load induced by RF radiation by distributing the heat, producing a "smearing" effect of the surface temperatures (44,60). However, there is a possibility that internal thermal "hot spots" may develop during an MR procedure. This issue needs to be thoroughly examined in human subjects undergoing MR procedures.

Shuman et al. (66) reported that significant temperature rises occur in internal organs of laboratory dogs produced during MR imaging performed high SARs. Of further note is that this study was conducted on anesthetized animals and is unlikely to be pertinent to conscious adult human subjects because of the previously discussed factors related to the physical dimensions of the animals, the fact that an anesthetic agent was used which may affect thermoregulation, as well as due to the dissimilar thermoregulatory systems of these two species. However, the data obtained by Shuman et al. (66) may have important implications for the use of MR procedures in pediatric patients because this patient population is typically sedated or anesthetized for MR examinations and certain physical dimensions of the dog are comparable to those of the pediatric population. Obviously, research is required to examine this issue more closely.

FUTURE STUDIES OF RF RADIATION–INDUCED HEATING DURING MR PROCEDURES

Several new pulse sequences and techniques have been developed and are currently undergoing clinical trials that use high levels of RF energy for their implementation (67,68). For example, the latest versions of the fast spin echo (FSE) and magnetization transfer contrast (MTC) pulse sequences may use SARs that easily exceed whole-body–averaged SARs ranging between 4.0 and 8.0 W/kg.

The FSE pulse sequences are hybrids of RARE (rapid acquisition relaxation enhanced) pulse sequences and have increased RF power depositions compared with conventional spin echoes (69). This is primarily due to the high density of 180° refocusing pulses used for these pulse sequences (69). MTC pulse sequences involve the use of selective and continuous saturation of macromolecular protons using an off-resonance RF pulse during the implementation of the technique (68). Again, the RF power deposition is of considerable concern. This is particularly a potential problem in MR imaging examinations that involve large body parts that require RF transmission using the body coil.

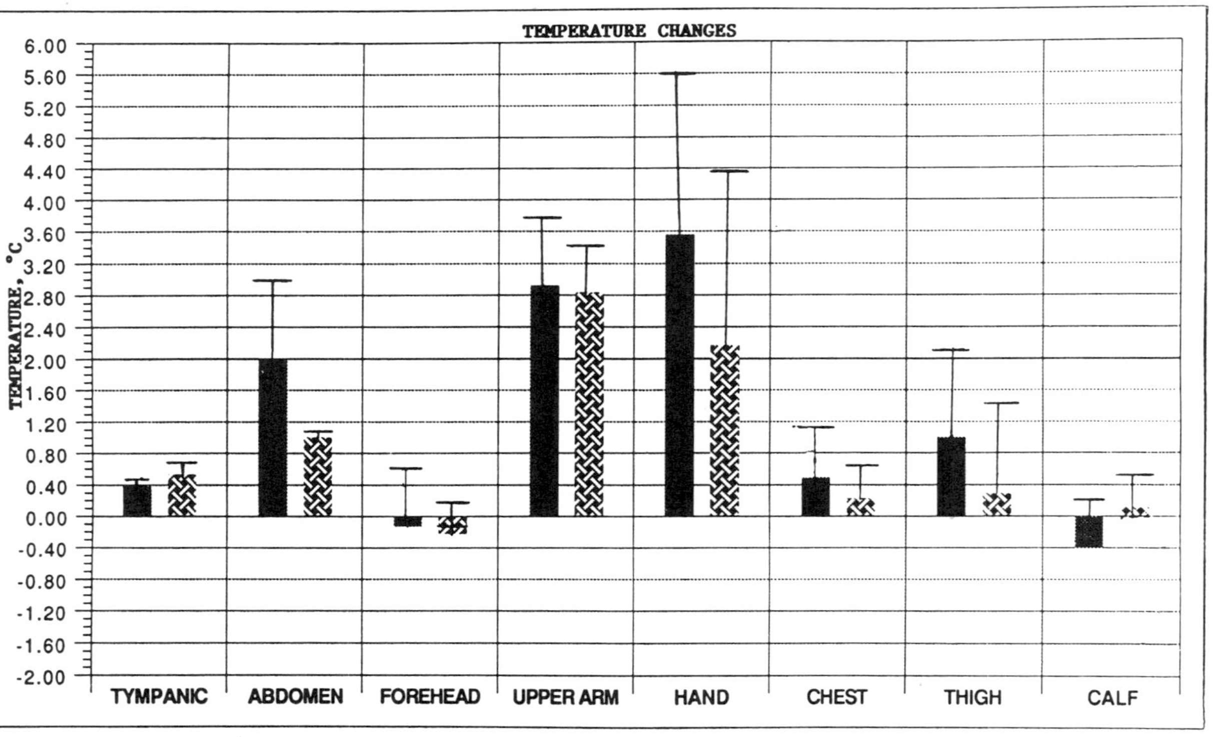

FIG. 3-8. Changes in body (tympanic membrane), abdomen, forehead, upper arm, hand, chest, thigh, and calf skin temperatures (**A**), systolic blood pressure, diastolic blood pressure, mean blood pressure, heart rate, oxygen saturation, and cutaneous blood flow (**B**) associated with MR imaging performed (n = 6 volunteer subjects) at a whole-body–averaged SAR of 6.0 W/kg in cool (22.5°C, closed bars) and warm (33.0°C, striped bars) environments (see ref. 53).

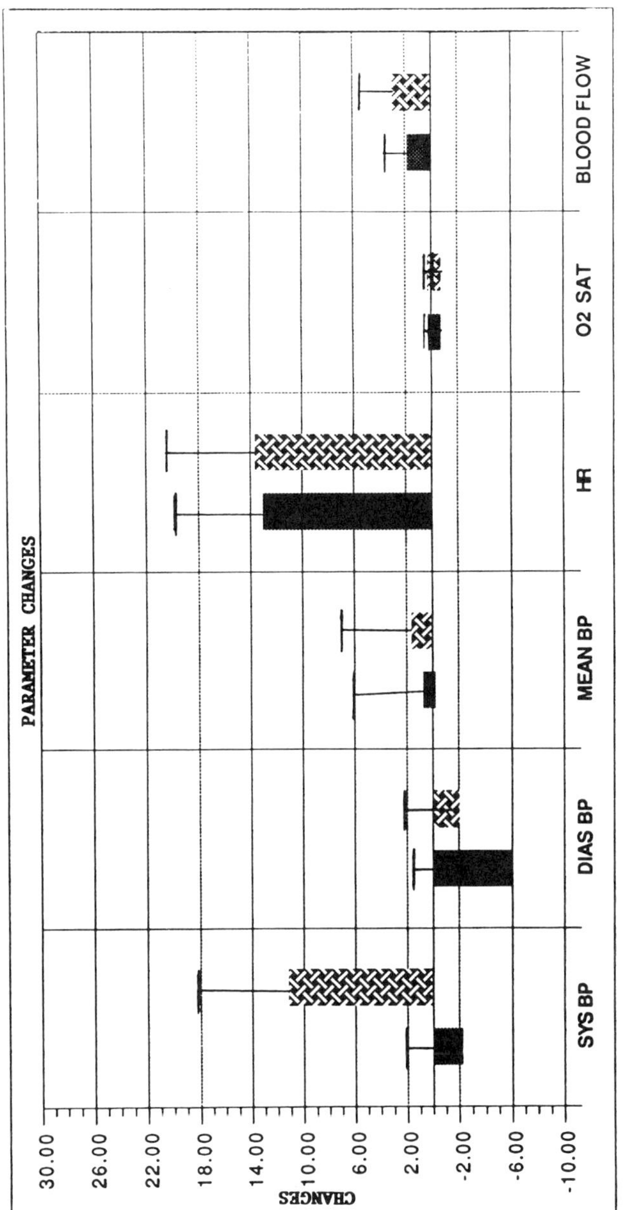

FIG. 3–8. *Continued.*

Both the FSE and MTC pulse sequences appear to offer important clinical advantages over conventional pulse sequences. However, before the FSE and MTC pulse sequences are routinely used for all clinical applications, investigations must be performed to assess and characterize thermal and other physiologic responses to the RF radiation–induced heating related to these new pulse sequences. Therefore, studies are currently examining the human thermoregulatory responses to SARs that are even higher than those that have been studied in recent years. Results from at least one investigation are encouraging with respect to the ability of individuals with normal thermoregulatory function to tolerate MR examinations that require high SARs (53).

Other MR procedures where RF radiation–induced heating may cause appreciable increases in tissue temperature include H-1 decoupling, Overhauser enhancement, and burst sequences used in MR spectroscopy. Therefore, these MR procedures will need to be evaluated to determine the relative safety of performing these applications in patient populations.

In addition, there are now several 3.0-, 4.0-, and one 4.57-T whole-body MR systems that are being used for a combination of imaging and spectroscopy applications in human subjects. These devices are capable of generating RF power depositions of approximately 7 to 15 times as much as that produced by a 1.5-T MR system for the same application (70,71). Investigations evaluating thermal responses in human subjects will also need to be performed to assess the safety of these powerful MR devices.

Additional studies are needed to assess thermal responses of patients with conditions or medications that may impair their ability to dissipate heat before subjecting them to MR procedures that require high SARs. There is currently an ongoing effort to characterize the thermal and other physiologic responses of these various patient groups to RF radiation–induced heating during MR examinations using high SARs.

Elevated body temperature is teratogenic in various animals, including primates (7,9,10). Research studies have shown that excessive heat may cause birth defects and prenatal mortality when the body temperature of the pregnant mother reaches 40 to 44°C (7,9,10). Lower, but still elevated, body temperatures may significantly increase the incidence of reduced body weight or cause physiologic changes or behavioral alterations (7,9,10). Increased temperatures that specifically result from exposure to RF radiation have been reported to adversely affect the developing embryo (7,9,10). To date there have been no studies designed to examine the thermal effects of RF radiation–induced heating during MR procedures performed in pregnant patients. Therefore, experiments will be needed to assess the potential adverse effects of RF radiation with respect to pregnant patients undergoing MR procedures.

REFERENCES

1. NCRP. Biological effects and exposure criteria for radiofrequency electromagnetic fields. Report No. 86. National Council on Radiation Protection and Measurements 1986. Bethesda, MD.

2. Gordon CJ. Thermal physiology. In: *Biological effects of radiofrequency radiation* 1984; 4-1–4-28. EPA-600/8-83-026A.
3. Gordon CJ. Effect of radiofrequency radiation exposure on thermoregulation. *ISI Atlas Sci Plants Anim* 1988;1:245–250.
4. Michaelson SM, Lin JC. *Biological effects and health implications of radiofrequency radiation.* New York: Plenum; 1987.
5. Adey WR. Tissue interactions with nonionizing electromagnetic fields. *Physiol Rev* 1981;61:435–514.
6. Elder JA. Special senses. In: *Biological effects of radiofrequency radiation,* 1984;5-64–5-78. EPA-600/8-83-026A.
7. Berman E. Reproductive effects. In: *Biological effects of radiofrequency radiation,* 1984;5-29–5-42. EPA-600/8-83-026A.
8. U.S. Environmental Protection Agency. Evaluation of Potential Electromagnetic Carcinogenicity. Office of Health and Environmental Assessment. U.S. Environmental Protection Agency, June 28, 1990 (EPA-600/6 90 005A).
9. O'Conner ME. Mammalian teratogenesis and radio-frequency fields. In: *Proceedings of the IEEE* 1980;68:56–60.
10. Lary JM, Conover DL. Teratogenic effects of radiofrequency radiatioin. *IEEE Eng Med Biol* 1987;44:42–46.
11. Edelman RR, Shellock FG, Ahladis J. Practical MRI for the technologist and imaging specialist. In: Edelman RR, Hesselink J, eds. *Clinical magnetic resonance.* Philadelphia: WB Saunders; 1990.
12. Persson BRR, Stahlberg F. *Health and safety of clinical NMR examinations.* Boca Raton, Fla: CRC Press; 1989.
13. Shellock FG, Crues JV. MRI: safety considerations in magnetic resonance imaging. *MRI Decisions* 1988;2:25–30.
14. Shellock FG. Biological effects and safety aspects of magnetic resonance imaging. *Magn Reson Q* 1989;5:243–261.
15. Kanal E, Shellock FG, Talagala L. Safety considerations in MR imaging. *Radiology* 1990;176:593–606.
16. Shellock FG, Crues JV. Biological effects and safety considerations of magnetic resonance imaging. In: *Magnetic resonance imaging syllabus.* American College of Radiology; 1991.
17. Shellock FG. MRI bioeffects and safety. In: Atlas S, ed. *Magnetic resonance imaging of the brain and spine.* New York: Raven Press; 1990.
18. Shellock FG. Thermal responses in human subjects exposed to magnetic resonance imaging. New York Academy of Sciences Symposium, Biological Effects and Safety Aspects of Nuclear Magnetic Resonance Imaging and Spectroscopy, Proceedings of the Meeting. 1992.
19. Bottomley PA, Redington RW, Edelstein WA, et al. Estimating radiofrequency power deposition in body NMR imaging. *Magn Reson Med* 1985;2:336–349.
20. Bottomley PA, Edelstein WA. Power deposition in whole body NMR imaging. *Med Phys* 1981;8:510–512.
21. Shellock FG, Litwer C, Kanal E. MRI bioeffects, safety, and patient management: a review. *Rev Magn Reson Imag* 1992;4:21–63.
22. Beers J. Biological effects of weak electromagnetic fields from 0 Hz to 200 MHz: a survey of the literature with special emphasis on possible magnetic resonance effects. *Magn Reson Imag* 1989;7:309–331.
23. Coulter S, Osbourne SL. Short wave diathermy in heating of human tissues. *Arch Phys Ther* 1936;17:679–687.
24. Gersten JW, Wakim KG, Herrick JF, Krusen FH. The effect of microwave diathermy on the peripheral circulation and on tissue temperature in man. *Arch Phys Med* 1949;30:7–25.
25. Gordon CJ. Normalizing the thermal effects of radiofrequency radiation: body mass versus total body surface area. *Bioelectromagnetics* 1987;8:111–118.
26. Athey TW. A model of the temperature rise in the head due to magnetic resonance imaging procedures. *Magn Reson Med* 1989;9:177–184.
27. Adair ER, Berglund LG. On the thermoregulatory consequences of NMR imaging. *Magn Reson Imag* 1986;4:321–333.
28. Adair ER, Berglund LG. Thermoregulatory consequences of cardiovascular impairment during NMR imaging in warm/humid environments. *Magn Reson Imag* 1989;7:25–37.

29. Burch GE, DePasquale NP. *Hot climates, man and his heart.* Springfield, Ill: Charles C Thomas Publishing; 1954.
30. Rowell LB. Cardiovascular aspects of human thermoregulation. *Circ Res* 1983;52:367–379.
31. Drinkwater BL, Horvath SM. Heat tolerance and aging. *Med Sci Sport Exer* 1979;11:49–55.
32. Fennel WH, Moore RE. Responses of aged men to passive heating. *Am J Physiol* 1969;67:118–119.
33. Kenny WL. Physiological correlates of heat intolerance. *Sports Med* 1985;2:279–286.
34. Barany FR. Abnormal vascular reaction in diabetes mellitus. *Acta Med Scand Suppl* 1955;304: 556–624.
35. Buskirk EF, Lundergren H, Magnussen L. Heat acclimation patterns in obese and lean individuals. *Ann NY Acad Sci* 1965;131:637–653.
36. Jauchem JR. Effects of drugs on thermal responses to microwaves. *Gen Pharmacol* 1985;16: 307–310.
37. Shellock FG, Drury JK, Meerbaum S, et al. Possible hypothalamic thermostat increase produced by a calcium blocker. *Clin Res* 1983;31:64A.
38. Food and Drug Administration. Magnetic resonance diagnostic device; panel recommendation and report on petitions for MR reclassification. *Fed Reg* 1988;53:7575–7579.
39. Shellock FG. Monitoring during MRI: an evaluation of the effect of high-field MRI on various patient monitors. *Med Electron* 1986;Sept:93–97.
40. Holshouser B, Hinshaw DB, Shellock FG. Sedation, anesthesia, and physiologic monitoring during MRI. *J Magn Reson Imag* 1993;3:553–558.
41. Kanal E, Shellock FG. Patient monitoring during clinical MR imaging. *Radiology* 1992;85: 623–629.
42. Wickersheim KA, Sun MH. Fluoroptic thermometry. *Med Electron* 1987;February:84–91.
43. Shellock FG, Crues JV. Temperature, heart rate, and blood pressure changes associated with clinical MR imaging at 1.5-T. *Radiology* 1987;163:259–262.
44. Shellock FG, Schaefer DJ, Grundfest W, et al. Thermal effects of high-field (1.5 Tesla) magnetic resonance imaging of the spine: clinical experience above a specific absorption rate of 0.4 W/kg. *Acta Radiol Suppl* 1986;369:514–516.
45. Shellock FG, Gordon CJ, Schaefer DJ. Thermoregulatory response to clinical magnetic resonance imaging of the head at 1.5 Tesla: lack of evidence for direct effects on the hypothalamus. *Acta Radiol Suppl* 1986;369:512–513.
46. Shellock FG, Crues JV. Corneal temperature changes associated with high-field MR imaging using a head coil. *Radiology* 1988;167:809–811.
47. Shellock FG, Crues JV. Temperature changes caused by clinical MR imaging of the brain at 1.5 Tesla using a head coil. *AJNR Am J Neuroradiol* 1988;9:287–291.
48. Shellock FG, Rothman B, Sarti D. Heating of the scrotum by high-field-strength MR imaging. *AJR Am J Roentgenol* 1990;154:1229–1232.
49. Shellock FG, Schatz CJ. Increases in corneal temperature caused by MR imaging of the eye with a dedicated local coil. *Radiology* 1992;185:697–699.
50. Shellock FG, Schaefer DJ, Crues JV. Alterations in body and skin temperatures caused by MR imaging: is the recommended exposure for radiofrequency radiation too conservative? *Br J Radiol* 1989;62:904–909.
51. Shellock FG, Rubin SA, Everest CE. Surface temperature measurement by IR. *Med Electron* 1986;86:81–83.
52. Shellock FG, Schaefer DJ, Crues JV. Evaluation of skin blood flow, body and skin temperatures in man during MR imaging at high levels of RF energy. *Magn Reson Imag* 1989;7(suppl 1): 335.
53. Shellock FG, Schaefer DJ, Kanal E. Physiologic responses to MR imaging performed at an SAR level of 6.0 W/kg. *Radiology* 1994;192:865–868.
54. Sperber D, Oldenbourg R, Dransfeld K. Magnetic field induced temperature change in mice. *Naturwissenschaften* 1984;71:100–101.
55. Gremmel H, Wendhausen H, Wunsch F. Biologische Effeckte Statischer Magnetfelder bei NMR-Tomographic Am Menshen. *Wiss Mitt Univ Kiel Radiol Klinik* 1983.
56. Shellock FG, Schaefer DJ, Gordon CJ. Effect of a 1.5 Tesla static magnetic field on body temperature of man. *Magn Reson Med* 1986;3:644–647.
57. Shellock FG, Schaefer DJ, Crues JV. Effect of a 1.5 Tesla static magnetic field on body and skin temperatures of man. *Magn Reson Med* 1989;10:371–375.

58. Tenforde TS. Thermoregulation in rodents exposed to high intensity stationary magnetic fields. *Bioelectromagnetics* 1986;7:341–346.
59. Schaefer DJ, Barber BJ, Gordon CJ, et al. Thermal effects of magnetic resonance imaging. In: *Book of Abstracts, Society of Magnetic Resonance in Medicine.* Berkeley, CA: Society of Magnetic Resonance in Medicine; 1985;2:925.
60. Schaefer DJ, Shellock FG, Crues JV, et al. Infrared thermographic studies of human surface temperature in magnetic resonance imaging. In: *Proceedings of the Bioelectromagnetics Society,* Eighth Annual Meeting, 1986; p. 68.
61. Vogl T, Krimmel K, Fuchs A, et al. Influence of magnetic resonance imaging of human body core and intravascular temperatures. *Med Phys* 1988;15:562–566.
62. Kido DK, Morris TW, Erickson JL, et al. Physiologic changes during high-field strength MR imaging. *AJNR Am J Neuroradiol* 1987;8:263–266.
63. Kurz KR, Goldstein M. Scrotal temperature reflects intratesticular temperature and is lowered by shaving. *J Urol* 1986;135:290–292.
64. Sacks E, Worgul BV, Merriam GR, et al. The effects of nuclear magnetic resonance imaging on ocular tissues. *Arch Ophthalmol* 1986;104:890–893.
65. Mapstone R. Measurement of corneal temperature. *Exp Eye Res* 1968;7:233–243.
66. Shuman WP, Haynor DR, Guy AW, et al. Superficial and deep-tissue increases in anesthetized dogs during exposure to high specific absorption rates in a 1.5-T MR imager. *Radiology* 1988;167:551–554.
67. Hennig J, Nauerth A, Friedburg H. RARE imaging: a fast imaging method for clinical MR. *Magn Reson Med* 1986;3:823–833.
68. Balaban RS, Ceckler TL. Magnetization transfer contrast in magnetic resonance imaging. *Magn Reson Q* 1992;8:116–117.
69. Melki PS, Mulkern RV, Panych LP, Jolesz FA. Comparing the FAISE method with conventional dual-echo sequences. *J Magn Reson Imag* 1991;1:319–326.
70. Redington RW, Dumoulin CL, Schenck F, et al. MR imaging and bioeffects in a whole body 4.0 Tesla imaging system. In: *Book of Abstracts, Society of Magnetic Resonance Imaging.* Berkeley, CA; Society of Magnetic Resonance Imaging; 1988;1:20.
71. Ortendahl DA. Whole-body MR imaging and spectroscopy at 4 Tesla: where do we go from here? *Radiology* 1988;169:864–865.

4

Magnetic Resonance Procedures and Pregnancy

Perhaps more than any other topic in MR safety discussions, the issue of possible adverse effects of the MR environment on pregnant individuals has caught the attention of all involved in this field. In 1988, 36% of all MR sites surveyed did not perform MR examinations on pregnant patients (1). This is unfortunate in consideration of the myriad of important clinical applications for MR procedures during pregnancy. Furthermore, there were markedly varied policies regarding the treatment of pregnant health care practitioners, from no pregnancy policy, to exclusion from the magnet room, to unrestricted activities. Some policies were dependent on the stage of gestation, whereas others were not.

The predominant issues related to MR procedures and pregnancy are: (a) the possible effects of the static magnetic field of the MR system, (b) the risks associated with exposure to the gradient magnetic fields, (c) the potential adverse effects of the radiofrequency (RF) electromagnetic fields, (d) possible adverse effects related to the combination of the three different electromagnetic fields, and (e) possible adverse effects related to the use of MR imaging contrast agents.

There are two primary differences between pregnant patients undergoing an MR examination and pregnant health care practitioners being exposed to the MR environment. First, one must be aware that exposure to gradient and/or RF electromagnetic fields requires that the pregnant individual be within the bore of the MR system, because the fields drop off so rapidly that all exposures outside the magnet bore become essentially insignificant. Thus, the safety considerations of the static, gradient, and RF electromagnetic fields and, of course, MR imaging contrast agents are the pertinent factors when discussing exposures relative to the pregnant patient. Health care practitioners rarely find themselves within the MR system room during data acquisition, which is the only time the gradient and/or RF electromagnetic fields are active and, therefore, of a potential concern.

Second, the exposure of a patient to the MR environment during pregnancy is an acute, short-term exposure. For the pregnant health care provider, however, the exposure to at least the static magnetic field (e.g., there may be exposure to the fringe field while sitting at the operator's console) is a chronic, low-level exposure. A pregnant technologist, for example, might find herself in static magnetic fields of several hundred or even several thousand gauss on a regular basis each working day for prolonged periods of time. Thus, the question of induced voltages from gradient magnetic field switching or RF power absorption really affects only the case of the pregnant patient and not the health care worker. The only exceptions are instances in which the nurse anesthetist or anesthesiologist needs to physically enter and stay within the bore of the magnet during an MR procedure or where the design features of an interventional MR system (e.g., MR systems that permit the MR user to have direct access to the patient) exposes the MR user to electromagnetic fields at levels that are used in patients.

It is difficult to assess the risks during pregnancy because of the many possible permutations of the various risk factors found in the MR environment. This becomes even more complicated because new hardware and software for MR systems is continually developed and implemented in the clinical setting. In other words, even if there are no demonstrated adverse effects from any one identifiable source, it is possible that some or all of these might work synergistically to produce an adverse outcome if they were applied simultaneously. In addition, although it is possible that some dose or frequency of exposure to the electromagnetic fields used for MR procedures might prove innocuous, other doses or frequencies might be deleterious.

Human subjects normally have a spontaneous abortion rate of more than 30%, which is relatively high (2). This increases the difficulty in identifying whether a spontaneous abortion is related to exposure to an MR procedure. At the very least for human subjects, assessing why a given pregnancy might have terminated with a less than optimal outcome can be a formidable task because of the exposures to various other non–MR-related risk factors that cannot be controlled during pregnancy.

Therefore, it is impossible to prove the safety of exposure to MR procedures with respect to human pregnancy. Instead, what might be successfully pursued are verifiable and reproducible data gleaned from experiments on cell preparations or laboratory animals and MR risk factors, keeping in mind the limitation of this form of data. Additionally, epidemiologic data from vast numbers of human subjects exposed to the MR environment during pregnancy may also be analyzed to address safety-related issues. On the basis of the interpretation of such data, one might arrive at a reasonable and logical conclusion regarding the risk of exposure of the pregnant patient, accompanying family member, technologist, nurse, physician, physicist, or other individual to the electromagnetic fields used for MR procedures.

PERTINENT LITERATURE RELATED TO MR PROCEDURES AND PREGNANCY

Several studies have investigated the possible adverse effects of the electromagnetic fields used for MR procedures and their effects on pregnancy. Some of these investigations report positive correlations and findings, whereas others directly contradict the findings of these studies or report negative results (3). For example, Barnothy (4) and LaForge et al. (5) concluded that exposure of mice and rats to strong static magnetic fields resulted in weight reduction, organ anomalies, and behavioral modifications. Strand et al. (6) found that there was a statistically significant enhancement in fertilization rates that resulted when rainbow trout sperm and/or ova were exposed to a 1-T magnetic field for 1 hour. Joshi et al. (7), examining white Leghorn chick morphogenesis after their exposure to a static magnetic field during early embryogenesis, found that there was a ". . .large incidence of malformations in structures such as brain, somites, heart and embryonic axis" (7). They further observed a more than doubling of the rate of mitosis in the neural region per cell population studied in the exposed versus the control groups. However, Ngo et al. (8) found DNA synthesis to be unaffected in Chinese hamster cells after prolonged exposure to a 0.75-T static magnetic field (8). Furthermore, Sutherland et al. (9) observed no effect on cell growth rates in tissue culture when Chinese hamster lung cells were exposed for more than 1 year to a static magnetic field of 10^{-7} T.

Exposure to low static magnetic fields have been implicated as being teratogenic under certain laboratory conditions. For example, there are data to suggest that there is an increased rate of developmental abnormalities observed in the newt embryo when the developing organism is shielded from the normal geomagnetic static magnetic fields (10). Low static magnetic fields of approximately 4.5 mT were also demonstrated to be associated with lower survival and decreased oviposition in *Drosophila* flies (11).

Enhanced DNA synthesis was observed by Liboff et al. (12) when exposed to time-varying magnetic fields ranging from 15 Hz to 4 kHz. Studying intrauterine development in Sprague-Dawley rats, Tofani et al. (13) found an increase in the incidence of fetal reabsorption, increased cranial abnormalities, and decreased total weight gain for dams exposed to chronic (multi-day) low-level 27-MHz RF irradiation (13). Although it is well documented that there is a dose-response relationship between body temperature and birth defects in RF-irradiated rats (14), the effect in this study seemed to be more than could be explained by power-heat deposition alone.

Peeling et al. (15) studied nematode survival, growth, and maturity in test animals exposed to static and time-varying magnetic fields. They found that although static magnetic fields up to 2.35 T seemed to have no effect on nematode survival, growth, and maturity, time-varying magnetic fields of the order typically used in MR imaging (6 mT/m and 5 T/s) alone or in conjunction with a static magnetic field seemed to induce some inhibition of growth and maturation of the test nematodes (15).

Magnetic field, constant current effects on the early embryonic development of frogs were studied by Ueno et al. (16). Various levels of gradient magnetic fields were tested, ranging up to as high as 1,000 T/m. Although there were no observed harmful or modifying effects on gastrulation or neurolation, there was an elevated rate of developmental anomalies in those embryos that had been exposed to these static gradient magnetic fields during the cleavage to the neurula stage (16). Conversely, Kay et al. (17), also studying the same species of frog, found no abnormalities in morphology, function, or developmental delay when they were exposed to MR imaging as embryos either intermittently or for prolonged periods.

Prasad et al. (18), studying a different species of frog, found no deleterious effect on its embryologic development when exposed to a 0.15- or 4.5-T MR system (the latter accompanied by 191 MHz RF pulses and gradient magnetic fields of 50 μT/cm) (18). Prasad et al. (19) also found no effect on early frog development when exposed for 20 min to 0.7 T static magnetic field and 30 MHz continuous wave RF electromagnetic radiation (19).

Data from early studies of cell transformation from exposure to 0.5-T magnetic fields (20) were shown to be artifactual as a result of unusual cell culture techniques (21). Geard et al. (22) reported no significant effects from prolonged MR exposure (static magnetic fields between 2.2 and 2.7 T, exposures ranging from 3 to 17 h in length, and RF levels from 25 to 30 MHz) on cell survival and transformation, cell kinetics, sister chromatid exchanges, or chromosomal aberrations. Cooke and Morris (23), examining human blood cells using MR imaging as well as static magnetic field exposures (up to 1 T), observed no significant effects on sister chromatid exchanges, chromatid lesions, chromosome lesions, or the number of cells with lesions. Similarly, Wolff et al. (24) studied Chinese hamster ovary cells exposed to a 0.35-T static magnetic field, pulsed RF at 15 MHz, and 2.35 G/cm pulsed gradient magnetic fields for 4 h. They reported no increased rate of chromosomal aberrations in the cells (24). Subsequently, Wolff et al. (25) again found no evidence of increased rates of sister chromatid exchange or chromosomal aberrations when examining Chinese hamster ovary cells and human lymphocytes exposed for more than 12 h to a 2.35-T static magnetic field and pulsed 100-MHz RF radiation. Schwartz and Crooks (26) also studied Chinese hamster ovary cells and reported similar results. Ardito et al. (27), however, found somewhat different results from those reported by others. Although there was no significant alteration in the frequency of sister chromatid exchanges after exposing human lymphocyte cultures to a static magnetic field of 740 G for 48 h, there was an increase in the total chromosomal aberrations seen (27).

Prasad et al. (28) did not observe any evidence of adverse cytogenetic effects when exposing mice for 1 hour to 0.7-T static magnetic fields along with continuous wave RF irradiation at 30 MHz (28). Sikov et al. (29) similarly found no increase in structural abnormalities when mice were exposed for 1 h to a 1-T magnetic field in utero (29). No increase in the abortion rate was observed after chronic exposure of male parent mice to magnetic fields (30). In addition, no effect was seen on mice spermatogenesis when male mice were exposed for 66 continuous h to a static magnetic field of 0.3 T (31). However, exposure of mice on the seventh gestational day to a 1.5-T static magnetic field with 64 MHz pulsed RF excitation pulses for 36 min resulted in a statistically significant increase in the rate of developmental abnormalities of the eye (32).

No effect was observed on the growth of seven generations of yeast cells exposed to a 1.5-T static magnetic field (33). Furthermore, there were no differences in the rate of mutations when *Drosophila* were exposed to 1.3-T static magnetic fields after exposure to a gaseous mutagen (34).

Heinrichs et al. (35) found no increase in teratogenesis of the musculoskeletal system in pregnant mice exposed for 16 consecutive hours (to either 0.35 T or 2 T) in mid-gestation. McRobbie et al. (36) examined the possible effects of the time-varying magnetic field component of MR imaging systems on pregnant mice. They observed no significant differences in the outcomes of the pregnancies, the number of litters, the weights of the pups, or the rates of growth between the exposed versus the nonexposed pup populations (36). Quail development was similarly found to be unaffected by prolonged (up to 16 days) exposure to even very strong (up to 6.4 T) static magnetic fields (37).

The most recent investigations that examined possible developmental changes associated with exposure to the electromagnetic fields used for MR procedures has been reported in a series of articles by Yip et al. (38–40). Yip et al. (38), using chick embryos exposed to simulated imaging conditions at 1.5 T found a trend toward higher abnormality and mortality rates when compared with controls. It was felt that more extensive studies are needed to confirm the positive findings from this particular study (38). In a follow-up study using similar experimental conditions, birth rates and the migration and proliferation of lateral motoneurons of chick embryos appeared to be unaffected by exposure to the electromagnetic fields (39). In another investigation of the effects of exposure to the MR environment, Yip et al. (40) reported that there was no effect on axonal growth in the sympathetic nervous system of the chick.

To our knowledge, there has been no prospective study performed involving a large population of pregnant human subjects exposed to MR procedures. However, one epidemiologic, retrospective study was performed to address the safety of MR procedures with respect to MR health care providers (41). Details of this study and the implications of the findings are discussed below.

In consideration of the data reviewed above, there apparently are discrepancies with respect to the experimental findings of the effects of electromagnetic fields used for MR procedures and the pertinent safety aspects of pregnancy. These discrepancies may be explained by a variety of factors, including the differences in the scientific methodology used for the experiment, the type of organism examined, and the variance in exposure duration as well as the conditions of the exposure to the electromagnetic fields. Obviously, additional investigations are warranted before the specific risks associated with exposure to MR procedures can be known and characterized.

MR PROCEDURES AND THE PREGNANT PATIENT

As noted in previous chapters of this book, there is a large and confusing body of data regarding the bioeffects of the electromagnetic fields used for MR procedures, especially with respect to effects on the development of organisms. The reader is referred to several excellent review articles on these topics (42,43), keeping in mind that much of the previous data were collected from investigations involving cell preparations or laboratory animals such that the information may not be directly applicable to human subjects.

There are many indications for the use of MR procedures in pregnant patients, besides for the more typical neurologic and musculoskeletal indications (44–58). However, for the case of the pregnant patient, there does not seem to be sufficient evidence supporting or refuting the overall safety of the electromagnetic fields used for MR procedures. Therefore, in cases where the referring physician and radiologist can defend that the outcome of the MR examination requested during pregnancy has the potential to change or alter the care or therapy of the mother or fetus, an MR procedure (i.e., MR imaging, angiography, or spectroscopy) may be performed with informed consent, regardless of the stage of trimester.

As stated in the Policies, Guidelines, and Recommendations for MR Imaging Safety and Patient Management issued by the Safety Committee of the Society for Magnetic Resonance Imaging in 1991 (59), "MR imaging may be used in pregnant women if other nonionizing forms of diagnostic imaging are inadequate or if the examination provides important information that would otherwise require exposure to ionizing radiation (e.g., fluoroscopy, CT, etc.). Pregnant patients should be informed that, to date, there has been no indication that the use of clinical MR imaging during pregnancy has produced deleterious effects." The above policy has been adopted by the American College of Radiology and is considered to be the "standard of care" with respect to the use of MR procedures in pregnant patients.

MR IMAGING CONTRAST AGENTS AND THEIR USE DURING PREGNANCY

As discussed in Chapter 8, Safety of MR Imaging Contrast Agents, the use of contrast media during pregnancy is a topic whose safety factors have not been defined clearly. For example, Magnevist (Berlex Laboratories, Wayne, NJ) readily crosses the placenta and is excreted by the fetal bladder (60). The contrast medium is then swallowed by the fetus, where it is once again filtered and excreted in the urine of the fetus. Obviously, this cycle will be repeated many times during the development of the fetus. The other gadolinium-based MR imaging contrast agents are assumed to act in a similar fashion.

The rates of clearance of MR imaging contrast agents from the amniotic fluid and the fetal circulation are unknown. At the present time, the product inserts for each commercially available gadolinium-based contrast agent does not support the use in pregnant patients because of the lack of studies to assess safety.

In certain cases, it may be necessary to use an MR imaging contrast agent to obtain crucial information in a pregnant patient undergoing an MR procedure (60). Therefore, we recommend that the risks versus the benefits of using the contrast agent during pregnancy be carefully considered in each case. The administration of an MR imaging contrast agent to a pregnant patient should occur only if the benefit justifies the potential risk to the fetus. Written, informed consent must be obtained from the patient with a specific indication that the associated risks are currently unknown (60). Refer to Chapter 8 for additional information on this topic.

MR PROCEDURES AND PREGNANT HEALTH CARE PERSONNEL

A survey of reproductive health among female MR operators was conducted in 1990 (41). Questionnaires were sent to all female MR technologists and nurses at most clinical MR facilities in the United States. The questionnaire addressed menstrual and reproductive experiences as well as work activities. This study attempted to account for known potential confounders (e.g., age, smoking, alcohol use) for this type of data. Of the 1,915 completed questionnaires analyzed, there were 1,421 pregnancies: 280 occurred while working as an MR employee (technologist or nurse), 894 while employed at another job, 54 as a student, and 193 as a homemaker.

Five categories were analyzed that included spontaneous abortion rate, preterm delivery (less than 39 weeks), low birth weight (less than 5.5 pounds), infertility (taking more than 11 months to conceive), and gender of the offspring (41). The data indicated that there were no statistically significant alterations in the five areas studied for MR workers relative to the same group studied when they were employed elsewhere, before becoming MR health care employees. Additionally, adjustment for maternal age, smoking, and alcohol use failed to markedly change any of the associations.

Menstrual regularity, cyclicity, and related topics were also examined in this study. These included inquiries regarding the number of days of menstrual bleeding, the heaviness of the bleeding, and the time between menstrual cycles. Admittedly, this is a difficult area to examine objectively, because it is depends entirely on both subjective memory and the memory of the respondent for a topic, where subjective memory is notoriously inadequate. Nevertheless, the data suggested that there was no clear correlation between MR workers and any specific modifications of the menstrual cycle (41).

The data from this extensive epidemiologic investigation were reassuring because there did not seem to be any deleterious effects from exposure to the static magnetic field component of the MR system. Therefore, we recommend a policy to permit pregnant health care workers to perform MR procedures, as well as to enter the MR system room, and to attend to the patient during their pregnancy, regardless of the trimester. We further recommend that the health care worker not remain within the MR system room or magnet bore during the actual operation of the device. This recommendation is especially important for those MR users involved in interventional MR-guided examinations and procedures to adhere to because it may be necessary for them to be exposed directly to the electromagnetic fields similar to those used for patients. This policy is not based on indications of adverse effects but, rather, from a conservative point of view and the feeling that there are insufficient data pertaining to the effects of the other electromagnetic fields of the MR system to support or allow unnecessary exposures.

REFERENCES

1. Kanal E, Shellock FG, Sonnenblick D. MRI clinical site safety survey: phase I results and preliminary data. *Magn Reson Imag* 1988;7(S1):106.
2. Wilcox A, Weinberg C, O'Connor J, et al. Incidence of early loss of pregnancy. *N Engl J Med* 1988;319:189–194.
3. Villa M, Mustarelli P, Caprotti M. Minireview: biological effects of magnetic fields. *Life Sci* 1991;49:85–92.
4. Barnothy J. Growth rate of mice in static magnetic fields. *Nature* 1963;200:86–87.
5. LaForge H, Sadeghi M, Seguin M. Magnetostatic field effect: stress syndrome pattern and functional relation with intensity. *J Psychol* 1986;120:299–304.
6. Strand J, Abernathy C, Sakalski J, Genoway R. Effects of magnetic field exposure on fertilization success in rainbow trout, Salmo gairdneri. *Bioelectromagnetics* 1983;4:295–301.
7. Joshi M, Kahn M, Damle P. Effect of magnetic field on chick morphogenesis. *Differentiation* 1978;10:39–43.
8. Ngo F, Blue J, Roberts W. The effect of a static magnetic field on DNA synthesis and survival of mammalian cells irradiated with fast neurons. *Magn Reson Med* 1987;5:307–317.
9. Sutherland R, Marton J, MacDonald J, Howell R. Effect of weak magnetic fields on growth of cells in tissue culture. *Physiol Chemistry Physics* 1978;10:125–131.
10. Asashima M, Shimada K, Pfeiffer C. Magnetic shielding induces early developmental abnormalities in the newt, Cynops pyrrhogaster. *Bioelectromagnetics* 1991;12:215–224.
11. Ramirez E, Monteagudo J, Garcia-Gracia M, Delgado J. Oviposition and development of Drosophilia modified by magnetic fields. *Bioelectromagnetics* 1983;4:315–326.
12. Liboff A, Williams T, Strong D, Wistar R. Time-varying magnetic fields: effect on DNA synthesis. *Science* 1984;223:818–820.
13. Tofani S, Agnesod G, Ossola P. Effects of continuous low-level exposure to radiofrequency radiation on intrauterine development in rats. *Health Physics* 1986; 51: 489–499.
14. Lary J, Conover D, Johnson P, Hornung R. Dose-response relationship between body temperature and birth defects in radiofrequency-irradiated rats. *Bioelectromagnetics* 1986;7:141–149.
15. Peeling J, Lewis J, Samoiloff M, Bock E, Tomchuk E. Biological effects of magnetic fields: chronic exposure of the nematode *Panagrellus redivivus*. *Magn Reson Imag* 1988;6:655–660.
16. Ueno S, Harada K, Shiokawa K. The embryonic development of frogs under strong DC magnetic fields. *IEEE Trans Magn* 1984;MAG-20:1663–1665.

17. Kay H, Herkens R, Kay B. Effect of magnetic resonance imaging on Xenopus Laevis embryogenesis. *Magn Reson Imag* 1988;6:501–506.
18. Prasad N, Wright D, Ford J, Thornby. Safety of 4-T MR imaging: study of effects on developing frog embryos. *Radiology* 1990;174:251–253.
19. Prasad N, Wright D, Forster J. Effect of nuclear magnetic resonance on early stages of amphibian development. *Magn Reson Imag* 1982;1:35–38.
20. Malinin G, Gregory W, Morelli L, Sharma V, Houck J. Evidence of morphological and physiological transformation of mammalian cells by strong magnetic fields. *Science* 1976;194:844.
21. Frazier M, Andrews T, Thompson B. In vitro evaluation of static magnetic fields. In: NTIS - Springfield, VA, 1979.
22. Geard C, Osmak R, Hall E, Simon H, Maudsley A, Hilal S. Magnetic resonance and ionizing radiation: a comparative evaluation in vitro of oncogenic and genotoxic potential. *Radiology* 1984;152:199–202.
23. Cooke P, Morris P. The effects of NMR exposure on living organisms. II. A genetic study of human lymphocytes. *Br J Radiol* 1981;54:622–625.
24. Wolff S, Crooks L, Brown P, Howard R, Painter R. Test for DNA and chromosomal damage induced by nuclear magnetic resonance imaging. *Radiology* 1980;136:707–710.
25. Wolff S, James T, Young G, Margulis A, Bodycote J, Afzal V. Magnetic resonance imaging: absence of in vitro cytogenetic damage. *Radiology* 1985;155:163–165.
26. Schwartz J, Crooks L. NMR imaging produces no observable mutations or cytotoxicity in mammalian cells. *AJR Am J Roentgenol* 1982;139:583–585.
27. Ardito G, Lamberti L, Bigatti P, Prono G. Influence of a constant magnetic field on human lymphocyte cultures. *Boll Soc It Biol Spec* 1984;60:1341–1346.
28. Prasad N, Bushong S, Thronby J, Bryan R, Hazelwood C, Harrell J. Effect of nuclear magnetic resonance on chromosomes of mouse bone marrow cells. *Magn Reson Imag* 1984;2:37–39.
29. Sikov M, Mahlum D, Montgomery L, Decker J. Development of mice after intrauterine exposure to direct current magnetic fields. Proceedings of the 18th Hanford Life Sciences Symposium. Richland, WA: Technical Information Center, US Department of Energy; 1979:462–473.
30. Mahlum D, Sikov M, Decker J. Dominant lethal studies in mice exposed to direct current magnetic fields. Proceedings of the 18th Hanford Life Sciences Symposium. Richland, WA: Technical Information Center, United States Department of Energy; 1979:474–484.
31. Withers H, Mason K, Davis C. MR effect on murine spermatogenesis. *Radiology* 1985;156: 741–742.
32. Tyndall D, Sulik K. Effects of magnetic resonance imaging on eye development in the C57BL/6J mouse. *Teratology* 1991;43:263–275.
33. Malko J, Constantinidus I, Dillehay D, Fajman W. Search for influence of 1.5 Tesla magnetic field on growth of yeast cells. *12th Annual Meeting of the Society for Magnetic Resonance in Medicine.* New York City: Society for Magnetic Resonance in Medicine; 1993:1370.
34. Kale P, Baum J. Genetic effects of strong magnetic fields in Drosophilia melanogaster. *Mutation Res* 1982;105:79–83.
35. Heinrichs W, Fong P, Flannery M, et al. Midgestational exposure of pregnant balb/c mice to magnetic resonance imaging. *Magn Reson Imag* 1988;6:305–313.
36. McRobbie D, Foster M. Pulsed magnetic field exposure during pregnancy and implications for NMR foetal imaging: a study with mice. *Magn Reson Imag* 1985;3:231–234.
37. Bouvet J, Maret G. Embryonic development of the quail in strong magnetic fields. In: Maret G, Kiepenheuer J, Boccarra N, eds. *Biophysical effects of steady magnetic fields.* Berlin: Springer-Verlag; 1988:138–143.
38. Yip YP, Capriotti C, Talagala SL, Yip JW. Effects of MR exposure at 1.5 T on early embryonic development of the chick. *J Magn Reson Imag* 1994;4:742–748.
39. Yip YP, Capriotti C, Norbash SG, Talagala SL, Yip JW. Effects of MR exposure on cell proliferation and migration of chick motoneurons. *J Magn Reson Imag* 1994;4:799–804.
40. Yip YP, Capriotti C, Yip JW. Effects of MR exposure on axonal outgrowth in the sympathetic nervous system of the chick. *J Magn Reson Imag* 1995;4:457–462.
41. Kanal E, Gillen J, Evans J, Savitz D, Shellock FG. Survey of reproductive health among female MR workers. *Radiology* 1993;187:395–399.
42. Adey W. Tissue interactions with nonionizing electromagnetic fields. *Physiol Rev* 1981;61: 435–514.

43. Beers J. Biological effects of weak electromagnetic fields from 0 Hz to 200 MHz: a survey of the literature with special emphasis on possible magnetic resonance effects. *Magn Reson Imag* 1989;7:309–331.
44. Smith F. The potential use of nuclear magnetic resonance imaging in pregnancy. *J Perinat Med* 1985;13:265–276.
45. Cohen J, Weinreb J, Lowe T, Brown C. MR imaging of a viable full-term abdominal pregnancy. *AJR Am J Roentgenol* 1985;145:407–408.
46. Johnson I, Symonds E, Kean D, et al. Imaging the pregnancy human uterus with magnetic resonance imaging. *Am J Obstet Gynecol* 1984;152:1136–1139.
47. McCarthy S, Stark D, Filly R, Callen P, Hricak H, Higgins C. Obstetrical magnetic resonance imaging: maternal anatomy. *Radiology* 1985;154:421–425.
48. McCarthy S, Filly R, Stark D, Callen P, Golbus M, Hricak H. Magnetic resonance imaging of fetal anomalies in utero: Early experience. *AJR Am J Roentgenol* 1985;154:677–682.
49. Powell M, Buckley J, Price H, Worthington B, Symonds E. Magnetic resonance imaging and placenta previa. *Am J Obstet Gynecol* 1986;154:565–569.
50. Stark D, McCarthy S, Filly R, Parer J, Hricak H, Callen P. Pelvimetry by magnetic resonance imaging. *AJR Am J Roentgenol* 1985;144:147–150.
51. Stark D, McCarthy S, Filly R, Callen P, Hricak H, Parer J. Intrauterine growth retardation: evaluation by magnetic resonance imaging. *Radiology* 1985;155:425–427.
52. Weinreb J, Brown C, Lowe T, Cohen J, Erdman W. Pelvic masses in pregnant patients: MR and US imaging. *Radiology* 1986;159:717–724.
53. Weinreb J, Lowe T, Cohen J, Kutler M. Human fetal anatomy: MR imaging. *Radiology* 1985;157:515–520.
54. Weinreb J, Lowe T, Santos-Ramos R, Cunningham F, Parkey R. Magnetic resonance imaging in obstetric diagnosis. *Radiology* 1985;154:157–161.
55. Smith FW, MacLennan F. NMR imaging in human pregnancy: a preliminary study. *Magn Reson Imag* 1984;2:57–64.
56. Hata T, Makihara K, Aoki S, Hata K, Kitao M. Magnetic resonance imaging of the fetus: initial experience. *Gynecol Obstet Invest* 1990;29:255–258.
57. Garden AS, Griffiths RD, Weindling AM, Martin PA. Fast-scan magnetic resonance imaging in fetal visualization. *Am J Obstet Gynecol* 1991;164:1190–1196.
58. Johnson IR, et al. Study of internal structure of the human fetus in utero by echo-planar magnetic resonance imaging. *Am J Obstet Gynecol* 1990;163:601–607.
59. Shellock FG, Kanal E. Policies, guidelines, and recommendations for MR imaging safety and patient management. *J Magn Reson Imag* 1991;1:97–101.
60. Kanal E, Shellock FG. *Safety manual on magnetic resonance imaging contrast agents.* New York: Lippincott-Raven Healthcare; 1996:21–22.

5

Auditory Effects of Magnetic Resonance Procedures

GRADIENT MAGNETIC FIELD-INDUCED ACOUSTIC NOISE

During the operation of MR systems various types of acoustic noises are produced. Some of these sounds may present minor or substantial problems to patients and health workers, including simple annoyance, difficulties in verbal communication, heightened anxiety, temporary hearing loss and, possibly, permanent hearing impairment (1–10).

The gradient magnetic field is the primary source of acoustic noise associated with MR procedures. This noise occurs during the rapid alterations of currents within the gradient coils. These currents, in the presence of a strong static magnetic field of the MR system, produce significant forces that act on the gradient coils (Fig. 5-1). Acoustic noise, manifested as loud tapping, knocking, or chirping sounds, is produced when the forces cause motion or vibration of the gradient coils as they impact against their mountings (3,7).

Gradient magnetic field–induced noise is enhanced by certain modifications of the parameters used for the MR procedure, including a decrease in section thickness, field of view, repetition time, and echo time (3–6). The physical features of the MR system, especially whether or not it has special sound insulation, also affects the transmission of the acoustic noise and its perception by the patient and MR system operator (3–6).

Gradient magnetic field–induced noise levels have been measured during a variety of pulse sequences for MR systems with static magnetic field strengths ranging from 0.35 to 1.5 T (3–6). Hurwitz et al. (3) published the first study of acoustic noise (3). This report indicated that the sound levels varied from 82 to 93 dB on the A-weighted scale and from 84 to 103 dB on the linear scale (3). Obviously, because the gradient magnetic field is primarily responsible for acoustic noise in the MR environment, the ability of the MR system to produce noise depends on the specifications for the gradients as well as the types of imaging parameters that are available on the MR system. The report by Hurwitz

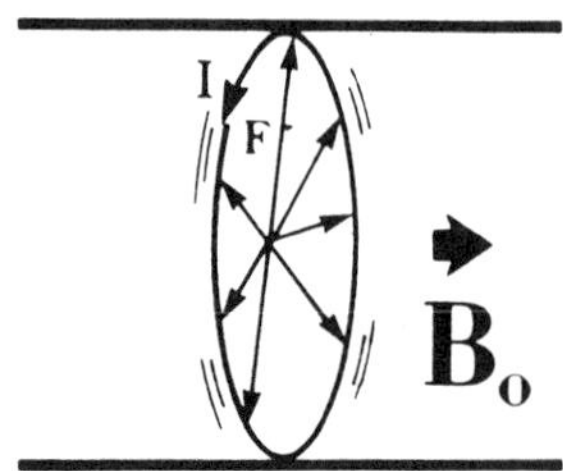

FIG. 5-1. A simplified explanation of gradient magnetic field–induced acoustic noise. Gradient coil is depicted as a single winding for illustrative purposes. When the gradient coil is pulsed by current, *I,* a brief force, *F,* is created in a radial direction. B_0, static magnetic field. From ref. 3.

et al. (3) concluded that gradient magnetic field–induced noise was an annoyance but well within recognized safety guidelines (3).

Later studies performed using other MR parameters, including "worst-case" pulse sequences, showed that fast gradient echo pulse sequences produced the greatest noise during MR imaging (4–6). Acoustic noise levels in these investigations did not exceed a range of 103 to 106 dB on the A-weighted scale and 106 dB on the linear scale (4–6). These acoustic noise levels are below those permissible by the Occupational Safety and Health Administration of the United States, especially when one considers that the duration of exposure is one of the most important physical factors that determines the effect of noise on hearing (11–13).

Other physical factors involved in hearing loss include the sound frequency, temporal pattern, and intensity of the noise (10–13). High frequencies tend to be more responsible for hearing loss than are low frequencies. Table 5-1 shows the relationship between the noise duration and recommended permissible sound levels for occupational exposures.

TABLE 5-1. *Permissible exposure levels to acoustic noise*

Noise duration per day (h)	Sound level (dB[a])
8.0	90
6.0	92
4.0	95
3.0	97
1.5	100
1.0	102
0.5	105
0.25	115

These federal guidelines refer to the upper limits for occupational exposures to acoustic noise. No recommendations exist for nonoccupational or medical exposure.

[a] A-weighted scale.

Data adapted from refs. 3 and 11.

The U.S. Food and Drug Administration indicates that the acoustic noise levels associated with the operation of MR systems must be shown to be below the level of concern established by pertinent federal regulatory or other recognized standards-setting organizations (14). If the acoustic noise is not below the level of concern, the sponsor (i.e., the manufacturer of the MR system) must recommend steps to reduce or alleviate the noise perceived by the patient.

These recommended limits for acoustic noise produced during MR procedures are based on recommendations for occupational exposures that are inherently chronic exposures with respect to the time duration (14). Comparable recommendations do not exist for nonoccupational exposure to relatively short-term noise produced by medical devices. Although the acoustic noise levels suggested for patients exposed during MR procedures on an infrequent and short-term temporal basis are considered to be highly conservative, they may not be appropriate for individuals with underlying health problems who may have problems with noise at certain levels or at particular frequencies.

The acoustic noise produced during MR procedures represents a potential risk to patients. Brummet et al. (1) reported temporary hearing loss in 43% of the patients that had MR imaging performed without ear protection. The possibility exists that significant gradient magnetic field–induced noise may produce substantial hearing problems in certain patients who are particularly susceptible to the damaging effects of loud noises. In fact, there have been unconfirmed claims of permanent hearing loss associated with MR examinations (10).

To date, there has been no evaluation of gradient magnetic field–induced noise associated with echo planar imaging (EPI) techniques. EPI techniques require significantly higher and more rapid gradient magnetic field transitions compared with conventional pulse sequences and, therefore, there are concomitant auditory effects that are obviously substantial. Because the EPI methods permit MR procedures to be accomplished with reduced acquisition times, the shorter time duration of exposure to the louder gradient magnetic field–induced acoustic noise may cause less of a problem with respect to alterations in hearing (3–6).

NOISE ABATEMENT TECHNIQUES

The safest and least expensive means of preventing problems associated with acoustic noise during MR procedures is to encourage the routine use of earplugs (1,7–9). Ear plugs, when properly used, can abate noise by 10 to 20 dB, which is an adequate amount of sound attenuation for the MR environment. The use of disposable earplugs has been shown to provide a sufficient decrease in acoustic noise that, in turn, would be capable of preventing the potential temporary hearing loss associated with MR procedures (1). Therefore, it behooves all MR centers to recommend these protective devices to patients before they undergo MR examinations. MR-compatible headphones that significantly muffle acoustic noise are also commercially available. Unfortunately, hearing protection devices hamper verbal communication with the patient during the operation of the MR system.

The effects of acoustic noise exposures on MR operators may be comparable to that experienced by patients if they remain in the room during MR procedures. Therefore, hearing protection should also be worn by these individuals, as well as by any others who stay in the room during the operation of the MR system.

A significant reduction in the level of acoustic noise caused by MR procedures has been accomplished by implementing the use of an active noise cancellation, or "antinoise," technique with the existing audio system (2). The antinoise technique consists of a real-time Fourier analysis of the noise emitted from the MR system (2). A signal possessing the same physical characteristics, but opposite phase than the sound generated by the MR system, is then produced. The opposite-phase signals are combined, resulting in a cancellation of the repetitive noise. The antinoise system involves a continuous feedback loop with constant monitoring of the sounds in the headphone earcovers so that the repetitive gradient magnetic field–induced noise is attenuated, while allowing the transmission of vocal communication or music to be maintained (2).

A reduction of as much as 50 to 70% in the sound level perceived by the ear has been reported using the antinoise system coupled to an MR system (2). This technique has not yet found wide-spread clinical application, but it has considerable potential for minimizing acoustic noise and its related problems.

OTHER ACOUSTIC NOISE ASSOCIATED WITH THE MR SYSTEM

Cryogen Reclamation Systems

Cryogen reclamation systems associated with superconducting magnets of MR systems are another source of acoustic noise found in the MR environment (7). These devices, which are effectively used to minimize the loss of cryogens, function on a continuous basis and produce a methodical, low frequency tapping or knocking noise. The magnitude of the sounds emanating from cryogen reclamation systems is considerably less than that caused by the activation of the gradient magnetic fields during MR procedures. Therefore, this acoustic noise, at the very least, may be only an annoyance to patients or MR operators in the MR environment.

Auditory Perception of Radiofrequency Electromagnetic Fields

When the human head is subjected to pulsed RF radiation at certain frequencies, an audible sound perceived as a click, buzz, chirp, or knocking noise may be heard (15–17). This acoustic phenomenon is referred to as "RF hearing," "RF sound," or "microwave hearing" (15–17).

Thermoelastic expansion is believed to be the mechanism responsible for the production of RF hearing, whereby there is absorption of RF energy that produces a minute temperature elevation (i.e., approximately 0.000001°C) over a brief time period (i.e., approximately 10 μs) in the tissue or matter of the head (15–17). Subsequently, a pressure wave is induced that is sensed by the hair cells of the cochlea via bone conduction (15–17). In this manner, the pulse of RF energy is transferred into an acoustic wave within the human head and sensed by the hearing organs (15–17).

The sounds that occur with RF hearing appear to originate from within or near the back of the human head, regardless of the orientation of the head in the RF field (15–17). The actual type of noise that is heard varies with the RF pulse width and repetition rate. The relative loudness depends on the total energy per pulse (15–17). RF energy–related acoustic noise has been observed at frequencies ranging from 216 to 7,500 MHz (15,17).

RF hearing is mathematically predictable from classical physics and has been studied and characterized in laboratory animals and human subjects (15–17). Individuals involved with the use of microwaves in industrial and military settings commonly experience RF hearing (15,17). With specific reference to the operation of MR scanners, RF hearing has been found to be associated with frequencies ranging from 2.4 to 170 MHz (15).

The gradient magnetic field–induced acoustic noise that occurs during MR procedures is significantly louder than the sounds associated with RF hearing. Therefore, noises produced by the RF auditory phenomenon are effectively masked and not perceived by patients or MR operators (15). Of further note is that there is no evidence of any detrimental health effects related to the presence of RF hearing (15). However, Roschman (15) recommends an upper level limit of 30 kW applied peak pulse power of RF energy for head coils and 6 kW for surface coils used during MR imaging or spectroscopy in order to avoid RF-evoked sound pressure levels in the head increasing above the discomfort threshold of 110 dB.

REFERENCES

1. Brummett RE, Talbot JM, Charuhas P. Potential hearing loss resulting from MR imaging. *Radiology* 1988;169:539–540.
2. Goldman AM, Gossman WE, Friedlander PC. Reduction of sound levels with antinoise in MR imaging. *Radiology* 1989;173:549–550.
3. Hurwitz R, Lane SR, Bell RA, Brant-Zawadzki MN. Acoustic analysis of gradient-coil noise in MR imaging. *Radiology* 1989;173:545–548.
4. Shellock FG, Morisoli SM, Ziarati M. Measurement of acoustic noise during MR imaging: evaluation of six "worst-case" pulse sequences. *Radiology* 1994;191:91–93.
5. McJury M, Blug A, Joerger C, Condon B, Wyper D. Acoustic noise levels during magnetic resonance imaging scanning at 1.5 T. *Br J Radiol* 1994;413–415.

6. McJury MJ. Acoustic noise levels generated during high field MR imaging. *Clin Radiol* 1995: 50:331–334.
7. Kanal E, Shellock FG, Talagala L. Safety considerations in MR imaging. *Radiology* 1990;176: 593–606.
8. Shellock FG, Kanal E. Policies, guidelines, and recommendations for MR imaging safety and patient management. *J Magn Reson Imag* 1991;1:97–101.
9. Shellock FG, Litwer CA, Kanal E. Magnetic resonance imaging: bioeffects, safety, and patient management. *Q Rev Magn Reson Med* 1992;4:21–63.
10. Kanal E, Shellock FG, Sonnenblick D. MRI clinical site safety survey: phase I results and preliminary data [Abstract]. *Magn Reson Imag* 1988;7(S1):106.
11. Miller LE, Keller AM. Regulation of occupational noise. In: Harris CM, ed. *Handbook of noise control.* New York: McGraw-Hill; 1979:2.
12. Melnick W. Hearing loss from noise exposure. In: Harris CM, ed. *Handbook of noise control.* New York: McGraw-Hill; 1979:1–16.
13. Robinson DW. Characteristics of occupational noise–induced hearing loss. In: Henderson D, Hamernik RP, Dosanjh DS, Mills JH, eds. *Effects of noise on hearing.* New York: Raven Press; 1976:383–405.
14. Food and Drug Administration. Magnetic resonance diagnostic device: panel recommendation and report on petitions for MR reclassification. *Fed Reg* 1988;53:7575–7579.
15. Roschmann P. Human auditory system response to pulsed radiofrequency energy in RF coils for magnetic resonance at 2.4 to 170 MHz. *Magn Reson Med* 1991;21:197–215.
16. Elder JA. Special senses. In: United States Environmental Protection Agency, Health Effects Research Laboratory. *Biological Effects of Radiofrequency Radiation.* EPA-600/8-83-026F, Research Triangle Park, 1984:570–571.
17. Postow E, Swicord ML. Modulated fields and "window" effects. In: Polk C, Postow E, eds. *CRC handbook of biological effects of electromagnetic fields.* Boca Raton: CRC Press; 1989: 425–462.

6

Claustrophobia, Anxiety, and Panic Disorders Associated with Magnetic Resonance Procedures

A patient undergoing an MR procedure may experience an acute or delayed psychological disturbance that, depending on the severity of the symptoms, can postpone or prevent completion of the examination (1–17). There are several ramifications when a patient experiences one of a spectrum of anxiety-related problems that may then lead to an incomplete or canceled MR study. These include clinical, medicolegal, and economic aspects and the fact that the patient may require an invasive diagnostic examination in place of the MR procedure.

Dysphoric psychological reactions have been reported to be encountered by as many as 65% of the patients examined by MR imaging (10,14,16). Of the various forms of psychological distress experienced by these patients, claustrophobia, anxiety, or panic attacks tend to be the most debilitating (9,10,12,14–18). As many as 20% of individuals attempting to undergo an MR procedure cannot complete it secondary to claustrophobia or other similar sensation (1,2). The referring physicians, radiologists, and technologists may be best prepared to manage affected patients if they understand the etiology of the problem and know the appropriate maneuver(s) or intervention(s) to implement for treatment of the condition (10,16).

The sensations of apprehension, tension, worry, claustrophobia, anxiety, fear, and panic attacks have been suggested to originate from one or more factors involved in the MR procedure, including the confining dimensions of the interior of the MR system (e.g., the patient's face may be 3 to 10 inches from the inner portion of the MR system), the prolonged duration of the examination, the gradient magnetic field–induced acoustic noise, the temperature and humidity within the MR system, the distress related to the restriction of movement, and the possible stress related to the administration of an MR imaging contrast agent (1–22). Additionally, the MR system may produce a feeling of sensory deprivation, which is also known to be a precursor of severe anxiety states (9).

MR systems that have an architecture that uses a vertical magnetic field offer a more open design that might reduce the frequency of some of the above problems associated with MR procedures. Fortunately, the latest versions of these MR systems, despite having static magnetic field strengths of 0.3 T or lower, have improved technology (i.e., better gradient field specifications, optimized surface coils, etc.) compared with older versions that provide acceptable image quality and are a suitable alternative for patients with respect to MR imaging. At least one preliminary report from a retrospective study suggested that a larger-sized MR system was associated with a reduction in claustrophobia (4). In addition, newly designed "extremity-only" MR devices that have no substantial confining features are further likely to be less prone to producing psychological problems in patients undergoing MR procedures (Fig. 6-1).

Adverse psychological reactions are sometimes associated with the MR procedures simply because the examination may be perceived by the patient as a "dramatic" medical test that has an associated uncertainty of outcome (i.e., there is a fear of the presence of disease or other abnormality) (9,10). According to one study, virtually every patient who undergoes MR imaging exhibits some degree of preimaging anxiety, usually related to a previous "unpleasant" imaging experience (5).

Any type of diagnostic imaging procedure may be responsible for producing a certain amount of anxiety or other psychological problem (5). For example, Thorp et al. (2) found that, with the exception of the MR system environment issue (i.e., the confined space), patients undergoing computed tomography compared with those undergoing MR imaging had similar feelings that the pro-

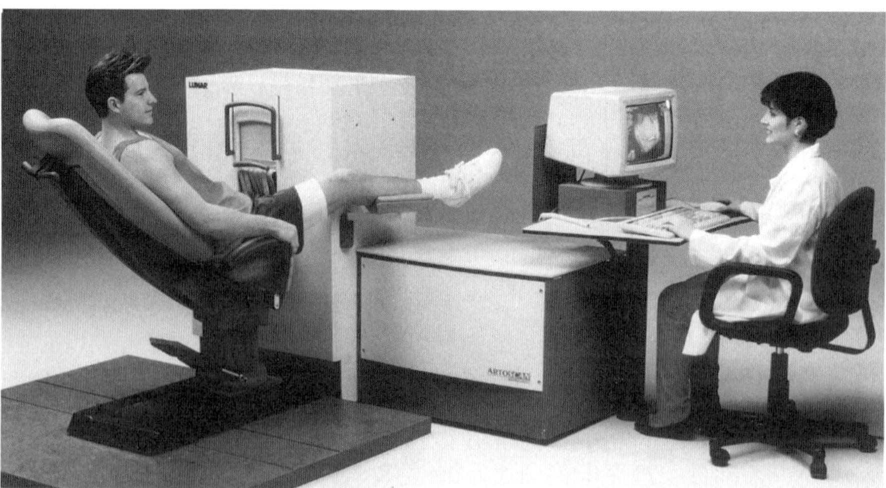

FIG. 6-1. A newly designed "extremity-only" MR device that has no substantial confining features is unlikely to produce psychological problems in patients undergoing MR procedures. (Courtesy of Lunar, Madison, WI.)

cedure was unpleasant. Patients finding the experience difficult tended to be those with high initial levels of anxiety, little experience with diagnostic procedures, and believed that they had cancer (2). The study by Thorp et al. (2) supports the need for direct professional interaction to prepare and educate the patient before any form of diagnostic imaging examination.

Some authors have proposed that it would be useful to identify patients at risk so that they could be handled more effectively before the MR examination (1–3,5). Performing a pre-procedure "fear assessment" may help predict patients who will experience psychological problems related to the MR procedure (1–3,5).

Although prescreening patients referred for MR procedures for the presence of claustrophobia or other forms of psychological distress has been recommended (10), it has been our experience that the suggestion of potential "claustrophobic surroundings" to the patient may serve to incite an anxious response that would not otherwise occur. For example, patients with no prior history of psychological problems have been unable to undergo examination by MR because of the acute onset of claustrophobia, anxiety, or panic. Conversely, patients known to have psychological disorders, including claustrophobia, have completed MR procedures without incident. Therefore, it is unlikely that predetermination of patients who may develop adverse psychological responses to MR procedures is a helpful or effective means of preparing for the situations that they present. We do not recommend asking if the patient is claustrophobic during the screening procedure.

Fishbain et al. (20,21) reported that two patients who tolerated MR imaging with great difficulty had persistent claustrophobia that required prolonged psychiatric intervention. It was felt that MR imaging triggered the persistent claustrophobia and, therefore, there is the potential for medicolegal problems to occur in certain cases (20,21). Fishbain et al. (20) proposed that if iatrogenic claustrophobia associated with MR imaging does ultimately become a medicolegal issue, MR sites may elect do the following: (a) ask if the patient has a history of claustrophobia, (b) ask if anyone in the patient's family has a history of claustrophobia, (c) warn the patient about the possible development of claustrophobia associated with MR imaging, and (d) have the patient sign a release form. The requirement for a release form is probably unwarranted considering the vast number of patients who have undergone MR procedures over the years compared with the cases of extreme claustrophobia, anxiety, or severe panic attacks.

Specific forms of psychological reactions to MR imaging, namely anxiety and panic attacks, are typically characterized by clinical symptoms that include fear of dying, nausea, paresthesia, palpitations, chest pain, faintness, dyspnea, and vertigo (18). Because many symptoms of panic attack represent overactivity of the sympathetic nervous system (18), there is a concern that catecholamine responses may precipitate cardiac arrhythmias and/or ischemia in susceptible patients during the MR procedure (19). However, this has not been reported in a clinical MR setting.

Several methods of handling patients who experience psychological difficulties related to MR procedures have been described and are summarized in Table 6-1 (10–13,15–24). Providing the patient with special preparation and education concerning the specific aspects of the MR examination, including the internal dimensions of the MR system, the level of gradient magnetic field–induced acoustic noise to expect, and the time duration of the examination, are believed to be among the more important means of preparing patients with potential adverse psychological reactions to MR procedures. This may be effectively accomplished by providing the patient time to view an educational video tape supplemented by a question and answer session with an MR-trained professional before the procedure.

Successful completion of MR examinations may be accomplished by allowing an appropriately screened relative or friend to remain with the patient during the procedure. A familiar person in the MR system room often helps patients who are anxious because they develop an increased sense of security (11,17). Simply maintaining verbal contact via the intercom system or physical contact by having an individual remain in the MR system room with the patient during the examination will frequently decrease psychological distress (11,16,17).

Electronic devices that use compressed air to transmit music or audio communication through headphones have been developed specifically for use with MR systems (7,24,25). MR-compatible music/audio systems may be acquired from a commercial vendor or can be made by adapting an airplane pneumatic earphone headset, as described by Axel (24). These MR-compatible music systems can be used to provide calming music to the emotionally distraught patient and, with the proper design, help to minimize exposure to gradient magnetic field–induced acoustic noise (Fig. 6-2). Reports have indicated that the

TABLE 6-1. *Recommended techniques for managing patients with psychological problems related to MR procedures*

1. Prepare and educate the patient concerning specific aspects of the MR examination (e.g., MR system dimensions, gradient noise, intercom system, etc.).
2. Allow an appropriately screened relative or friend to remain with the patient during the MR procedure.
3. Maintain physical or verbal contact with the patient during the MR procedure.
4. Use MR-compatible headphones to provide music to the patient and to minimize gradient magnetic field-induced noise.
5. Use an MR-compatible television monitor to provide a visual distraction to the patient.
6. Place the patient in a prone position inside the MR system.
7. Place the patient feet first instead of head first into the MR system.
8. Use special mirrors or prism glasses.
9. Use a blindfold so that the patient is not aware of the close surroundings.
10. Use bright lights at inside and at either end of the MR system.
11. Use a fan inside of the MR system to provide adequate air movement.
12. Use relaxation techniques such as controlled breathing or mental imagery.
13. Use systematic desensitization.
14. Use medical hypnosis.
15. Use a sedative or other similar medication.

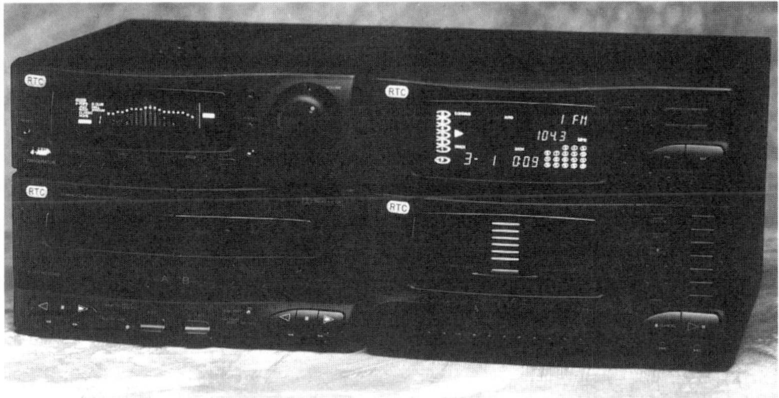

FIG. 6-2. MR-compatible projection television used for patients during MR procedures. (Courtesy of Resonance Technology, Van Nuys, CA.)

use of these devices has been successful in reducing symptoms of anxiety in patients during MR procedures (7,25). In addition, it is now possible to provide visual stimulation to the patient via a projection television (Fig. 6-3). Using music and/or television typically serves as a useful technique to distract potentially upset patients during MR procedures.

Placing the patient in a prone position inside the MR system so that the patient can visualize the opening of the bore provides a sensation of being inside a device that is more spacious and alleviates the "closed-in" feeling associated with the supine position (11). Prone positioning of the patient may not be a practical alternative in many cases, especially when MR imaging is performed on anatomic regions that require the use of flat local coils, such as examinations of the spine or if the patient has underlying medical conditions (e.g., shortness of breath, the presence of chest tubes, etc.) that prevent this placement scheme (1). Another patient positioning method that helps in some patients is to place the individual feet-first instead of head-first into the MR system.

MR system–mounted mirrors or prism glasses can be used to permit the patient to maintain a vertical view of the outside of the MR system in order to minimize phobic responses. Using a blindfold so that the patient is not aware of the close surroundings has also been suggested to be an effective technique for enabling anxious patients to successfully undergo MR procedures (11,17).

The overall environment of the MR system may be changed to optimize the management of apprehensive patients (17). For example, the presence of higher lighting levels tends to make most individuals feel less anxious. Therefore, the use of bright lights at either end and inside the MR system can produce a less imposing environment for the patient. In addition, using a fan inside the MR system to provide more air movement will help reduce the sensation of confinement (17) and lessen any tissue heating that may result when high levels of RF power are used for MR imaging.

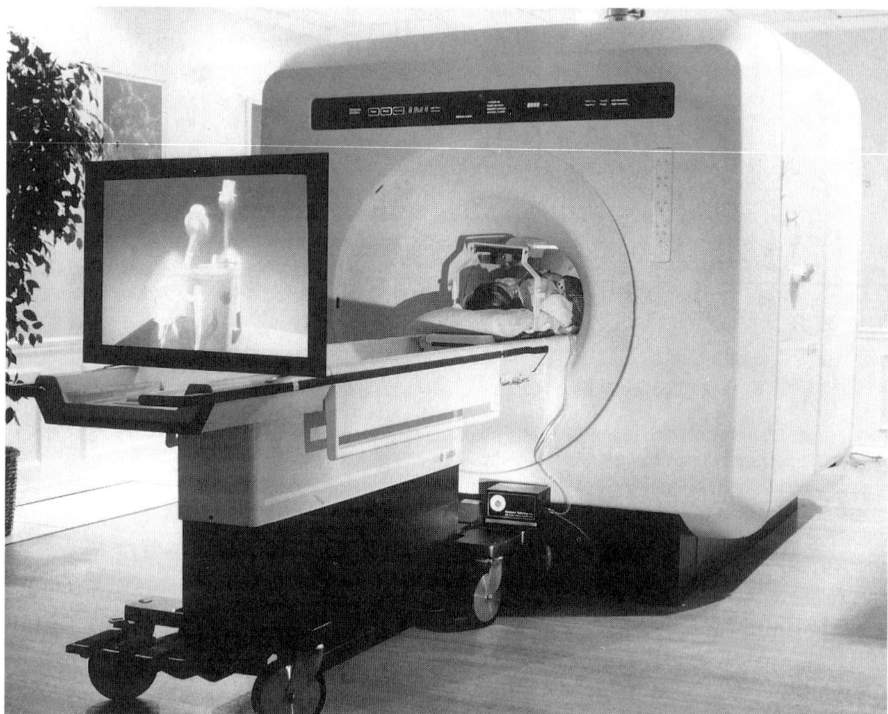

FIG. 6-3. Example of MR-compatible stereo system used to provide music to patients during MR procedures. (Courtesy of Resonance Technology, Van Nuys, CA.)

Educating the patient with regard to the aspects of the examination by providing detailed information about the structure of the MR system and other features of the procedures to expect may not be entirely sufficient for alleviating psychological distress. Quirk et al. (15) reported that psychological preparation that included information about the examination and the use of relaxation strategies (i.e., breathing relaxation techniques, visualization of pleasant images, performance of mental exercises, etc.) was shown to be more effective for reducing anxiety in patients compared with providing information alone.

Klonoff et al. (12) suggested that educating patients along with providing systematic desensitization exercises may be useful for minimizing psychological disorders related to MR procedures. Because the spatial aspects of the MR system and duration of the examination were felt to be important factors involved in the systematic desensitization process, a special protocol was developed and used to treat a single patient with psychological distress (12).

In one case, systematic desensitization was conducted before the MR procedure and involved having the patient place her head in a box. The size of the box was incrementally decreased until it approximated the internal dimensions of the MR system (12). Additionally, the patient was required to increase gradually the amount of time she could tolerate the box over her head, until it equaled 50 to 60 min, to approximate the maximum time needed for MR imaging (12). The patient also wore prism glasses that permitted her to have a direct view in the vertical plane during MR imaging (12). After four treatment sessions, the patient was able to successfully undergo MR imaging (12).

Medical hypnosis has been demonstrated to be a successful means of treating phobias (23) and, not surprisingly, has been used as an effective intervention to enable a claustrophobic or anxious patient to complete examination by MR imaging (13,22). Successful hypnotherapy requires a trained medical hypnotist and a willing, trance-susceptible patient (13,22). Therefore, identifying the appropriate patient that would benefit from being hypnotized during the MR procedure and having a hypnosis therapist available for treatment are prerequisites for instituting this technique of patient management.

There is a secondary effect of using hypnosis for patients with psychological disorders undergoing MR procedures insofar as patients have reported feeling a general reduction in anxiety in their everyday lives after undergoing hypnosis for MR imaging (22). Unfortunately, time constraints in the clinical MR setting do not always permit adequate attention to the patient's emotional problems (22), such that patients with claustrophobia or other forms of psychological distress may not be easily managed using behavioral therapy or medical hypnosis techniques, especially considering that multiple treatment sessions with a trained therapist may be required.

In most MR facilities, patients who are severely affected by claustrophobia, anxiety, or panic attacks in response to MR procedures are usually sedated when other proposed attempts to counteract their psychological problems fail. Using short-acting sedatives such as diazepam, alprazolam, intranasal midazolam, or one of the newer anxiolytic medications may be the only means of managing patients with a high degree of anxiety related to the MR procedure.

A study conducted by Avrahami (18) in patients with panic attacks who were unable to undergo MR imaging reported that treatment with intravenous diazepam caused the symptoms to disappear rapidly and permitted completion of the examination in every case. However, the use of sedatives in patients before and during MR procedures may not be required in all instances, nor is it practical (10,12,13,15,22). We suggest that one or a combination of the suggested nonmedication techniques indicated in Table 6-1 be attempted before immediately electing to use a sedative.

If a sedative or other similar drug is used in a patient in preparation for an MR procedure, the use of this medication in the MR setting involves several important considerations (6). For example, the time when the patient should be administered the medication for optimal effect before the examination should be considered along with the possibility that there may be an adverse reaction to the drug (6). Provisions should also be available for an area to permit adequate recovery of the patient after the MR procedure. The patient should also have someone available to provide transportation from the MR facility after receiving medication. Additional details related to the proper protocol to implement and support sedation of patients in the MR environment are provided in Chapter 7.

REFERENCES

1. Melendez C, McCrank E. Anxiety-related reactions associated with magnetic resonance imaging examinations. *JAMA* 1993;270:745–747.
2. Thorp D, Owens RG, Whitehouse G, Dewey ME. Subjective experiences of magnetic resonance imaging. *Clin Radiol* 1990;41:276–278.
3. Kilborn LC, Labbe EE. Magnetic resonance imaging scanning procedures: development of phobic response during scan and at one-month follow-up. *J Behav Med* 1990;13:391–401.
4. Dantenforfer K, Wimberger D, Katschnig H, Imhoff H. Claustrophobia in MRI scanners. *Lancet* 1991;338:761–762.
5. MacKenzie R, Sims C, Owens RG, Dixon AK. Patient's perceptions of magnetic resonance imaging. *Clin Radiol* 1995;50:137–143.
6. Moss ML, Boungiorno PA, Clancy VA. Intranasal midazolam for claustrophobia in MRI. *J Comp Assist Tomogr* 1993;17:991–992.
7. Slifer KJ, Penn-Jones K, Cataldo MF, Conner RT, Zerhouni EA. Music enhances patient's comfort during MR imaging. *AJR Am J Roentgenol* 1991;156:403.
8. Duluca SA, Castronovo FP. Hazards of magnetic resonance imaging. *Am Family Phys* 1990;41:145–146.
9. Flaherty JA, Hoskinson K. Emotional distress during magnetic resonance imaging. *N Engl J Med* 1989;320:467–468.
10. Granet RB, Gelber LJ. Claustrophobia during MR imaging. *N Engl J Med* 1990;87:479–482.
11. Hricak H, Amparo EG. Body MRI: alleviation of claustrophobia by prone positioning. *Radiology* 1984;152:819.
12. Klonoff EA, Janata JW, Kaufman B. The use of systematic desensitization to overcome resistance to magnetic resonance imaging (MRI) scanning. *J Behav Ther Exp Psychiatry* 1986;17:189–192.
13. Phelps LA. MRI and claustrophobia. *Am Family Phys* 1991;42:930.
14. Quirk ME, Letendre AJ, Ciottone RA, Lingley JF. Anxiety in patients undergoing MR imaging. *Radiology* 1989;170:463–466.
15. Quirk ME, Letendre AJ, Ciottone RA, Lingley JF. Evaluation of three psychological interventions to reduce anxiety during MR imaging. *Radiology* 1989;173:759–762.
16. Shellock FG, Kanal E. Policies, guidelines, and recommendations for MR imaging and patient management. *J Magn Reson Imag* 1991;1:97–101.
17. Weinreb J, Maravilla KR, Peshock R, Payne J. Magnetic resonance imaging: improving patient tolerance and safety. *AJR Am J Roentgenol* 1984;143:1285–1287.
18. Avrahami E. Panic attacks during MR imaging: treatment with IV diazepam. *AJNR Am J Neuroradiol* 1990;11:833–835.
19. Brennan SC, Redd WH, Jacobsen PB, et al. Anxiety and panic during magnetic resonance scans. *Lancet* 1988;2:512.
20. Fishbain D, Goldberg M, Labbe ED, et al. MR imaging as a trigger for persistent claustrophobia. *AJR Am J Roentgenol* 1989;152:653.
21. Fishbain D, Goldberg M, Labbe ED, et al. Long-term claustrophobia following magnetic resonance imaging. *Am J Psychiatry* 1988;145:1038–1039.
22. Friday PJ, Kubal WS. Magnetic resonance imaging: improved patient tolerance utilizing medical hypnosis. *Am J Clin Hypnosis* 1990;33:80–84.
23. McGuinness TP. Hypnosis in the treatment of phobias: a review of the literature. *Am J Clin Hypnosis* 1984;26:261–272.
24. Axel L. Simpler music/audio system for patients having MR imaging. *AJR Am J Roentgenol* 1988;151:1080.
25. Miyamoto AT, Kasson RT. Simple music/audio system for patients having MR imaging. *AJR Am J Roentgenol* 1988;151:1060.

7

Physiologic Monitoring During Magnetic Resonance Procedures

Monitoring vital signs during an MR procedure is indicated whenever a patient requires observations of physiologic parameters as part of routine management because of an underlying health problem or whenever a patient is unable to respond or alert the health care practitioner performing the MR procedure regarding pain, respiratory problem, cardiac distress, or other difficulty that might arise during the examination (1). In addition, a patient should be monitored if there is a greater potential for a change of physiologic status during the MR procedure (1–3). With the advent of newer types of MR applications, such as MR-guided surgery and therapy, there is also an increased need to monitor patients in the MR environment. Additionally, MR systems that use echo planar imaging (EPI) techniques or with static magnetic fields greater than 2 T may also need to monitor patients continuously to ensure their safety because of the potential risks that may be encountered with these MR devices.

Because of the widespread use of MR imaging contrast agents and the potential for adverse effects or idiosyncratic reactions related to the use of these drugs, it is prudent to have MR-compatible monitoring devices readily available in the MR setting for proper management of patients who may experience side effects (1). This is emphasized because side effects related to the use of MR contrast agents, although extremely rare, may be quite serious or even fatal.

Fatalities and severe injuries have occurred in association with MR procedures, which may have been prevented with the proper use of monitoring equipment and devices (1,3–32). Therefore, MR users must carefully consider the ethical and medicolegal ramifications of providing adequate patient care, which includes identifying those patients who require monitoring in the MR setting and after a proper protocol to ensure their safety using appropriate devices (1–3). Table 7-1 lists examples of patients who may require monitoring during MR procedures.

In 1992, the Safety Committee of the Society for Magnetic Resonance Imaging published guidelines and recommendations concerning the monitoring of

TABLE 7-1. *Examples of patients that may require monitoring during MR procedures*

Patients who are physically or mentally unstable.
Patients who have their normal physiologic function(s) compromised in any way.
Patients who are unable to communicate.
Neonatal and pediatric patients.
Sedated or anesthetized patients.
Patients undergoing MR-guided interventional procedures.
Patients undergoing MR procedures using advanced MR systems (e.g., echo planar imaging systems, MR systems with static magnetic field strengths that exceed 2 T, etc.).
Patients who may have a reaction to an MR imaging contrast agent.

patients during MR procedures (2). This information indicates that all patients undergoing MR procedures should, at the very least, be visually (e.g., using a camera system) and/or verbally (e.g., intercom system) monitored, and that patients who are sedated, anesthetized, or are unable to communicate should be physiologically monitored and supported by the appropriate means (2). Of note is that recent guidelines issued by the Joint Commission on Accreditation of Healthcare Organizations indicate that all patients who receive sedatives or anesthetics require monitoring during the administration and recovery from these medications (33). This includes similar types of patients in the MR environment.

POTENTIAL HAZARDS ASSOCIATED WITH THE USE OF PHYSIOLOGIC MONITORS DURING MR PROCEDURES

Several hazards are associated with the performance of patient monitoring during MR examinations. Physiologic monitors that contain ferromagnetic components (i.e., transformers, outer casings, etc.) can be strongly attracted by the static magnetic field used by the MR system, posing a serious "missile" hazard to patients and MR operators. In addition, they have the potential of damaging the MR system (11,13,14,21,26).

In certain cases, securing the MR-compatible monitor a suitable distance (e.g., approximately 8 feet from the opening of the bore of a 1.5-T magnet or according to the specifications of the manufacturer of the monitor) from the MR system is sufficient to prevent it from becoming a potential projectile and to protect the operation of the monitoring device. If possible, devices with ferromagnetic components should be permanently fixed and properly labeled with warning information to prevent them from being moved too close to the MR system. All personnel involved with MR procedures should be aware of the importance of the placement of monitoring equipment and of the hazards related to moving portable equipment too close to the MR system of any static magnetic field strength.

Radiofrequency (RF) fields from the MR system can affect the operation of the monitor. In addition, the monitor may emit spurious noise that, in turn, distorts the MR image during MR procedures. For example, RF interference can be leaked by monitors that contain microprocessors or other similar components. This electromagnetic noise may be so severe that moderate to severe imaging artifacts are produced (Fig. 7-1). To prevent adverse radiofrequency-related interactions between the MR system and monitor, the addition of RF-shielded cables, RF filters, special outer "shielding" casings, or fiberoptic transmission of the signals can be used to modify the monitors to work properly during MR procedures. This is only one of the considerations to address compatibility of the monitor with the MR system.

Electrical currents may be generated during the operation of MR systems in the conductive materials used to construct monitors (1,11,21,26). These currents may be of sufficient magnitude to cause thermal injury to the patient (1,34–38). Numerous first, second, and third degree burns have occurred in association with MR procedures that were directly attributed to the use of monitoring devices (1,34–38). These thermal injuries have been associated with the

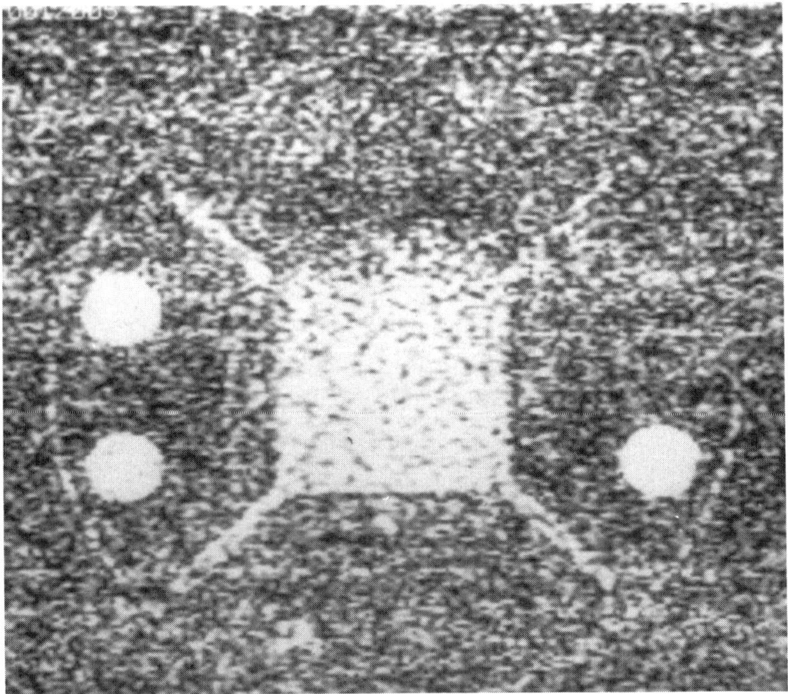

FIG. 7-1. Example of severe image distortion caused by spurious RF noise from a monitor operating within the MR system room. A fluid-filled Plexiglas phantom was scanned with a T1-weighted pulse sequence during the operation of the monitor.

use of electrocardiographic lead wires, plethysmographic gating systems, pulse oximeters, and other types of monitors that require the use of wires or cables made from conductive materials (1,34–38). Several safety procedures should be followed to prevent burns from occurring in association with the use of monitors and other devices during MR procedures (Table 7-2).

EVALUATING PHYSIOLOGIC MONITORS FOR MR COMPATIBILITY

Conventional monitoring equipment was not designed to operate in the harsh MR environment where static, gradient, and RF electromagnetic fields can adversely affect the operation of these devices. Fortunately, MR-compatible monitors and other devices have been developed and can be used routinely in inpatient and outpatient MR facilities (1–32).

TABLE 7-2. *Recommendations for the prevention of burns associated with the use of physiologic monitoring equipment during MR procedures*

1. Use only monitoring equipment that has been tested and determined to be MR compatible.
2. Permit only individuals that have been properly-trained for work on the MR system and properly-trained to operate monitors to be responsible for patients in the MR environment.
3. Check the integrity (e.g., cracking, fraying, etc.) of the electrical insulation of each monitoring lead, cable, or wire before using the device during an MR procedure.
4. Remove all electrically conductive material from the bore of the MR system that is not required for the MR procedure (i.e., unused surface coils, cables, etc.).
5. Keep all electrically conductive material(s) that must remain in the bore of the MR system from directly contacting the patient by placing thermal and/or electrical insulation (including air) between the conductive material and the patient. For example, place EKG leads underneath the patient comfort pads and/or use additional foam pads between the patient and cables to prevent direct contact with the patient's tissue.
6. Keep electrically conductive material (EKG leads, cables, etc.) that must remain within the bore of the MR system from forming large diameter, conductive loops (remember, the patient's tissue may be involved in the formation of the conductive loop).
7. Position all cables to prevent "cross points". A cross point is the point where a cable crosses another cable, a cable loops across itself, or a cable touches either the patient or sides of the magnetic bore more than once.
8. Do not cross cables inside or outside of the bore of the magnet of the MR system (note that loops can be closed, U-shaped, or S-shaped).
9. Position all EKG cables so that they exit down the center of the patient table of the MR system.
10. Position the patient so that there is no direct contact between the patient's skin and the bore of the magnet of the MR system.
11. Use only MR system manufacturer approved EKG wires, leads, and electrodes and appropriate application techniques.
12. Do not position conductive leads or cables across a metallic prosthesis.
13. Remove any monitor that does not appear to be operating properly during the MR procedure.
14. Discontinue the MR procedure immediately if the patient reports feeling warm or hot.
15. Follow the instructions for proper operation of the monitoring equipment provided by the manufacturer of the device.

Preclinical testing is required for all monitoring devices that are intended for use in the MR setting. This is usually accomplished by the manufacturer in conjunction with MR users who are interested in using a particular type of device. The testing process for determining the compatibility of a monitoring device with MR procedures is usually performed by initially calibrating the monitor and checking its operation outside of the MR area to determine that it is functioning properly. Next, an evaluation is made using a hand-held magnet to assess the presence of ferromagnetic components. This procedure should be performed on all metallic components of the device. If the monitor has ferromagnetic components (which is the case for most devices), it should be placed in a position that is a suitable distance from the MR system to avoid attraction of the ferromagnetic components by the magnetic fringe field, and labeled accordingly.

A phantom is then imaged using examples of each of the various pulse sequences that are typically used in the clinical setting, while the monitor is operating. This allows a determination of whether the device produces any spurious electromagnetic noise that would distort the image quality or other aspects of the MR procedure. Finally, the monitor is applied to volunteer subjects and patients and observed during operation of the MR system to determine if it is functioning in an acceptable manner. Because of the extensive testing required for this preclinical evaluation, most MR users rely on published reports or information provided to them by MR manufacturers regarding the use of physiologic monitors in the MR environment.

TECHNIQUES FOR PHYSIOLOGIC MONITORING AND PROVIDING OTHER PATIENT SUPPORT DURING MR PROCEDURES

Various monitors and other patient support devices have been developed or specially modified to perform during MR procedures (1–32). Table 7-3 lists examples of MR-compatible devices that have been successfully tested and operated during MR procedures performed using MR systems with static magnetic field strengths up to 1.5 T. The following are descriptions of important physiologic parameters that may be assessed using MR-compatible devices and the appropriate methods to record them during MR procedures.

Electrocardiogram

Monitoring the EKG in the MR environment is particularly challenging because of inherent distortion of the EKG waveform. This effect is seen primarily when blood, a conductive fluid, flows through the static magnetic field of the MR system (39). The induced biopotential is seen primarily as an augmentation of T-wave amplitude, although other nonspecific waveform changes are also

TABLE 7-3. *Examples of MR-compatible monitors, devices, and ventilators*[a]

Device and manufacturer:	Function
MR-Compatible Pulse Oximeter Invivo Research, Inc. Orlando, FL	Oxygen saturation, heart rate
MRI Fiber-optic Pulse Oximeter Nonin Medical Inc. Plymouth, MN	Oxygen saturation, heart rate
MR-Compatible Pulse Oximeter Magnetic Resonance Equipment Corp. Bay Shore, NY	Oxygen saturation, heart rate
Omega 1400 Invivo Research, Inc. Orlando, FL	Blood pressure, heart rate
Omni-Trak 3100 MRI Vital Signs Monitor Invivo Research, Inc. Orlando, FL	Heart rate, EKG, oxygen saturation, respiratory rate, gas exchange, blood pressure
MR Equipment Vital Signs Monitor[b] Model 6500 Bay Shore, NY	Heart rate, EKG, oxygen saturation, respiratory rate, gas exchange, blood pressure
Laserflow Blood Perfusion Monitor Vasomed, Inc. St. Paul, MN	Cutaneous blood flow
Medpacific LD 5000 Laser-Doppler Perfusion Monitor Medpacific Corporation Seattle, WA	Cutaneous blood flow
Respiratory Rate Monitor, Models 515 and 525 Biochem International Waukesha, WI	Respiratory rate, apnea
MicroSpan Capnometer 8800 Biochem International Waukesha, WI	Respiratory rate, end tidal carbon dioxide, apnea
Aneuroid Chest Bellows Coulborun Instruments Allentown, Pennsylvania	Respiratory rate
Fluoroptic Thermometry System, Model 3000 Luxtron Santa Clara, CA	Temperature
Omni-Vent, Series D Columbia Medical Marketing Topeka, KS	Ventilator
Ventilator, Models 225 and 2500 Monaghan Medical Corporation Plattsburgh, PA	Ventilator
Anesthesia Ventilator Ohio Medical Madison, WI	Ventilator
Infant Ventilator MVP-10 Bio-Med Devices, Inc. Madison, WI	Ventilator

TABLE 7-3. *Continued.*

Device and manufacturer:	Function
Ohmeda Excel MRI Anesthesia Delivery System Ohmeda, Inc. Madison, WI	Delivery of gas anesthesia
Siemens-Elema Model 900C Iselin, NJ	Ventilator

[a] Note that these devices may require modifications to make them MR-compatible and none of them should be positioned closer than 8 feet from the entrance of the bore of a 1.5 T MR system. Also, monitors with metallic cables, leads, probes or other similar patient interfaces may cause mild-to-moderate artifacts if placed near the imaging area of interest. Consult manufacturers to determine additional information related to compatibility with specific MR systems.

[b] This multi-parameter monitoring device has not received U.S. Food and Drug Administration recognition as of 8/96.

apparent on the EKG. Because an elevated T wave or ST segment may be associated with true physiologic disorders, the static magnetic field–induced EKG distortions may be problematic. For this reason, a baseline recording of the EKG before placing the patient inside the MR system may be necessary.

Additional artifacts caused by the static, gradient, and RF electromagnetic fields can severely distort the EKG, making observation of morphologic changes and detection of arrhythmia quite difficult (Fig. 7-2). To minimize some of these artifacts, a variety of filtering techniques—active and passive—may be used.

Active techniques involve the use of low-pass filters or the electronic suppression of noise, which decrease the artifacts that occur from the gradient and RF electromagnetic fields while maintaining the intrinsic qualities of the EKG (18,29,39–41). Passive techniques include proper lead placement and special cable and lead preparation methods that tend to minimize the artifacts seen on the EKG (40). Rokey et al. (18) described the use of a specially designed time-varying filter developed to reduce the artifacts associated with the gradient magnetic field during the operation of the MR system. This device used a telemetry system to preserve the low-frequency isolation between the inside and outside of the RF shield of the room (18).

EKG artifacts that occur in the MR environment may also be decreased substantially by implementing several simple techniques (1,40), including using EKG electrodes that have minimal metal, selecting electrodes and cables that contain no ferromagnetic metals, placing the limb electrodes in close proximity to one another, placing the line between the limb electrodes and leg electrode parallel to the magnetic field flux lines, keeping the area between the limb electrodes and leg electrode small, placing the area of the electrodes near or in the center of the MR system, and twisting or braiding the cables.

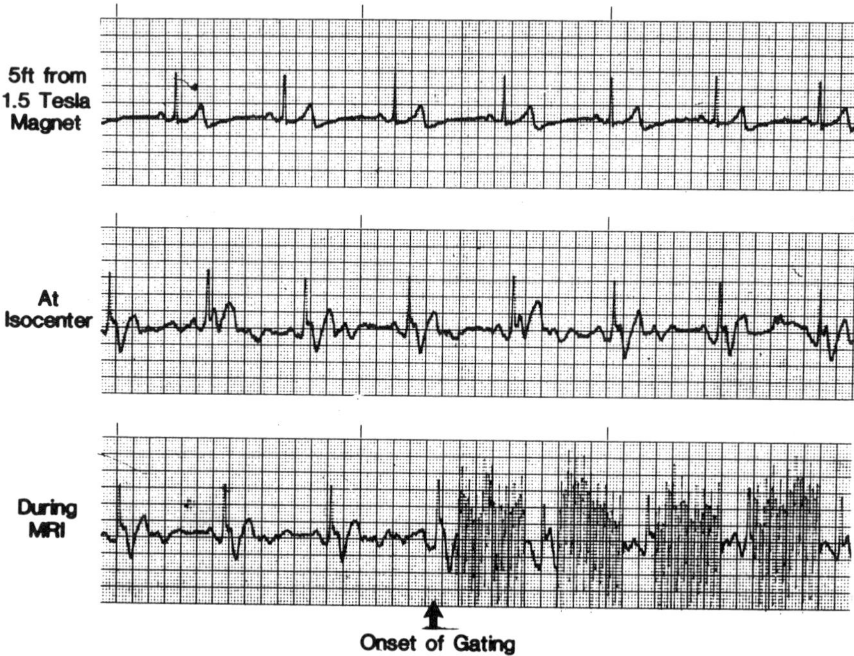

FIG. 7-2. Electrocardiogram recorded outside, inside, and during the operation of a 1.5-T MRI scanner. Note the augmented T wave resulting from the induced flow potential as well as the other nonspecific changes caused by the static magnetic field. In addition, during MRI (onset of gating) there is severe distortion of the electrocardiographic waveform.

Heart Rate

Heart rate may be determined continuously in patients during MR procedures using various types of appropriate equipment including an EKG, photoplethysmograph, or pulse oximeter monitor (1,4,7,11,14,21,26). A noninvasive heart rate and blood pressure monitor (see section below) may also be used to obtain intermittent recordings of heart rate during MR procedures (1,11,21).

Respiratory Rate and Apnea

Because respiratory depression and upper airway obstruction are frequent complications associated with the use of sedatives and anesthetics, monitoring techniques that detect a decrease in respiratory rate, hypoxemia, or airway obstruction should be used during the administration of these agents (1,11,42–46). This is particularly important in the MR setting because simple visual observation of the patient's respiratory efforts is difficult because of the configuration of most MR systems.

Respiratory rate monitoring may be accomplished during MR procedures by various techniques. An impedance method that uses chest leads and electrodes similar to those used to record the EKG can be used to record the respiratory rate. This technique of respiratory monitoring measures a difference in electrical impedance induced between the leads that correspond to changes in respiratory movements.

Proper placement of the electrodes to record respiratory rate often precludes the ability to obtain a useful EKG for heart rate because of the differing positioning patterns required to acquire each of these parameters. In addition, the electrical impedance method of assessing respiratory rate may be inaccurate in pediatric patients because of the small volumes and associated motions of the relatively small thorax area.

Respiratory rate may also be monitored during MR procedures using a rubber bellows placed around the patient's thorax or abdomen (i.e., for "chest" or "belly" breathers) (1,11,47). The bellows is attached to a remote pressure transducer that records body movement changes associated with inspiration and expiration (47). This bellows monitoring technique, like the electrical impedance method, is capable of recording only body movements associated with respiratory efforts. Therefore, these techniques of monitoring respiratory rate do not detect apneic episodes related to upper airway obstruction (i.e., absent airflow despite respiratory effort) and may not provide sufficient sensitivity for assessing patients during MR procedures. For this reason, assessment of respiratory rate and identification of apnea should be accomplished using other, more appropriate monitoring devices.

Respiratory rate and apnea may be monitored during MR procedures with an end-tidal carbon dioxide monitor or a capnometer, as previously described (1,11,21) (see Table 7-3). These devices measure the level of carbon dioxide during the end of the respiratory cycle (i.e., end-tidal carbon dioxide), when carbon dioxide is at its maximum level. Additionally, capnometers provide quantitative data with respect to end-tidal carbon dioxide, which is important for determining certain aspects of gas exchange in patients (Fig. 7-3). The waveform provided on the end-tidal CO_2 monitors is also useful for assessing whether the patient is having any difficulties with breathing. The interface between the patient and the end-tidal carbon dioxide monitor and capnometer is a plastic nasal or oronasal cannula. This interface prevents any potential adverse interaction between the monitor and the patient during an MR procedure.

Pulse Oximetry

Pulse oximetry is a monitoring technique that assesses the oxygenation of tissue and a pulse oximeter is used for this measurement. This device deter-

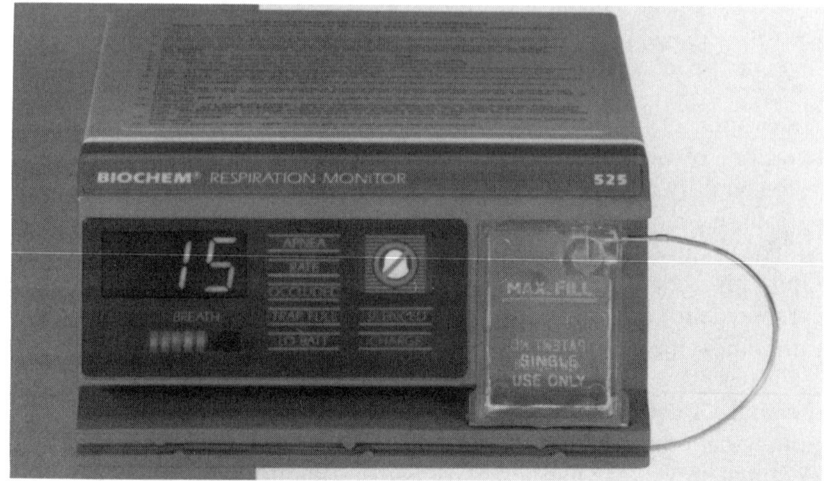

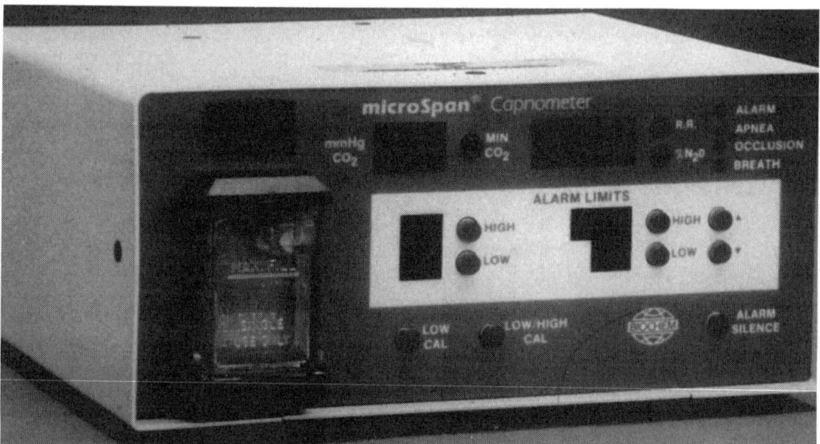

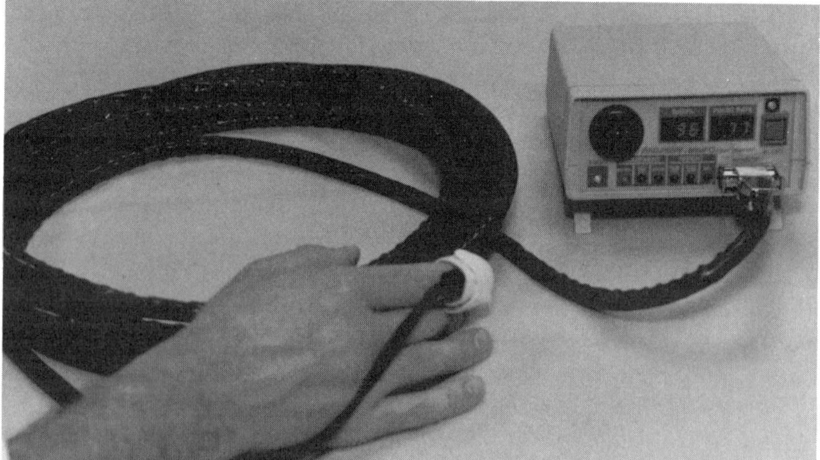

FIG. 7-3. Examples of MR-compatible equipment. Respiratory monitor (**A**), capnometer (**B**), fiberoptic pulse oximeter (**C**), noninvasive heart rate and blood pressure monitor (**D**), cutaneous blood flow monitor (**E**), multiparameter physiologic monitor (**F**), fluoroptic thermometer with multiple sensors (**G**), and portable respirator (**H**).

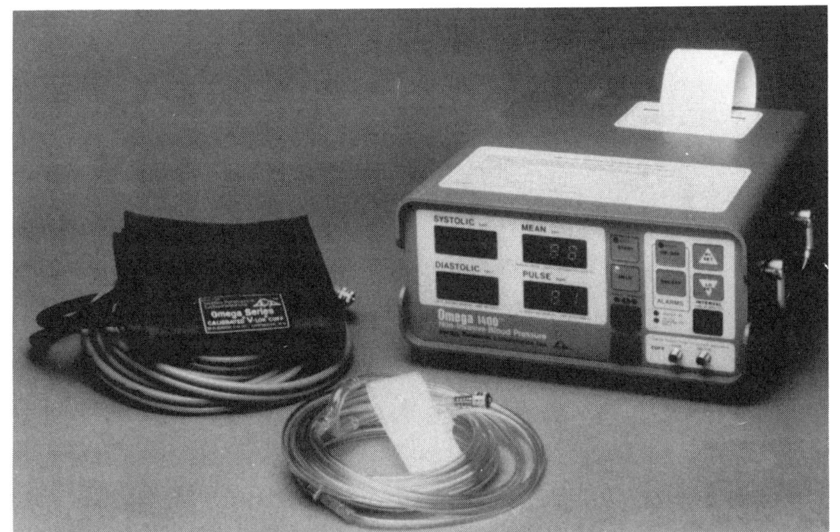

D

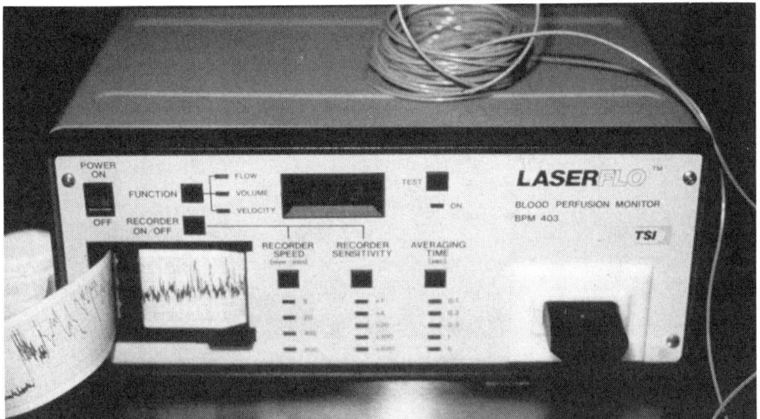

E

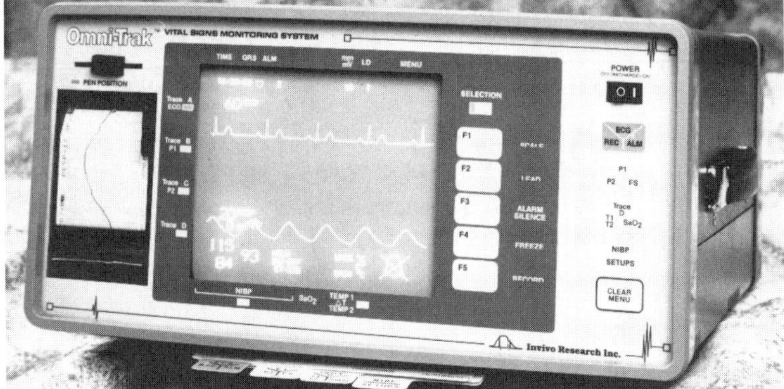

F

FIG. 7-3. *Continued.*

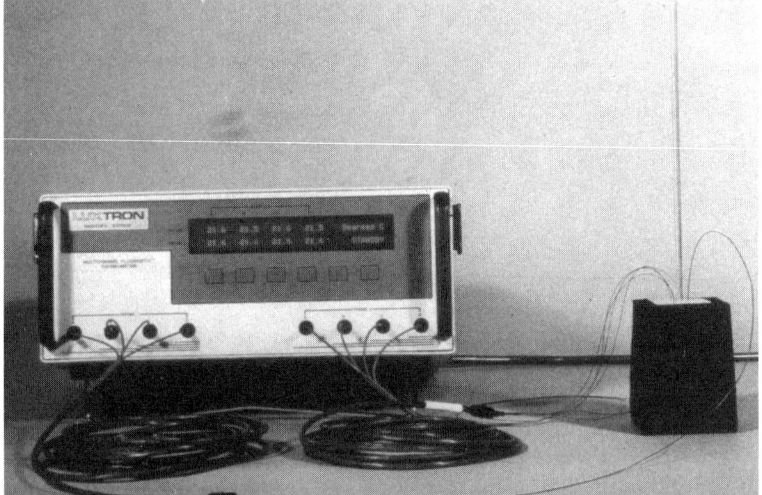

G

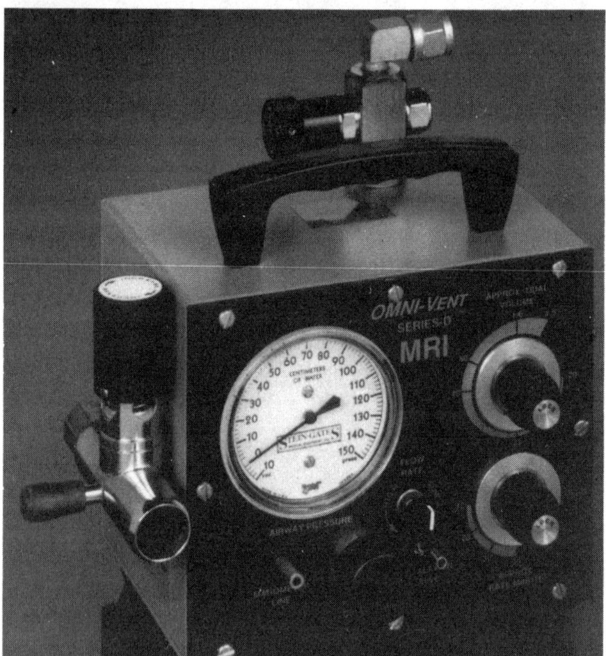

H

FIG. 7-3. *Continued.*

mines oxygen saturation and pulse rate on a continuous basis by measuring the transmission of light through a vascular measuring site such as the earlobe, fingertip, or toe. Because oxygen-saturated blood absorbs differing quantities of light compared with unsaturated blood, the amount of light absorbed by the blood can be used to calculate the ratio of oxygenated hemoglobin to total hemoglobin and displayed as the oxygen saturation.

The patient's heart rate is calculated by measuring the frequency with which the pulsations occur as the blood pulsates through the vascular bed. Pulse oximetry is considered by anesthesiologists as the standard practice for monitoring sedated or anesthetized patients (33,42–46). Therefore, using a pulse oximeter to monitor all patients who require continuous assessment during MR procedures is highly recommended. Commercially available, specially modified pulse oximeters using hard wire cables have been used, with moderate success, to monitor sedated and anesthetized patients during the MR procedures (see Fig. 7-3). Unfortunately, these pulse oximeters tend to work intermittently during the operation of the MR system, primarily because of interference from the gradient and/or radiofrequency electromagnetic fields. Of greater concern is the fact that many patients have been burned using pulse oximeters with hard wire cables during MR procedures, presumably as a result of excessive current being induced in inappropriately looped conductive cables attached to the patient probes of the pulse oximeters (1,35,37,38).

Pulse oximeters have been developed that use fiberoptic technology to obtain and transmit the physiologic signals from the patient (1,26) (see Table 7-3). These devices operate without interference by the electromagnetic fields used for MR procedures. It is physically impossible for a patient to be burned by the use of a fiberoptic pulse oximeter during an MR procedure because there are no conductive pathways formed by any metallic materials that connect to the patient (1,26).

Blood Pressure

A conventional, manual sphygmomanometer may be adapted for use during MR procedures by lengthening the tubing from the cuff to the device so that the mercury column may be positioned an acceptable distance from the magnetic fringe field of the MR system (1,11,13,14). Blood pressure equipment that incorporates a spring gauge instead of a mercury column may be adversely affected by magnetic fields, causing this type of device to be inaccurate in the MR setting (1,11). Therefore, spring-gauge blood pressure devices should undergo prior testing before being used to monitor patients undergoing MR procedures (1,11).

Blood pressure monitors that use noninvasive techniques, such as the oscillometric method, may be used to obtain semicontinuous recordings of systolic, diastolic, and mean blood pressures as well as pulse rate (1,11,21). These devices can be used to monitor systemic blood pressure in adult, pediatric, and neonate patients by selecting the appropriate size of blood pressure cuff (see Fig. 7-3).

Noninvasive blood pressure monitors may be modified for use during MR procedures by lengthening the hose or tubing that connects the blood pressure cuff to the monitor in order to position the monitor a suitable distance from the static magnetic field of the MR system (1,11,21). Any metallic connectors between the cuff and hose should be removed and replaced with plastic fittings. These modifications are typically performed by the commercial manufacturers.

The inflation of the blood pressure cuff using automated, noninvasive blood pressure monitors may disturb lightly sedated patients, especially pediatric or neonate patients, causing them to move and disrupt the MR procedure. For this reason, a noninvasive blood pressure monitor may not be the best instrument to perform physiologic monitoring in every type of patient.

Intravascular, Intracardiac, and Intracranial Pressures

Direct monitoring of intravascular, intracardiac, or intracranial pressures may be accomplished in patients during MR procedures using a specially designed fiberoptic pressure transducer or a nonferromagnetic, micromanometer-tipped catheter (6,9). These monitoring devices are unaffected by the electromagnetic fields used for MR procedures and are capable of invasively recording pressures that are comparable to those obtained using conventional pressure transducers (6,9).

Invasive pressure monitoring may also be accomplished using conventional techniques whereby an additional length of pressure tubing is applied to place the transducer in an acceptable position relative the MR system (11,17,27,32). Other modifications of the MR environment may also be required to prevent distortion of MR images when this type of monitoring technique is used to record pressures invasively (32).

Cutaneous Blood Flow

Monitoring blood flow through the cutaneous capillaries provides a means of assessing tissue perfusion, which is an indirect method of determining the circulatory status of the patient (see Fig. 7-3). Cutaneous blood flow may be noninvasively monitored during MR procedures using the laser Doppler velocimetry method (1,11,21,22,23).

A low power beam of laser light is delivered to the tissue via a fiberoptic probe. As the light moves through the tissue, the moving red blood cells impart a Doppler frequency shift of photons. A pair of separate optical fibers collect the light signals carrying information on the velocity and density of red blood cells in the cutaneous capillary bed. Cutaneous blood flow, blood volume, and velocity may be monitored using this technique (1).

Monitors that record cutaneous blood flow use fiberoptic cables along with a special probe that is attached to the patient using double-sided adhesive tape. Skin surface areas that have a relatively high cutaneous blood flow such as the toe, foot, finger, hand, or ear provide the best results for monitoring this physiologic parameter during MR procedures.

Temperature

There are several occasions when monitoring skin and/or body temperature during an MR procedure is important: in neonates with inherent problems retaining body heat (a tendency that is augmented when accompanied by sedation or anesthesia), during delivery of high levels of RF power to patients whenever certain pulse sequences or MR spectroscopy with proton decoupling procedures are performed, and in patients with underlying health conditions or who are taking drugs that impair their ability to dissipate heat (1,23,24,36).

Skin and body temperatures may be monitored during MR procedures using a variety of techniques (1,11,14,24,28). Using hard-wire, thermistor, or thermocouple techniques in the MR environment may cause artifacts or erroneous temperature measurements because of direct heating of the temperature probe. Nevertheless, if properly modified, temperature recordings may be accomplished in the MR setting using specialized hard-wire leads and thermistors (28).

A more effective means of monitoring temperatures during MR procedures is by use of a fluoroptic thermometry system (1,11,24,30,31). Experiments have shown that this method is both safe and reliable and can be used with MR systems that have static magnetic field strengths up to 12 T (24,30,31).

A fluoroptic monitoring system has several additional features that make it acceptable for temperature monitoring during MR procedures (see Fig. 7-3). For example, this device incorporates fiberoptic probes that are small but efficient in carrying optical signals over long paths, it provides noise-free applications in electromagnetically hostile environments, and has fiberoptic components that will not pose a risk to patients (1,24,30,31).

Multiparameter, Physiologic Monitors

In certain cases, it may be necessary to monitor several different physiologic parameters during MR procedures. For example, multiparameter monitors are particularly useful for monitoring high-risk patients or patients who require general anesthesia. In addition, the physiologic signals obtained using these devices are often useful, and in many instances more effective, for performing MR procedures that require synchronization or gating with cardiac and/or respiratory motion. The most efficient means of performing the task of obtaining multiple physiologic parameters is by using a monitoring system that permits simultaneous recordings of several different physiologic functions such as heart rate, respiratory rate, blood pressure, and oxygen saturation (see Fig. 7-3).

To date, only one multiparameter monitoring system is recognized for use in the MR environment by the U.S. Food and Drug Administration (see Table 7-2). This device is designed to have components positioned within the MR system room and incorporates special circuitry to reduce substantially the artifacts that affect the recording of EKG and other physiologic variables. Recent testing has demonstrated that this multiparameter monitoring system is also capable of operating properly in conjunction with the use of EPI MR systems and MR systems developed specifically for performance of MR-guided interventional procedures (unpublished observations, 1994, 1995).

Ventilators

Devices used for mechanical ventilation of patients typically contain mechanical switches, microprocessors, and ferromagnetic components that could be adversely affected by the electromagnetic fields used by MR systems (1,4,5,8,10,11,13,15–17). Ventilators that are activated by high pressure oxygen and controlled by the use of fluidics (and, therefore, do not require electricity) may still have ferromagnetic parts that can malfunction as a result of interference by MR systems.

MR-compatible ventilators have been modified or specifically designed for use during MR procedures performed in adult as well as neonate patients (4,5,8,10,11,13,15–17) (see Fig. 7-3). These devices are constructed of nonferromagnetic materials and have been evaluated to ensure that they do not produce imaging artifacts.

Additional Devices

Oxygen may be provided to patients in the MR room using various mechanisms. In the simplest set-up, an oxygen tank (which is typically made from ferromagnetic metal; however, nonferromagnetic oxygen tanks are also commercially available) may be positioned at a remote site and extension tubing can be passed through a small opening or port in the Faraday shield to the patient in the MR room. Other MR sites may elect to build special outlets that provide oxygen or other gases, as well as suction, to the MR room.

An MR-compatible anesthesia system has been specially designed for use in the MR environment that is a three-gas machine and can accommodate two vaporizers (see Table 7-3). This device is constructed primarily of nonferromagnetic materials and operates without producing distortion of MR images, according to tests conducted using a 1.5-T MR system.

SELECTION OF PHYSIOLOGIC PARAMETERS TO MONITOR DURING MR PROCEDURES

Which physiologic parameter(s) should be monitored during the MR procedure? The answer to this question depends on the patient's history, present condition, and what is being done to the patient during the MR procedure. For example, if the patient has had medication administered that has a known side effect of respiratory depression, it would be desirable to monitor respiratory rate, apnea, and/or oxygen saturation (1,42–47). If the patient requires general anesthesia during the MR procedure, extensive monitoring of multiple physiologic parameters will typically be required. Management of the patient in the MR environment should be comparable to that used in the operating room setting with respect to the monitoring requirements. Specific recommendations for physiologic monitoring of patients during MR procedures should be developed in consideration of "standard of care" issues as well as in consultation with anesthesiologists or other similar specialists (33,42–46).

PERSONNEL INVOLVED IN MONITORING PATIENTS DURING MR PROCEDURES

Specially trained individual(s) at each MR facility (e.g., the risk manager or anesthesiologist) should determine the type of monitoring required and ensure that electrical and/or mechanical monitoring devices are compatible with the MR system (1–30). Only those individuals with appropriate training should be responsible for monitoring patients during MR procedures. This includes several facets of monitor-related training. For example, the individual must be well acquainted with the operation of the monitoring devices used in the MR environment and should be able to recognize equipment malfunctions and recording artifacts (1,46). In addition, they need to be appropriately trained to recognize normal versus abnormal readings for each physiologic parameter monitored. The monitoring of physiologic parameters during an MR procedure should be the responsibility of one or more individuals, including technologists, nurses, nurse anesthetists, radiologists, or anesthesiologists, depending on the medical history, condition of the patient, and physiologic parameters that are being monitored (1,46).

At minimum, the individual should be aware of whom to contact in the event that an adverse effect is experienced by the patient. Ideally, the person responsible for monitoring the patient should also be well versed in treating and attempting to correct any significant abnormality of the physiologic parameter being monitored. For example, if an anesthetized patient undergoing an MR procedure suddenly exhibits a rapid decline in oxygen saturation, the individual should be able to deal with any of its potential causes, whether they are related to the ventilation equipment, endotracheal tube placement, or a condition intrinsic to the patient.

At no time should a patient undergoing the MR procedure be in a position in which there is no one to detect and respond to any problem that might arise (46). Furthermore, arrangements must be made to continue appropriate physiologic monitoring of the patient by trained personnel after the MR procedure is performed, while the patient recovers from the effects of the sedative or anesthetic agent.

REFERENCES

1. Kanal E, Shellock FG. Patient monitoring during clinical MR imaging. *Radiology*. 1992;185: 623–629.
2. Kanal E, Shellock FG. Policies, guidelines, and recommendations for MR imaging safety and patient management. *J Magn Reson Imag* 1992;2: 247–248.
3. Schiebler M, Kaut-Watson C, Williams DL. Both sedated and critically ill require monitoring during MRI. *MR* 1994;Winter:34–38.
4. Barnett GH, Roper AHD, Johnson AK. Physiological support and monitoring of critically ill patients during magnetic resonance imaging. *J Neurosurg* 1988;68:246–250.
5. Boutros A, Palicek W. Anesthesia for magnetic resonance imaging. *Anesth Analg* 1987;66:367–374.
6. Dell'Italia LJ, Carter B, Millar H, Pohost GM. Development of a micromanometer-tip catheter to record high-fidelity pressures during cine-gated NMR without significant image distortion. *Magn Reson Med* 1991;17:119–125.
7. Fisher DM, Litt W, Cote CJ. Use of oximetry during MR imaging of pediatric patients. *Radiology* 1991;178:891–892.
8. Dunn V, Coffman CE, McGowan JE, Ehrardt JC. Mechanical ventilation during magnetic resonance imaging. *Magn Reson Imag* 1985;3:169–172.
9. Roos CF, Carrol FE. Fiber-optic pressure transducer for use near MR magnetic fields. *Radiology* 1985; 156: 548.
10. Geiger RS, Cascorbi HF. Anesthesia in an NMR scanner. *Anesth Analg* 1984;63:619–625.
11. Holshouser B, Hinshaw DB, Shellock FG. Sedation, anesthesia, and physiologic monitoring during MRI. *J Magn Reson Imag* 1993;3:553–558.
12. Hubbard A, Markowitz R, Kimmel B, Kroger M, Bartko M. Sedation for pediatric patients undergoing CT and MRI. *J Comp Assist Tomogr* 1992;16:33–6.
13. Karlik S, Heatherley T, Pavan F, et al. Patient anesthesia and monitoring at a 1.5 T MRI installation. *Magn Reson Med* 1988;7:210–211.
14. McArdle C, Nicholas D, Richardson C, Amparo E. Monitoring of the neonate undergoing MR imaging: technical considerations. *Radiology* 1986;159:223–226.
15. McGowan JE, Erenberg A. Mechanical ventilation of the neonate during magnetic resonance imaging. *Magn Reson Imag* 1989;7:145–148.
16. Mirvis SE, Borg U, Belzberg H. MR imaging of ventilator-dependent patients: preliminary experience. *AJR Am J Roentgenol* 1987;149:845–846.
17. Rejger VS, Cohn BF, Vielvoye GJ, De-Raadt FB. A simple anesthetic and monitoring system for magnetic resonance imaging. *Eur J Anesthesiol* 1989;6:373–378.
18. Rokey RR, Wendt RE, Johnston DL. Monitoring of acutely ill patients during nuclear magnetic resonance imaging: use of a time-varying filter electrocardiographic gating device to reduce gradient artifacts. *Magn Reson Med* 1988;6:240–245.
19. Roth JL, Nugent M, Gray JE, et al. Patient monitoring during magnetic resonance imaging. *Anesthesiology* 1985;62:80–83.
20. Selden H, De Chateau P, Ekman G, et al. Circulatory monitoring of children during anesthesia in low-field magnetic resonance imaging. *Acta Anesthesiol* 1990;34:41–43.
21. Shellock FG. Monitoring during MRI. An evaluation of the effect of high-field MRI on various patient monitors. *Med Electron* 1986:93–97.

22. Shellock FG. Monitoring vital signs in conscious and sedated patients during magnetic resonance imaging: experience with commercially available equipment. In: *Book of Abstracts, Society of Magnetic Resonance in Medicine.* Berkeley, CA: Society of Magnetic Resonance in Medicine; 1986;3:1030–1031.
23. Shellock FG, Schaefer DJ, Crues JV. Evaluation of skin blood flow, body and skin temperatures in man during MR imaging at high levels of RF energy. *Magn Reson Imag* 1989;7(suppl 1): 335.
24. Shellock FG, Schaefer DJ, Crues JV. Alterations in body and skin temperatures caused by MR imaging: is the recommended exposure for radiofrequency radiation too conservative? *Br J Radiol* 1989;62:904–909.
25. Shellock FG. Monitoring sedated patients during MRI [Letter]. *Radiology* 1990;177:586.
26. Shellock FG, Myers SM, Kimble K. Monitoring heart rate and oxygen saturation during MRI with a fiber-optic pulse oximeter. *AJR Am J Roentgenol* 1991;158:663–664.
27. Smith DS, Askey P, Young ML, Kressel HY. Anesthetic management of acutely ill patients during magnetic resonance imaging. *Anesthesiology* 1986;65:710–711.
28. Taber K, Layman H. Temperature monitoring during MR imaging: comparison of fluoroptic and standard thermistors. *J Magn Reson Imag* 1992;2:99–101.
29. Wendt RE, Rokey R, Vick GW, Johnston DL. Electrocardiographic gating and monitoring in NMR imaging. *Magn Reson Imag* 1988;6:89–95.
30. Wickersheim KA, Sun MH. Fluoroptic thermometry. *Med Electron* 1987;Feb:84–91.
31. Wickersheim KA, Sun MH. Fiberoptic thermometry and its applications. *J Microwave Power* 1987;1987:85–94.
32. Taber KH, Thompson J, Coveler LA, Hayman LA. Invasive pressure monitoring of patients during magnetic resonance imaging. *Can J Anesth* 1993;40:1092–1095.
33. Joint Commission on Accreditation of Healthcare Organizations. *Accreditation Manual for Hospitals.* 1993.
34. ECRI. Thermal injuries and patient monitoring during MRI studies. *Health Devices Alert* 1991;20:362–363.
35. Kanal E, Shellock FG. Burns associated with clinical MR examinations. *Radiology* 1990;175: 585.
36. Kanal E, Shellock FG, Talagala L. Safety considerations of magnetic resonance imaging. *Radiology* 1990;176:593–606.
37. Shellock FG, Slimp G. Severe burn of the finger caused by using a pulse oximeter during MRI [Letter]. *AJR Am J Roentgenol* 1989;153:1105.
38. Shellock FG, Kanal E. Burns associated with the use of monitoring equipment during MR procedures. *Radiology* 1995;6:271–271.
39. Teneforde TS, Gaffey CT, Moyer BR, Budinger TF. Cardiovascular alterations in Maccaca moneys exposed to stationary magnetic fields. Experimental observations and theoretical analysis. *Bioelectromagnetics* 1983;4:1–9.
40. Dimick RN, Hedlund LW, Herfkens RF, et al. Optimizing electrocardiographic electrode placement for cardiac-gated magnetic resonance imaging. *Invest Radiol* 1987;22:17–22.
41. Damji AA, Snyder RE, Ellinger DC, et al. RF interference suppression in a cardiac synchronization system operating in a high magnetic field NMR imaging system. *Magn Reson Imag* 1988:637–640.
42. Nuzzo PF. Anesthesia monitoring. *Med Electron* 1987;April:92–95.
43. Cohen MD. Pediatric sedation. *Radiology* 1990;175:611–612.
44. Committee on Drugs SoA. Guidelines of the elective use of conscious sedation, deep sedation and general anesthesia. *Pediatrics* 1985;76:317–321.
45. Fisher DM. Sedation of pediatric patients: an anesthesiologists' perspective. *Radiology* 1990;175:613–615.
46. Practice Guidelines for Sedation and Analgesia by Non-Anesthesiologists. *Anesthesiology* 1996;84:459–471.
47. Ehman RL, McNamara MT, Pallack ZM, Hricak H. Magnetic resonance imaging with respiratory gating: techniques and advantages. *AJR Am J Roentgenol* 1984;143:1175–1182.

8

Safety of Magnetic Resonance Imaging Contrast Agents

The advances in MR imaging techniques over the past decade have been accompanied by the introduction of MR imaging contrast agents. These have had great value in detecting and identifying pathologic processes, especially those involving the central nervous system. Utility in clinical MR imaging of abdominal, breast, and musculoskeletal conditions has been demonstrated with some of these agents and may be indicated with others after further clinical experience (1).

At present, three MR imaging contrast agents are approved by the FDA for intravenous use: Magnevist (gadopentetate dimeglumine; Berlex Laboratories, Wayne, NJ), Omniscan (gadodiamide; Nycomed Salutar, Oslo, Norway), and ProHance (gadoteridol injection; Bracco Diagnostics, Princeton, NJ).

Approximately 30% to 40% of the more than 7 million MR examinations performed in the United States each year are accompanied by administration of one of these MR imaging contrast agents (1–3). Therefore, the MR practitioner must be aware of the mechanisms of action of these agents, their route(s) of administration, their pharmacokinetics, their side effects, and their potential for adverse events. In addition, the practitioners must know how to handle side effects and adverse events if they occur and must know the contraindications, if any, to administration of these drugs. It is also important to be acquainted with the various safety issues associated with the use of MR imaging contrast agents. Each of the above-mentioned issues and topics is discussed in this chapter. However, this discussion does not cover any of the new MR imaging contrast agents that are currently in various stages of pre-market–approval testing. As new advances occur, including those for specialized studies such as MR angiography and functional MR examinations, our knowledge base will have to be updated to incorporate the latest data available for these new contrast agents.

Adapted from *Safety Reference Manual on Magnetic Resonance Imaging Contrast Agents* by Emanuel Kanal and Frank G. Shellock.

MECHANISMS OF ACTION

All diagnostic MR examinations attempt to differentiate tissues from each other by taking advantage of differences in their intrinsic magnetic properties. Such differences are predominantly based on one of four main categories: (a) their hydrogen or proton densities; (b) their T1 constants at a given field strength (defining their longitudinal or vertical magnetization recovery rates); (c) their T2(*) constants (defining their horizontal or transverse magnetization decay rates); and (d) their motion or flow profiles (if any).

All the intravenously administered MR imaging contrast agents currently in use have similar, if not identical, mechanisms of action. All are based on gadolinium chelates and, therefore, are paramagnetic agents that develop a magnetic moment when placed in a magnetic field.

The gadolinium chelates possess seven unpaired electrons in the outer electron shell of the gadolinium ion. The resultant, rather large magnetic moment produced by such paramagnetic agents whose ions are tumbling through their molecular environment produces a relatively large, time-varying magnetic field in the vicinity of the paramagnetic molecule that can enhance the relaxation rates (both longitudinal and horizontal) of nearby water protons (2). In this manner, MR imaging contrast agents predominantly decrease the T1 constants of the tissues that take them up, and do so in a roughly dose-dependent manner.

As with any paramagnetic agent and as noted above, there is always some accompanying T2(*) shortening (i.e., increased rate of transverse magnetization decay) for the tissues that take up the contrast agent; this also is dose-dependent. Nevertheless, with the MR imaging parameters currently in routine clinical use and at the doses and timing of administration currently used, the predominant clinical effect noted on most MR imaging sequences is T1 shortening (i.e., increased rate of longitudinal magnetization recovery) rather than T2(*) shortening. Therefore, these MR imaging contrast agents are usually of greatest benefit when the target tissue of interest has an intrinsic T1 value similar to that of the background tissue against which it must be differentiated, but which takes up the contrast agent while the background tissue does not. The reason for this is that contrast in MR imaging, by definition, is the difference between the signal strengths of two tissues. It is therefore important that the target tissue take up the contrast agent and that the background tissue against which it is to be contrasted does not, or does so at substantially different rates and/or concentrations (or vice versa). If both the target and background tissues reacted in the same way to the MR imaging contrast agent, there would be little benefit to its use because little to no gain in signal contrast would be achieved.

With some tissues, time-uptake curves have been measured such that the rate of uptake of the contrast agent from the bloodstream after bolus administration can be roughly predicted. This assists in the decision-making process regarding time to image after administration of the agent, to identify a time at which concentration differences, and therefore T1 values, between target and background tissues are greatest. Thus, MR imaging can differentiate between recurrent herniated lumbar disks versus scar tissue, or can detect pituitary microadenomas if the imaging is completed shortly after administration of the agent instead of waiting 15 min or more for contrast agent concentration equilibration to take place.

Considering their mechanisms of action, it is reasonable to assume that the type of MR imaging most likely to display successfully the tissue that takes up the contrast agent at a high intensity (i.e., strongly magnetized) is one that emphasizes T1 differences between tissues. Therefore, the pulse sequences that successfully differentiate tissues predominantly by their T1 differences, such that the short T1 tissues would be intense relative to those with longer T1 values, would be ideal for application after such MR contrast administration. Short TR (roughly less than three times the longer tissue's T1 value) studies with large flip angles and moderately short TE values are ideal for MR imaging after administration of contrast agents.

Conversely, studies with moderately long TR values, with very low excitation flip angles, and/or with long TE values may not adequately demonstrate the tissue that takes up the contrast agent. Furthermore, these pulse sequences may fail to demonstrate the tissue taking up the agent as a high signal intensity, because the sequence itself is one that minimizes the role of longitudinal magnetization recovery rates in determining ultimate tissue signal intensity values.

Finally, for similar reasons, a short TI inversion recovery (STIR) or a fast spin-echo STIR pulse sequence would inherently decrease the signal from any tissue with a relatively short T1, compared with the relatively greater signal still present from tissues with longer T1 values. Therefore, STIR pulse sequences performed after contrast administration can be expected to yield images in which the tissue(s) that take(s) up the agent are, if anything, actually darker than they would be if the contrast agent had not been administered or if a more standard short TR and short TE (i.e., T1-weighted) partial saturation spin-echo imaging pulse sequence had been performed. Both fat (with its intrinsically short T1 value) and the enhancing mass would darken on such a sequence, whereas in a chemical-specific saturation sequence (e.g., CHESS, frequency specific saturation, fat saturation, fat sat), the fat alone would be darkened and the enhancing mass would remain intense. Such fat saturation sequences are most helpful after administration of MR imaging contrast agents, especially in the skull base, spine, musculoskeletal system, and abdomen. For similar reasoning, however, fluid-attenuating inversion recovery (the so-called FLAIR) techniques should generally provide images of which the tissue taking up the contrast agent should demonstrate good to excellent contrast enhancement, as long as the TE is not prohibitively long.

PHARMACOKINETICS

The pharmacokinetics of contrast imaging agents depend on the state of the gadolinium complex. Free gadolinium has a biologic half-life of several weeks, with uptake and excretion of gadolinium taking place predominantly via the kidneys and liver. Unfortunately, free gadolinium ion is also quite toxic (4). Gadolinium is therefore chelated to another structure that restricts the ion and thus markedly decreases its toxicity. However, chelation also alters the pharmacokinetic profile of the complex (2). Chelation also decreases the efficiency with which the gadolinium complex can accomplish its primary diagnostic task, that is, decreasing the T1 rate constant of the tissues that take up the MR imaging contrast agent. Inherent to these pharmacokinetics is a tradeoff between the relaxivity of the agent (i.e., the efficiency with which it speeds up, per given concentration of the agent, longitudinal magnetization recovery of tissues that take up the agent) and its safety profile.

As noted above, chelation alters the pharmacokinetics of the MR imaging contrast agent. One of the most significant aspects of this altered pharmacokinetic profile is manifest in the excretion pathway. After chelation, the gadolinium complex exhibits a roughly 500-fold increase in the rate of renal excretion compared with pre chelation values (5,6). It is the chelating agent itself, attached to the gadolinium ion, that differentiates these agents from one another.

All the MR imaging contrast agents currently approved for intravenous administration are based on gadolinium and have similar mechanisms of action, biodistributions, pharmacokinetics, and half-lives (2,3,7,8). Drug equilibration and physiologic biodistribution for each of these agents occur within the extracellular fluid space, with biologic elimination half-lives of roughly 1.5 h (2). If these agents are taken orally, there is very low absorption of gadolinium from the gastrointestinal tract (2,9). One study demonstrated that 99.2% of orally administered Magnevist was fecally excreted and not absorbed (10).

For Magnevist, the chelating agent is the DTPA molecule. For Omniscan it is DTPA-BMA, and for ProHance it is the HP-DO3A molecule. Magnevist has a linear structure and is an ionic compound; Omniscan has a linear structure and is non-ionic; ProHance is also non-ionic, with a macrocyclic (ring) structure (Fig. 8-1). Despite the marked differences between these chelating molecules, their ionic versus non-ionic nature, and their linear versus ring-like molecular structure, they appear to have remarkably similar effectiveness and safety profiles. Some differences do exist, but most appear to be of minor clinical significance. These are listed and discussed separately below.

As previously noted, free gadolinium ion is rather toxic. Therefore, concerns about toxicity increase with increased dissociation of the gadolinium ion from its chelate. Increased dissociation may be caused either by high concentrations of other molecules that compete with the gadolinium for the chelate (e.g., zinc or copper) and/or by any situation that causes the gadolinium-chelate complex to remain within the body for a prolonged period of time. The dissociation of the chelate from the gadolinium ion is determined in part by the concentration of competing ions and by the time that it is allowed to remain in solution. In human subjects both these conditions are of potential concern. For example, increased concentration of competing moieties and/or increased time during

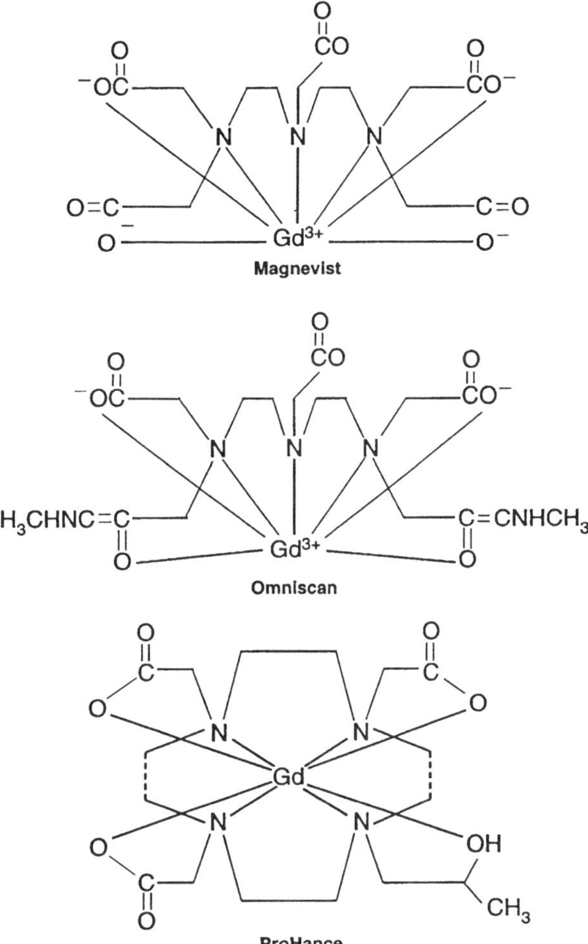

FIG. 8-1. Molecular structures of the three MR imaging contrast agents currently approved for intravenous administration in the United States.

which the gadolinium chelate complex remains within the body are situations that would increase concerns about potential safety of use in those patients.

After intravenous administration of gadolinium-based contrast agents, copper and zinc (normally present in small amounts within the bloodstream), which have a competing affinity for the chelate, displace some of the gadolinium from the chelating molecule, which is released as free gadolinium ion (Gd3^{+}). Although gadolinium is a toxic substance, the total concentration of the released free gadolinium is very low and is cleared rapidly, enabling a low concentration of free ion to be maintained. As new physiologic sources of copper and zinc ions are "leaked" into the intravascular space to reestablish their concentration equilibrium, they displace more gadolinium from its chelate, which continues to be rapidly cleared by the kidneys.

This cycle continues until all the gadolinium chelate is cleared from the body via the kidney by glomerular filtration. In patients with normal renal function, the rate of dissociation is slower than that of clearance, thus preventing the occurrence of any accumulation phenomena (6). Some authors have conjectured and have subsequently demonstrated that the macrocyclic molecules tend to bind gadolinium more tightly than do the linear ones (8,11,12).

ROUTE(S) OF ADMINISTRATION

Omniscan and ProHance were each approved to be administered as an intravenous bolus. Although Magnevist was initially applied and approved for slow intravenous administration at a rate not to exceed 10 ml/min, later studies using rapid intravenous administration of Magnevist have indicated no significant differences in the incidence of adverse effects compared with slow intravenous administration (13–15). Accordingly, all three MR imaging contrast agents are now approved by the FDA for rapid bolus administration (e.g., 10 ml/15 s).

TOXICITY

There are several ways to assess the toxicity of a drug, including determination of its LD_{50} and of the incidence and type(s) of adverse events encountered with its administration at routine doses and by routine routes.

The LD_{50}, or 50% lethal dose, denotes the dose of a drug that, when administered to test animals, results in the acute death of half of the test population. The reported LD_{50} values of the MR imaging contrast agents, as studied in rodents, is quite high, being highest for Omniscan (>30 mmol/kg), followed by ProHance (12 mmol/kg), and lowest for Magnevist (6–7 mmol/kg). This yields LD_{50} values more than approximately 300, 120, and 60 times the typical diagnostic dose of 0.1 mmol/kg, respectively, for Omniscan, ProHance, and Magnevist (2,16). There are also data suggesting that fewer acute cardiodepressive effects are encountered with the use of a non-ionic than of an ionic agent when it is injected rapidly and into a central vein (17). Even if this is true, however, its clinical applicability at present may be quite limited, as MR imaging contrast agents are typically injected into peripheral veins and only small total volumes are administered (2).

CONTRAINDICATIONS

There are no known specific contraindications to the administration of Magnevist, Omniscan, and ProHance, although certainly care must be taken with patients who have experienced an adverse reaction to a previous dose of one of these contrast agents. Close observation of certain patients by an appropriate physiologic monitoring technique (e.g., pulse oximetry) and frequent verbal and visual contact throughout the examination, as well as for a short time after its completion, are advisable to ensure patient safety during contrast-enhanced MR imaging (18,19).

There have been rare reported incidents of laryngospasm and/or anaphylactoid reactions (requiring therapeutic interventions) associated with the administration of each of the MR imaging contrast agents (personal communication, Dr. Reich, 1993) (14,20–28).

In consideration of the above, it is advisable to continue a prolonged observation period of all patients with a history of allergy or drug reaction. As stated in the package insert for all these contrast agents:

> The possibility of a reaction, including serious, fatal, life-threatening, anaphylactoid, or cardiovascular reactions or other idiosyncratic reactions should always be considered especially in those patients with a known clinical hypersensitivity or history of asthma or other allergic respiratory disorders.

Therefore, MR facilities should be prepared and equipped to manage any adverse effects caused by a patient's reaction to a contrast agent.

The question is often asked as to whether a radiologist/physician needs to be on hand for the intravenous administration of any of these MR contrast agents. It is also often quoted that nurses or similar paramedical personnel administer agents, including antibiotics and chemotherapy, which are associated with a substantially greater incidence of adverse and serious adverse events yet have no physician in immediate attendance. However, the argument has been made that those medications are for therapeutic interventional objectives, whereas the MR imaging contrast agents are for diagnostic purposes and may be argued to be of less substantial immediate patient benefit. Nevertheless, as a matter of opinion only, it might be reasoned that the key factors are that the radiologist needs to demonstrate that he or she:

1. was involved in the decision, with appropriate clinical indications, to administer the contrast agent to this patient in the first place (please recall that these agents, as with the MR examination itself, are to be administered only by the prescription of an appropriately licensed professional);
2. was in a position to be notified immediately in the unlikely event of an untoward adverse reaction (i.e., that it was clear to the health care professionals performing the examination, contrast administration, and patient monitoring who was the physician responsible for this patient and who was to be notified in case of an emergent or adverse event);
3. was able to, and indeed did, respond, either in person or by adequately skilled representation, in a timely fashion; and
4. did administer appropriate supportive care upon arrival.

Furthermore, it is good advice that each site ensure that not only is a written policy clearly in place regarding this issue, but that the site can demonstrate that this policy was adhered to in the case being questioned.

However, the above also assumes several points. For example, it is assumed that the patients being imaged without the immediate physical presence of a physician in direct attendance are all stable outpatients—and are neither unstable nor inpatients. Further, it is assumed that such patients do not fall into any of the known higher risk groups for adverse or serious reactions to the administration of gadolinium based MR contrast agents. For example, it would be assumed that these patients have no known history of hypersensitivity or adverse event to a previously administered dose of any of this category of MR contrast agent, nor any known history of hypersensitivity or adverse event to a previously administered dose of an iodinated contrast agent (as these patients seem also to have a somewhat higher rate of adverse reactions to such agents), nor any known history of asthma or other such allergic respiratory disorder (who also seem to have a somewhat elevated incidence of untoward events to the administration of such gadolinium-based MR contrast agents). Clearly, were any of the above to be the case for the patient at hand, it would be more difficult to defend the lack of a physician in direct attendance, if an adverse event occurs.

Given that anaphylactoid reactions are among the worst of the adverse events that one might experience and anticipate with these agents, one might design anticipated response times (from onset of symptomatology to arrival on scene with appropriate medical personnel) to be on the order of less than 60 to 90 s. This would enable timely response to cardiovascular collapse. It is appropriate to ensure that all who administer these MR imaging contrast agents be skilled in basic cardiopulmonary resuscitation to assist in life support until the arrival of appropriate medical personnel. Please note that these are only opinions, which may well differ from those of others in your particular site. In any case, it is strongly suggested that, whatever time frame within which one wishes to constrain their response times, it should be clearly demonstrable as to why these times were selected—and that they were indeed adhered to in the case in question.

In the opinion of a (plaintiff's) medical malpractice attorney contacted regarding the above, the above seemed reasonable. He further recognized that the cost of medical care would skyrocket if society would demand that a physician be present in person for each and every drug administered with such impressive safety profiles as those of these gadolinium-based MR contrast agents. What is expected, rather, is reasonable standard of care.

OSMOLALITY AND OSMOTIC LOAD

Many studies have documented the impressively high safety index of MR imaging contrast agents, especially as compared with the iodinated contrast media used for computed tomography (3,13,14,29–44). However, one should bear in mind the considerably different volumes of the agents administered for MR contrast compared with those used for typical CT contrast doses. Indeed, from a safety-profile standpoint, it is inappropriate to compare ionic and non-ionic MR imaging contrast agents to ionic and non-ionic CT contrast agents because of the drastically different osmotic loads associated with each of these drugs. Table 8-1 compares standard osmotic loads delivered by standard doses of MR and CT contrast agents for a typical 70-kg patient.

The osmolality of these agents ranges from 630 mmol/kg of water, or roughly twice that of plasma (approximately 285 mmol/kg of water) for ProHance, to 789 mmol/kg of water (roughly three times that of plasma) for Omniscan, to 1,960 mmol/kg of water (roughly six to seven times that of plasma) for Magnevist (45).

The lower osmolality of ProHance compared with Magnevist was the subject of an investigation in the rat model into the effect of extravasation of this agent versus extravasation of Magnevist (46). The findings indicated that extravasation of Magnevist was associated with a higher incidence of necrosis, hemorrhage, and edema compared with ProHance, although this report cautioned about extrapolating the results to extravasation of MR imaging contrast agents in human subjects.

CLINICAL SAFETY PROFILES

The availability of data regarding the incidence of adverse events from clinical administration of these agents varies according to the length of time that they have been in clinical use. The first MR imaging contrast agent to receive FDA approval and, therefore, the one for which there is the greatest amount of clinical experience and information, is Magnevist. Approximately 7 million doses have been administered in the United States since its approval in June 1988. This compares with approximately 1 million total administered doses for

TABLE 8-1. *Osmotic load comparisons between MR imaging contrast agents and CT contrast media for a 70-kg patient*

	Osmotic load (mOsm)
MR imaging contrast agent[a]	
ProHance	8.8
Omniscan	11.1
Magnevist	27.4
CT contrast agent	
Iohexol	105.0
Iopamidol	119.0
Diatrizoate	255.0

[a] Dose of 0.1 mmol/kg (14-ml volume administered).

ProHance since its FDA approval in November 1992 and approximately 1.2 million doses for Omniscan since its approval by the FDA in January 1993 (Arlington Medical Resources data, August 1995). The total incidence of adverse reactions of all types for each of the MR imaging contrast agents ranges from approximately 2% to 5% (3,20,37,47).

The most common reactions are nausea, emesis, hives, and headache. Local injection site symptoms, including irritation, focal burning, or a cool sensation, are also among the most commonly reported. With the use of Magnevist, transient elevations in serum bilirubin (3–4% of patients) have been reported, and with both Magnevist and Omniscan a transient elevation in iron (15–30% of patients) appears to reverse spontaneously within 24 to 48 h (3,14). Delayed reactions including hypertension, vasovagal responses, and syncope have also been reported with the use of MR imaging contrast agents. Accordingly, the product inserts for these drugs advise that all patients should be observed for several hours after drug administration. Unfortunately, this recommendation is seldom followed in clinical practice.

SPECIFIC ADVERSE EVENTS

For the sake of accuracy and consistency, it is helpful to clarify some commonly used (and misused) terminology pertaining to adverse events that occur with medications. As defined by the FDA, a "serious reaction" is one in which an adverse experience from a drug proves fatal or life-threatening, is permanently disabling, requires inpatient hospitalization, or is an overdose (Code of Federal Regulations, Title 21, Part 314). A "life-threatening reaction" in FDA terminology is one in which the individual initially reporting the incident believes that the patient was at immediate risk for death from the event. This makes it clear that individual interpretation of a given adverse event may differ from that defined by the FDA, which considers all other events to be nonserious.

Despite the high degree of safety of these agents, various adverse reactions have been reported in association with their administration. Overall, remarkably similar types and rates of adverse reactions have been reported for each of the currently approved MR imaging contrast agents (although not every adverse reaction has been reported with each of these agents). The total incidence of adverse events for any of these agents appears to be less or far less than 5%. The incidence of any single adverse event is approximately 1% of all patients, or even lower. By far the most common events are nausea, headache, and emesis. Other reactions have also occurred, although at frequencies of 1% or less. These can be broken down by organ system (as they are treated in the package inserts accompanying these drugs). Nonspecific, general adverse reactions are numerous, although still relatively rare.

Reported reactions involving the site of injection have included pain, warmth, localized edema, and/or a localized burning sensation. Rarely, regional lymphangitis has been reported. Therefore, one might expect local irritative reactions as potential adverse responses, especially with the use of the more hyperosmolar agent. Indeed, there has been at least one incident of possible phlebitis, requiring hospitalization, that was temporally related to administration of an intravenous dose of one of these agents (personal communication, Dr. LaFlore, 1990).

Several delayed-onset cases of erythema, swelling, and pain at and proximal to the site of administration have been reported, typically appearing 1 to 4 days after intravenous administration. This typically progressed for several days, plateaued, and then resolved over several more days (15). In addition, some objective studies have demonstrated that tissue sloughing can be caused by extravasation of gadolinium dimeglumine (46,48). Nevertheless, doses greater than or more than double that used in the United States (i.e., up to 0.5 mmol/kg) have already been investigated in the clinical setting (14,49–51; Frank G. Shellock, personal communication, 1995) and have been used for quite some time in Europe, with no apparent significant adverse effects. Omniscan, Magnevist, and ProHance are indicated in the United States for a dose of 0.1 mmol/kg.

The recommended dose for Omniscan or ProHance is 0.1 mmol/kg, although in patients suspected of having poorly enhancing lesions, in the presence of negative or equivocal scans, a second dose of 0.2 mmol/kg may be given for a cumulative dose of 0.3 mmol/kg. It can be safely stated that severe adverse local reactions to even considerable amounts (>10 ml) of extravasation of these agents appear to be quite rare.

More generalized, nonspecific adverse reactions that have also been reported include headache, chest pain and/or tightness, fever, fatigue, arthralgias, rigors, asthenia, hot flashes, flushed feeling, malaise, weakness, facial edema, neck rigidity, abdominal cramps, fever, itching, watery eyes, a tingling sensation in the throat, and generalized coldness. Cardiovascular symptoms reported after the administration of these agents include hypotension, hypertension, vasodilatation, pallor, nonspecific EKG changes, chest pain, phlebitis, warmth, prolonged P–R interval, tachycardia, and A–V nodal rhythm.

Adverse gastrointestinal reactions reported after MR imaging contrast agent administration include nausea, emesis, nonspecific gastrointestinal distress and/or abdominal pain, tooth pain, increased salivation, diarrhea, eructation, melena, itching and/or edema of tongue, gingivitis, and dry mouth.

Adverse neurologic reactions reported in association with the administration of these agents include headache, agitation, paresthesia, abnormal coordination, anorexia, anxiety, syncope, tremor, ataxia, dry mouth, thirst, taste abnormality, personality disorder, mental status decline, somnolence, dizziness, tinnitus, conjunctivitis, lacrimation disorder (tearing), eye irritation, and staring episodes. Seizures (including grand mal) after administration of these agents have been reported (14,32,52). In at least one case, injection of an MR imaging contrast agent was believed to induce a seizure in a patient with a history of grand mal seizures.

Adverse respiratory system events reported with the use of these agents include throat irritation, rhinorrhea/rhinitis, sneezing, dyspnea, wheezing, laryngismus, and cough.

Reported dermatologic adverse events include rash, pruritus, urticaria (hives), flushing, bruising, erythema, myalgia, skin discoloration, sweating, swelling, and tingling sensations in the extremities and digits.

Although (reversible) renal failure has been reported with the administration of these contrast agents (as noted in the package insert), no objectively documented and reproducible nephrotoxicity has been reported (53–56).

An anaphylactoid reaction is one that involves respiratory, cardiovascular, cutaneous, and possibly gastrointestinal and/or genitourinary manifestations (57). This is not to say that all events characterized by these symptoms are by definition anaphylactoid. However, it does become more difficult to make the diagnosis of anaphylaxis without these symptoms, especially the classic triad of upper airway obstructive symptomatology, decreased blood pressure (or other similar severe cardiovascular symptoms), and cutaneous manifestations, such as urticaria.

Anaphylactoid reactions have also been reported with the use of each of these agents. In many of these instances the patient had a history of respiratory difficulty or an allergic respiratory problem, such as asthma. As previously mentioned, the current package inserts for these agents warn that caution should be exercised in administering them to patients with known allergic respiratory disease. The true incidence of such anaphylactoid reactions is unclear, but certainly appears to be well above 1:100,000 for each of these agents and may, in fact, be closer to 1:500,000 for some.

CROSS-REACTIVITY

An interesting question, without a clear-cut answer, is whether a patient who reacts adversely to one drug may experience cross-reactivity with the other imaging contrast agent. It is unclear why two patients recently experienced presumed anaphylactoid-like reactions to ProHance after having previously received Magnevist without difficulty (58; R. J. Witte, personal communication, 1994). To date, no trend or explanation appears to be available that might explain this unusual set of circumstances, let alone why they occurred in patients of the same investigator, at the same site, and with the same agents and similar prior histories of exposure. It is similarly unclear why another patient who experienced nausea-emesis on each occasion of having received Magnevist experienced no adverse events in the following 11 studies for which ProHance was administered (P. Vagelgang, personal communication, 1995).

Omniscan and ProHance are the only MR imaging contrast agents with FDA approval to be administered for specific clinical indications and via a specific methodology up to a total dose of 0.3 mmol/kg, or a total of three times the (standard) dose for each of these FDA-approved agents. Here, too, the incidence of adverse effects of any type for ProHance appears to be less than 4%, with nausea and taste disturbance each having an incidence of roughly 1.4% and all other adverse reactions being less than 1% each (A.Y. Olukotun, personal communication, 1993) and for Omniscan being less than 3%, excluding local injection site reactions.

A recent prospective study of bolus administration of ProHance at standard doses in a clinical setting to 3,558 patients over a 9-month period revealed a total adverse event incidence of 2.1% (59), with most such adverse events being nausea (0.98%) and emesis (0.34%).

TREATMENT OF ADVERSE EVENTS AND REACTIONS

In 1991, the American College of Radiology published the *Manual on Iodinated Contrast Media* as a guide for radiologists who use contrast agents (57). This useful guide includes information concerning the latest forms of treatment for various types of adverse events or reactions to contrast agents. It is recommended that radiologists and their staff review this manual, as well as other recently published articles, which will prepare them to respond appropriately to any adverse event(s) that may occur (57–62). Table 8-2 indicates the recommended management of acute reactions to contrast agents as indicated by the manual, which can also be used in treating patients who experience adverse events or other reactions to MR imaging contrast agents. Mild reactions such as nausea, vomiting, headache, dizziness, altered taste, or anxiety typically require only observation, with little or no treatment other than possible alleviation of the symptoms.

SUMMARY OF SIMILARITIES AND DIFFERENCES

Although much of the data in this section is covered elsewhere in this chapter, it will serve to centralize much of the discussion regarding how these agents compare and in what areas differences do exist.

Similarities

The adverse reaction rate for any of these agents seems to hover at less than 5%. The more commonly experienced adverse reactions from these agents may be nausea, emesis, hives, headache, and local injection site reactions. Allergic and true anaphylactoid reactions have been reported with all three of these FDA-approved intravenous MR contrast agents. When the incidence of such

TABLE 8-2. *Management of acute reactions to contrast agents*

REACTION

Urticaria

No treatment needed in most cases

H_1-receptor blocker

Diphenhydramine (Benadryl) p.o./i.m./i.v. 50 mg or hydroxyzine (Vistaril) p.o./i.m./i.v. 25–50 mg

H_2-receptor blocker may be added

Cimetidine (Tagamet) 300 mg p.o. or i.v. slowly, diluted in 10 ml D_5W solution, or ranitidine (Zantac) 50 mg p.o. or i.v. slowly, diluted in 10 ml D_5W solution

If severe/widely disseminated

α-Agonist (arteriolar and venous constriction), epinephrine s.c. (1:1,000) 0.1–0.3 m (if not cardiac contraindication)

Facial/laryngeal edema

α-Agonist (arteriolar and venous constriction)

Epinephrine 0.1–0.3 ml 1:1,000 s.c., or if s.c. route fails or if peripheral vascular collapse, then 1.0–3.0 ml, 1:10,000 slowly i.v.

May repeat $\times$ 3 p.r.n. up to a maximal dose of 1.0 mg

Oxygen 2–6 L/min

If not responsive to therapy or for obvious laryngeal edema (acute)

Call anesthesiologist/Code Blue team

Consider intubation

Bronchospasm

Oxygen 2–6 L/min

Monitor ECG, O_2 saturation (pulse oximeter), blood pressure

Epinephrine 0.1–0.3 ml 1:1,000 s.c. or β-agonist inhalers [bronchiolar dilators, i.e., metaproteranol (Alupent), terbutaline (Brethaire), albuterol (Proventil)]

If s.c. route fails or if peripheral vascular collapse, then 1.0–3.0 ml, 1:10,000 slowly i.v.

May repeat $\times$ 3 p.r.n. up to a maximum of 1.0 mg

Alternatively

Aminophylline 6.0 mg/kg i.v. in D_5W over 10–20 min (loading dose); then 0.4–1.0 mg/kg/h p.r.n.

Or terbutaline 0.25–0.5 mg i.m./s.c.

Call Code Blue for severe bronchospasm (or if oxygen saturation $\leq$88%)

Hypotension with tachycardia

Legs up, Trendelenburg position; monitor ECG, pulse oximeter, blood pressure

Oxygen 2–6 L/min

Rapid administration of large volumes of isotonic lactated Ringer's solution (Ringer's lactate $>$ normal saline $>$ D_5W)

If poorly responsive

Epinephrine 0.1–0.3 ml 1:1,000 s.c. or if s.c. route fails or if peripheral vascular collapse, then 1.0—3.0 ml, 1:10,000 slowly i.v.

Can repeat $\times$ 3 p.r.n. up to a maximum of 1.0 mg

If still poorly responsive

Transfer to intensive care unit for further management

Hypotension with bradycardia: vagal reaction

Legs up, Trendelenburg position, secure airway, give oxygen

Secure i.v. access, give atropine 0.6–1.0 mg i.v. slowly

Monitor vital signs, repeat atropine up to 2.0 mg total dose

Push fluid replenishment i.v. (Ringer's lactate $>$ normal saline $>$ D_5W

Hypertension, severe

Monitors in place: ECG, pulse oximeter, blood pressure

Apresoline 5.0 mg i.v.

Sodium nitroprusside, arterial line; infusion pump necessary to titrate

For pheochromocytoma, phentolamine 5.0 mg (1.0 mg in children) i.v.

TABLE 8-2. *Continued.*

REACTION

Seizures/convulsions

Oxygen 2–6 L/min
Consider diazepam (Valium) 5.0 mg or midazolam (Versed) 2.5 mg i.v.
If longer effect needed, obtain consultation; consider phenytoin (Dilantin) infusion 15–18 mg/kg at 50 mg/min
Careful monitoring of vital signs required

Pulmonary edema

Elevate torso; apply rotating tourniquets (venous compression)
Oxygen 2–6 L/min
Diuretics: furosemide (Lasix) 40 mg i.v. slowly
Consider morphine/meperidine (Demerol)
Corticosteroids (optional)

Adapted from American College of Radiology, ref. 57.
H, histamine.

anaphylactoid reactions is so exceedingly rare as it is with each of these agents, it is difficult to place any significance on relative anaphylactoid reaction rates. It is safe to say that, at worst, the rate of true anaphylactoid reaction from any of these agents is probably in the 1:100,000 range, and may be as high as 1: 500,000. Nevertheless, in terms of total adverse reactions as well as serious adverse reaction rates, it is clear that any of these contrast agents are among the statistically safest drugs with which diagnostic radiologists have had the opportunity to use. Although initially this was not the case, at this point in time all three of the commercially available MR imaging contrast agents have approval for bolus intravenous administration.

Standard doses for these agents are the same (i.e., the same volume of each of these agents would be administered to any given individual), being 0.1 mmol/kg. [As they are all distributed as 500 mM (0.5 mol) solutions, this translates into 0.2 ml/kg for each of these contrast agents for the standard dose].

The relaxivities (i.e., the degree to which each of these agents shortens the T1 and the T2 of tissues that take up the agent at any given concentration and at any given field strength) are extremely comparable. In other words, after administering a standard dose of any of these contrast agents to a given patient in a given magnet on a given imaging sequence, it should not be possible for a blinded researcher to determine which of the three agents was the one that had been administered, as they would all be expected to produce substantially similar results, or effects, on the final image. Routes of administration and clearance as well as clearance rates are quite similar for all three of these agents.

None of these contrast agents appears to be nephrotoxic. There are no known contraindications to any of these agents, although caution should be exercised for all these agents in patients with either known hypersensitivity to the agent or a history of asthma or other allergic respiratory disorders where there is a higher incidence of adverse reactions.

Differences

Especially as there is a 4+-year time period in which Magnevist was the only FDA-approved MR imaging contrast agent for intravenous application, there have been quite a few million doses of Magnevist distributed to this point with (very roughly) more than 1 million of each of the other agents distributed to date. There are osmolality differences between these agents as well, with the osmolality of Magnevist being 1,960 mmol/kg of water, Omniscan 789 mmol/kg of water, and ProHance 630 mmol/kg of water. (Plasma has an osmolality of roughly 285 mmol/kg of water.)

The clinical significance of this difference is diminished by the fact that the total volume of administered standard dose is generally quite small. Thus, unless the patient is in severe congestive heart failure and/or fluid overload status, it may well be reasonable to expect to administer safely any of these contrast agents. Admittedly, a lower osmolarity agent might well be preferable if the patient were, for example, in florid pulmonary edema/fluid overload. Furthermore, for rapid hand injections of these contrast agents for a bolus dynamic MR examination that may require a tight bolus of the agent within the vascular system, a lower osmolarity/viscosity agent would enable the agent to be more readily injected over a shorter time/tighter bolus. (For sites with an MR-compatible injector such as the recently approved Medrad Spectris MR injection system, this is less of a consideration.)

Currently, Omniscan and ProHance are approved for higher dose administration (a total of triple dose, or 0.3 mmol/kg) in specific clinical applications and settings where, for example, the lesion is suspected as being otherwise poorly enhancing. Magnevist (as per the package insert from 4/94 revision) is approved for use in adults and children over 2 years of age with central nervous system lesions and for body applications (excluding the heart) in adults. Omniscan (as per the new 2/96 package insert revision) is now approved for use in adults and children over age 2 with central nervous system lesions and for body applications (excluding the heart) in adults.

Incidentally, the recommended dosage for renal imaging with Omniscan is half the standard dose, or 0.05 mmol/kg (0.1 ml/kg). ProHance (as per package insert from the 12/94 revision) is approved for imaging adults and children over age 2 with intracranial and spine lesion and adults with head and neck lesions.

SPECIAL PATIENT POPULATIONS

Renal Insufficiency/Renal Failure/Wilson's Disease

As previously mentioned, there are potential concerns regarding the level of, or the accumulation of, free gadolinium ion in patients with renal failure. Although the safety of administering MR imaging contrast agents to patients with impaired renal function or overt renal failure has not been clearly established, several studies suggest that these agents should be well tolerated (14,32,52,53,63–66). Although there is a theoretic concern that decreasing the rate of clearance of the gadolinium chelate might increase the concentration of free gadolinium within the body, the data suggest that, for a given level of renal function, administration of lower volume doses may be safer than administration of standard doses of iodine-based contrast agents to that same patient (65). Similarly, the safety of administering one of the MR imaging contrast agents to patients with elevated levels of copper (as in Wilson's disease) or zinc has not been firmly established, and will depend on such factors as the glomerular filtration and renal clearance rates, as well as the blood copper levels, of such patients (6). It has also been shown that Magnevist and ProHance are dialyzable, with more than 95% of the administered dose being removed by the third dialysis treatment (14,67,68). It is presumed that Omniscan would be similarly dialyzable, but to date we have been unable to find any peer-reviewed, citable data to support this.

Chronic or Repeat Administration

There are concerns about total storage or accumulation of the MR imaging contrast agents, or even of free gadolinium ion, after multiple doses administered over a patient's lifetime (this may be particularly true for pediatric patients, who are often followed clinically for routine follow-up contrast-enhanced MR examinations for many years in the care of certain conditions). The amount of detectable drug remaining in the liver, kidneys, and bone days after administration appears to be higher for Omniscan than for Magnevist (3), and both appear to be higher than for ProHance (8,11,12). Even though these data might be considered preliminary, no data are currently available regarding the safety of long-term cumulative exposure to low doses of free gadolinium ion. Therefore, there may be a clinical limitation to the number of times a patient can be safely scanned with gadolinium-based contrast agents. At present, this question remains unanswered and is a topic that warrants further investigation.

Sickle Cell Anemia

The FDA has indicated concern in the package insert information regarding the use of gadolinium-based MR imaging contrast agents in patients with sickle cell anemia. According to the package inserts for these agents, the enhancement of magnetic moment may potentiate sickle erythrocyte alignment. This information was based on in vitro studies that clearly documented the alignment of deoxygenated sickle erythrocytes perpendicular to an externally applied magnetic field (69,70). Therefore, there is a theoretic potential for inducing vaso-occlusive complications in vivo. However, no studies to date have demonstrated such effects in vivo or have shown any basis for increased clinical concern regarding the administration of any of these contrast agents to patients with sickle cell anemia or other hemoglobinopathy. Finally, there have been no reports to date of sickle crisis being precipitated by administration of any of these drugs.

Pregnancy

Magnevist crosses the placental barrier and appears within the fetal bladder only moments after intravenous administration. It is assumed that the other MR imaging contrast agents behave in a similar fashion and cross the placental barrier easily. From the fetal bladder, these contrast agents would then be excreted into the amniotic fluid and subsequently swallowed by the fetus, after which they would either pass unaltered into and/or through the fetal gastrointestinal tract and/or would be filtered and excreted in the fetal urine, with the entire cycle being repeated innumerable times.

To date, no data are available that permit evaluation of the clearance rate of MR imaging contrast agents from the amniotic fluid. In view of the paucity of information supporting the use of these agents in pregnant patients, a conservative approach is recommended against administration of any of the gadolinium-based agents to pregnant patients (at least until more data become available), unless there is a compelling clinical reason for their use. Simply restated, it would be prudent to administer these drugs to pregnant patients only when the potential benefit of so doing justifies the potential risk to the fetus. If it is decided to administer contrast agents to pregnant patients to facilitate MR imaging, it is appropriate to first obtain (if clinically possible in nonemergent cases) written, informed patient consent, specifically stipulating that the risk associated with the use of these drugs during pregnancy is unknown.

Lactation

Concerning the use of contrast agents during lactation, once again there appear to be more studies and data available for Magnevist than for the other agents. Magnevist is excreted in very low concentrations (i.e., 0.011% of the total dose) in human breast milk over approximately 33 h (71,72). The concentration of this contrast agent in breast milk peaks at approximately 4.75 h and decreases to less than a fifth of this level (to less than 1 μmol/L) 22 h after injection (71,72). For this reason, and as an extra precaution, it is recommended that nursing mothers express their breasts and not breastfeed for 36 to 48 h after administration of an MR imaging contrast agent, to ensure that the nursing child does not receive the drug in any appreciable quantity. However, it should be noted that the LD_{50} value of intravenous gadolinium chloride or gadolinium acetate (both of which easily release free gadolinium ions) is lowered by approximately 1,000-fold compared with when the agent is administered orally, because of the very low absorption of gadolinium from the gastrointestinal tract (2,9). This supports other data showing that 99.2% of orally administered Magnevist was fecally excreted and not absorbed (10).

USE OF MR IMAGING CONTRAST AGENTS IN PEDIATRIC PATIENTS

At present, the use of MR imaging contrast agents in pediatric patients over 2 years of age is approved for all three agents for brain and spine lesions at a dose of 0.1 mmol/kg. For children under 2 years of age, the safety of these agents has not been established. Additional studies are ongoing to address the use of the various MR imaging contrast agents in pediatric patients (31).

FUTURE ISSUES

Several new ionic and non-ionic MR imaging contrast agents are now being developed and investigated, which are based on other chelates of gadolinium or on other paramagnetic/superparamagnetic ions. Therefore, safety issues pertaining to the use of the gadolinium chelates may have no bearing on the safety, or even the efficacy, of any of these other media, as they may be unrelated in mechanism of action, form of administration, toxicology, and pharmacokinetics. As new MR imaging contrast agents are developed, we should not feel that we can simply apply safety guidelines developed for gadolinium to the use of the newer agents.

REFERENCES

1. Runge V, ed. *Enhanced magnetic resonance imaging.* St. Louis: CV Mosby; 1989.
2. Oksendal A, Hals P. Biodistribution and toxicity of MR imaging contrast media. *J Magn Reson Imag* 1993;3:157–165.
3. Harpur E, Worah D, Hals P, Holtz E, Furuhama K, Nomura H. Preclinical safety assessment and pharmacokinetics of gadodiamide injection, a new magnetic resonance imaging contrast agent. *Invest Radiol* 1993;28:S28–43.
4. Tweedle MF, Eckelman SC, et al. Effect of free Gd on distribution and pharmacokinetics. Book of Abstracts, Society for Magnetic Resonance in Medicine, Berkeley, CA; 1986;3:1047.
5. Chang C. Magnetic resonance imaging contrast agents. Design and physiochemical properties of gadodiamide. *Invest Radiol* 1993;28(suppl 1):S21–7.
6. Cacheris W, Quay S, Rocklage S. The relationship between thermodynamics and the toxicity of gadolinium complexes. *Magn Reson Imag* 1990;8:467–481.
7. Tweedle M, Eaton S, Eckelman W, et al. Comparative chemical structure and pharmacokinetics of MRI contrast agents. *Invest Radiol* 1988;23(suppl 1):S236–239.
8. Tweedle M. Physiochemical properties of gadoteridol and other magnetic resonance contrast agents. *Invest Radiol* 1992;27(suppl 1):S2–6.

9. Nell G, Rummel W. Pharmacology of intestinal permeation. In: Csaky T, ed. *Handbook of experimental pharmacology*, vol. 70, pt II. Berlin: Springer-Verlag; 1984;489:461–508.
10. Weinmann H, Brasch R, Press W, Wesbey G. Characteristics of gadolinium-DTPA complex: a potential NMR contrast agent. *AJR Am J Roentgenol* 1984; 142:619–624.
11. Wedeking P. Kumar K, Tweedle M. Dissociation of gadolinium chelates in mice: relationship to chemical characteristics. *Magn Reson Imag* 1992; 10:641–648.
12. Gibby WA, Puttagunta NR, Smith GT, et al. Human comparative studies of zinc and copper transmetallation in serum and urine of MRI contrast agents. In: *Book of Abstracts, Society for Magnetic Resonance in Medicine.* Berkeley, CA Society for Magnetic Resonance in Medicine; 1994; 1:389.
13. Kashanian F, Goldstein H, Blumetti R, Holyoak W, Hugo F, Dolker M. Rapid bolus injection of gadopentetate dimeglumine: absence of side effects in normal volunteers. *AJNR Am J Neuroradiol* 1990; 11:853–856.
14. Niendorf H, Dinger J, Haustein J, Cornelius I, Alhassan A, Clauss W. Tolerance data of Gd-DTPA: a review. *Eur J Radiol* 1991; 13:15–20.
15. Kanal E, Applegate G, Gillen C. Review of adverse reactions, including anaphylaxis, in 5260 cases receiving gadolinium-DTPA by bolus injection. *Radiology* 1990; 177(P):159.
16. Weinmann H-J, Gries H, Speck U. Gd-DTPA and low osmolar Gd chelates. In: Runge V, ed. *Enhanced magnetic resonance imaging.* St. Louis: CV Mosby; 1989:74–86.
17. Muhler A, Saeed M, Brasch R, Higgins C. Hemodynamic effects of bolus injection of gadodiamide injection and gadopentetate dimeglumine as contrast media at MR imaging in rats. *Radiology* 1992; 183:523–538.
18. Kanal E, Shellock F. Patient monitoring during clinical MR imaging. *Radiology* 1992; 185: 623–629.
19. Kanal E, Shellock F. Policies, guidelines, and recommendations for MR imaging safety and patient management. *J Magn Res Imag* 1992;2:247–248.
20. LaFlore J, Goldstein H, Rogan R, Keelan T, Ewell A. A prospective evaluation of adverse experiences following the administration of Magnevist (gadopentetate dimeglumine) injection. In: *Book of Abstracts, Society of Magnetic Resonance in Medicine.* Berkeley, CA: Society of Magnetic Resonance in Medicine; 1989:3:1067.
21. Takebayashi S, Sugiyama M, Nagase M, Matsubara S. Severe adverse reaction to IV gadopentetate dimeglumine. *AJR Am J Roentgenol* 1993; 160:659.
22. Shellock F, Hahn P, Mink J, Itskovich E. Adverse reactions to intravenous gadoteridol. *Radiology* 1993; 189:1–2.
23. Salonen O. Case of anaphylaxis and four cases of allergic reaction following Gd-DTPA administration. *J Comput Assist Tomogr* 1990; 14:912–913.
24. Tishler S, Hoffman J. Anaphylactoid reactions to IV gadopentetate dimeglumine. *AJNR Am J Neuroradiol* 1990; 11:1167.
25. Weiss K. Severe anaphylactoid reaction after IV Gd-DTPA. *Magn Reson Imag* 1990;8:817–818.
26. Tardy B, Guy C, Barral G, Page Y, Ollagnier M, Bertrand C. Anaphylactic shock induced by intravenous gadopentetate dimeglumine. *Lancet* 1992; 339:494.
27. Omohundro J, Elderbrook M, Ringer T. Laryngospasm after administration of gadopentetate dimeglumine. *J Magn Reson Imag* 1992; 1:729–730.
28. Chan C, Bosanko C, Wang A. Pruritis and paresthesia after IV administration of Gd-DTPA. *AJNR Am J Neuroradiol* 1989; 10:S53.
29. Felix R, Schorner W. Intravenous contrast media in MRI: clinical experience with gadolinium-DTPA over four years. *Proc Second European Congress of NMR in Medicine in Biology.* Berlin: 1988.
30. Niendorf H, Valk J, Reiser M. First use of Gd-DTPA in pediatric MRI. *Proc Second European Congress of NMR in Medicine in Biology.* Berlin: 1988.
31. Ball WJ, Nadel S, Zimmerman R, et al. Phase III multicenter clinical investigation to determine the safety and efficacy of gadoteridol in children suspected of having neurologic disease. *Radiology* 1993; 186:769–774.
32. Niendorf H, Haustein J, Cornelius I, Alhassan A, Claus W. Safety of gadolinium-DTPA: extended clinical experience. *Magn Reson Med* 1991;22:222–228.
33. Sullivan M, Goldstein H, Sansone K, Stoner S, Holyoak W, Wiggins J. Hemodynamic effects

of Gd-DTPA administered via rapid bolus or slow infusion: a study in dogs. *AJNR Am J Neuroradiol* 1990;11:537–540.
34. Goldstein H, Kashanian F, Blumetti R, Holyoak W, Hugo F, Blumenfield D. Safety assessment of gadopentetate dimeglumine in US clinical trials. *Radiology* 1990;174:17–23.
35. Hajek P, Sartoris D, Gylys-Morin V, et al. The effect of intra-articular gadolinium-DTPA on synovial membrane and cartilage. *Invest Radiol* 1990;25:179–183.
36. Brasch R. Safety profile of gadopentetate dimeglumine. *MRI Decisions* 1989;3:13–19.
37. McLachlan S, Lucas M, DeSimone D, et al. Worldwide safety experience with gadoteridol injection (ProHance). In: *Book of Abstracts, Society of Magnetic Resonance in Medicine.* Berkeley, CA: Society of Magnetic Resonance in Medicine; 1992;3:1426.
38. Berlex Laboratories. A two year report on the safety and efficacy of Magnevist (gadopentetate dimeglumine) injection. Wayne, NJ: Berlex Laboratories, 1990.
39. DeSimone D, Morris M, Rhoda C, et al. Evaluation of the safety and efficacy of gadoteridol injection (a low osmolal MR contrast agent): clinical trials report. *Invest Radiol* 1991;26(suppl 1):S212–216.
40. Carvlin M, DeSimone D, Meeks M. Phase II clinical trial of gadoteridol injection, a low osmolal magnetic resonance imaging contrast agent. *Invest Radiol* 1992;27:S16–21.
41. Runge V, Bradley W, Brant-Zawadski M, et al. Clinical safety and efficacy of gadoteridol: a study in 411 patients with suspected intracranial and spinal disease. *Radiology* 1991;181:701–709.
42. McLachlan S, Eaton S, DeSimone D. Pharmakokinetic behavior of gadoteridol injection. *Invest Radiol* 1992;27(suppl 1):S12–125.
43. Soltys R. Summary of preclinical safety evaluation of gadoteridol injection. *Invest Radiol* 1992;27(suppl 1):S7–11.
44. Shellock FG, Kanal E. *Magnetic resonance: bioeffects, safety, and patient management.* New York: Raven Press; 1994.
45. Watson A, Rocklage S, Carvlin M. Contrast agents. In: Stark D, Bradley W, eds. *Magnetic resonance imaging,* vol. 1. St. Louis: Mosby Yearbook: 1992:372–437.
46. Cohan R, Leder R, Herzberg A, et al. Extravascular toxicity of two magnetic resonance contrast agents: preliminary experience in the rat. *Invest Radiol* 1991;26:224–226.
47. Olukoton A, Parker J, Meeks M, et al. The safety of gadoteridol injection: US clinical trial experience. *J Magn Reson Imag* 1994;4:105.
48. McAlister W, McAlister V, Kissane J. The effect of Gd-dimeglumine on subcutaneous tissues: a study with rats. *AJNR Am J Neuroradiol* 1990;11:325–327.
49. Niendorf H, Haustein J, Louton T, Beck W, Laniado M. Safety and tolerance after intravenous administration of 0.3 mmol/kg Gd-DTPA. *Invest Radiol* 1991;26:S221–223.
50. Niendorf H, Laniado M, Semmler W, Schomer W, Felix R. Dose administration of gadolinium-DTPA in MR imaging of intracranial tumors. *AJNR Am J Neuroradiol* 1987;8: 803–815.
51. Haustein J, Bauer W, Hibertz T, et al. Double dosing of Gd-DTPA in MRI of intracranial tumors. In: *Book of Abstracts, Society for Magnetic Resonance in Medicine.* Berkeley, CA: Society of Magnetic Resonance in Medicine; 1990;1:258.
52. Harbury O. Generalized seizure after IV gadopentetate dimeglumine. *AJNR Am J Neuroradiol* 1991;12:666.
53. Rofsky NM, Weinreb JC, Bosniak MA, Libes RB, Birnbaum BA. Renal lesion characterization with gadolinium-enhanced MR imaging: efficacy and safety in patients with renal insufficiency. *Radiology* 1991;180:85–89.
54. Munechicka H, Sullivan DC, Hedlund LW, et al. Evaluation of acute renal failure with magnetic resonance imaging using gradient-echo and Gd-DTPA. *Invest Radiol* 1991;26:22–27.
55. Leander P, Allard M, Caille J, Golman K. Early effect of gadopentetate and iodinated contrast media on rabbit kidneys. *Invest Radiol* 1992;27:922–926.
56. Prince MR, Arnoldus C, Frisoli JK. Nephrotoxicity of high-dose gadolinium compared with iodinated contrast. *J Magn Reson Imag* 1996;6:162–166.
57. American College of Radiology. *Manual on iodinated contrast media.* American College of Radiology, 1991.
58. Witte R, Anzai L. Life threatening anaphylactoid reaction after intravenous gadoteridol administration in a patient who had previously received gadopentetate dimeglumine. *AJNR Am J Neuroradiol* 1994;15:523–524.

59. Hieronim DE, Kanal E, Swanson DP. Dosage of gadoteridol and adverse reactions related to gadopentate. *Am J Health-Syst Pharm* 1995;52:2556–2559.
60. Atkinson T, Kaliner M. Anaphylaxis. *Clin Allergy* 1992;76:841–855.
61. Fiddian-Green R, Haglund U, Gutierrez G, Shoemaker W. Goals for the resuscitation of shock. *Crit Care Med* 1993;21:S25–31.
62. Yunginger J. Anaphylaxis. *Ann Allergy* 1992;69:87–96.
63. Haustein J, Niendorf H, Krestin G, et al. Renal tolerance of gadolinium-DTPA dimeglumine in patients with chronic renal failure. *Invest Radiol* 1992;27:153–156.
64. Frank J, Choyke P, Girton M, Morrison P, Diggs R, Skinner M. Gadopentetate dimeglumine clearance in renal insufficiency in rabbits. *Invest Radiol* 1990;25:1212–1216.
65. Haustein J, Niendorf H, Louton T. Renal tolerance of Gd-DTPA. A retrospective evaluation of 1,171 patients. *Magn Reson Imag* 1990;8(suppl 1):43.
66. Runge V, Rocklage S, Niendorf H, et al. Discussion: gadolinium chelates. Workshop on Contrast Enhanced Magnetic Resonance. Napa, CA; 1991:229–232.
67. Lackner K, Krahe T, Gotz R, Haustein J. The dialysability of Gd-DTPA. In: Bydder G, Felix R, Bucheler E, eds. *Contrast media in MRI.* Bussum: Medicom Europe; 1990:321–326.
68. Tweedle MF, Eckelman WC, Wedeking P. Pharmacokinetics and metabolism of 153 gadolinium complexes. *Labelled Comp Radiopharm* 1986;23(10–12):1347–1348.
69. Brody A, Sorette M, Gooding C, et al. Induced alignment of flowing sickle erythrocytes in a magnetic field. *Invest Radiol* 1985;20:560–566.
70. Brody A, Embury S, Mentzer W, Winkler M, Gooding C. Preservation of sickle cell blood flow patterns during MR imaging. An in vivo study. *AJR Am J Roentgenol* 1988;151:239–241.
71. Schmiedl U, Maravilla K, Gerlach R, Dowling C. Excretion of gadopentetate dimeglumine in human breast milk. *AJR Am J Roentgenol* 1990;154:1305–1306.
72. Rofsky N, Weinreb J, Litt A. Quantitative analysis of gadopentetate dimeglumine excreted in breast milk. *J Magn Reson Imag* 1993;3:131–132.

9

Screening Before Magnetic Resonance Procedures

All individuals, including patients, volunteer subjects, visitors, MR health care providers, and custodial workers, must be thoroughly screened by qualified personnel before being exposed to the static, gradient, or radiofrequency electromagnetic fields of the MR system (1–17). Conducting a careful screening procedure is crucial to ensure the safety of anyone who enters the area of the MR system. Most instances associated with MR-related injuries have been a direct result of deficiencies in screening methods (1,6,11,13,14,16,18–21). Unfortunately, not all MR users perform a rigorous screening procedure and there tends to be a lack of consensus on what constitutes an appropriate or necessary protocol that will ensure the safety of individuals and patients in the MR setting (1,6). Therefore, this chapter presents and discusses the various important components involved in the screening process that should be performed before allowing individuals to undergo MR procedures or to enter into the MR environment.

MR SCREENING QUESTIONNAIRE

The initial screening process should involve completion of a questionnaire that is specifically designed to determine if there is any reason that the individual would have an adverse reaction to the electromagnetic fields used for the MR procedure (1–3,6,15). The questionnaire should include important queries concerning previous surgery, prior injury from a metallic foreign body, and whether the individual is pregnant. In addition, the questionnaire should contain a means of determining if the individual has any of the various implants, materials, devices, or objects that are considered to be a contraindication or problematic (i.e., as a result of producing imaging artifacts) for the MR procedure (1–28). This includes any device that is electrically, magnetically, or mechanically activated (please refer to Chapters 10 and 11 for a more thorough discussion of these topics).

MR PROCEDURE SCREENING FORM

Date ____________________
Name ____
Sex ________ Age ______ Physician ____________________ Patient No. __________
Date of Birth ______________ Height ____________ Weight ______________
Procedure ________________________________ Outpatient ____Inpatient ______
Diagnosis ____
Clinical History ____
____
____

	YES	NO
Have you ever had a surgical procedure or operation of any kind?........................	___	___
If yes, please list all prior surgeries and approximate dates: _______________		
Have you ever been injured by any metallic foreign body (e.g., bullet, BB, shrapnel, etc.)?........................	___	___
Please describe: ____________________________		
Have you ever had an injury to the eye involving a metallic object (e.g., metallic slivers, shavings, foreign body, etc.)?........................	___	___
Please describe: ____________________________		
Do you have anemia or diseases that affect your blood?........................	___	___
Do you have a history of renal disease, seizure, asthma, or allergic respiratory disease?........................	___	___
Do you have any drug allergies?........................	___	___
If yes, please list: ____________________________		
Have you ever had a reaction to a contrast medium used for MRI or CT?.............	___	___
Are you pregnant or do you suspect that you are pregnant?........................	___	___
Are you breast feeding?........................	___	___
Last menstrual period: ____________________ Post-menopausal?..........	___	___
Are you taking oral contraceptives or receiving hormone treatment?.....................	___	___

PERTINENT PREVIOUS STUDIES:

	BODY PART	DATE
X-rays	____________	_____
Computed tomography	____________	_____
Ultrasound	____________	_____
Nuclear Medicine	____________	_____
MRI	____________	_____

We STRONGLY recommend using the ear plugs or headphones we supply for your MRI examination since some patients may find the noise levels unacceptable and the noise levels may temporarily affect your hearing.

FIG. 9-1. Example of questionnaire used for screening individuals before undergoing MR procedures or entering the MR environment.

THE FOLLOWING ITEMS MAY BE HAZARDOUS OR MAY INTERFERE WITH THE MRI EXAMINATION BY PRODUCING AN ARTIFACT.

Please mark on this drawing the location of any metal inside your body.

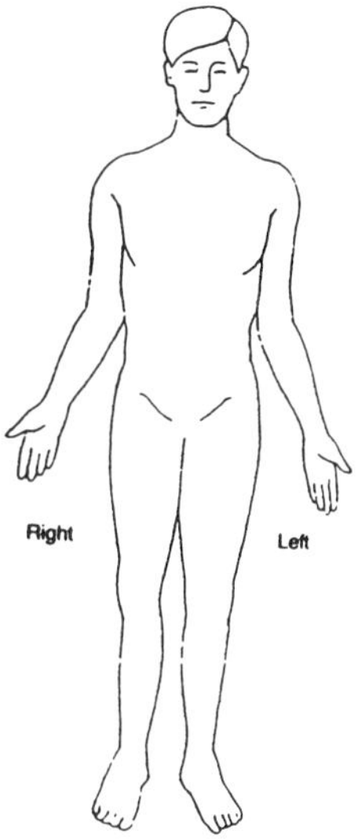

Right Left

PLEASE INDICATE IF YOU HAVE ANY OF THE FOLLOWING:

YES	NO	
___	___	Cardiac pacemaker
___	___	Aneurysm clip(s)
___	___	Implanted cardiac defibrillator
___	___	Neurostimulator
___	___	Any type of biostimulator Type: ______________
		Any type of internal electrode(s), including:
___	___	Pacing wires
___	___	Cochlear implant
___	___	Other: ______________
___	___	Implanted insulin pump
___	___	Swan-Ganz catheter
___	___	Halo vest or metallic cervical fixation device
___	___	Any type of electronic, mechanical, or magnetic implant Type: ______________
___	___	Hearing aid
___	___	Any type of intravascular coil, filter, or stent (e.g., Gianturco coil,Gunther IVC filter, Palmaz stent, etc.)
___	___	Implanted drug infusion device
___	___	Any type of foreign body, shrapnel, or bullet
___	___	Heart valve prosthesis
___	___	Any type of ear implant
___	___	Penile prosthesis
___	___	Orbital/eye prosthesis
___	___	Any type of implant held in place by a magnet
___	___	Any type of surgical clip or staple(s)
___	___	Vascular access port
___	___	Intraventricular shunt
___	___	Artificial limb or joint
___	___	Dentures
___	___	Diaphragm
___	___	IUD
___	___	Pessary
___	___	Wire mesh
___	___	Any implanted orthopedic item(s) (i.e., pins, rods, screws, nails, clips, plates, wire, etc.) Type: ______________
___	___	Any other implanted item Type: ______________
___	___	Tattooed eyeliner*

* A SMALL PERCENTAGE OF PATIENTS WITH TATTOOED EYELINER HAVE EXPERIENCED TRANSIENT SKIN IRRITATION IN ASSOCIATION WITH MRI. THEREFORE, YOU MUST DECIDE IF THIS SLIGHT RISK WARRANTS UNDERGOING YOUR EXAMINATION. YOU MAY WANT TO DISCUSS THIS MATTER WITH YOUR REFERRING PHYSICIAN.

I attest that the above information is correct to the best of my knowledge. I have read and understand the entire contents of this form and I have had the opportunity to ask questions regarding the information on this form.

Patient's signature ______________________________

MD / RN / RT signature ______________________ Date __________

Print MD / RN / RT name ______________________________

page 2

FIG. 9-1. *Continued.*

A diagram of the human body should be provided on the questionnaire so that the individual being screened may specifically indicate the position of any object that would be potentially hazardous or that would interfere with or confuse the interpretation of the MR procedure by causing an artifact (1,3,6,22,23). The screening questionnaire should also be used to obtain additional pertinent information related to the safe performance of the MR procedure. For example, questions may be asked concerning previous adverse reactions to contrast media that should alert the health care provider to potential problems associated with the administration of an MR imaging contrast agent, should it be required for the examination (1,3,6). Finally, pertinent questions may be included related to the phase of the menstrual cycle and the use of oral contraceptives and/or hormone treatment relevant to patients undergoing MR studies for suspected gynecologic abnormalities (3).

In 1994, the Safety Committee of the Society for Magnetic Resonance (previously designated at the Society for Magnetic Resonance Imaging and currently called the International Society for Magnetic Resonance in Medicine) published screening recommendations and a questionnaire that encompassed all the important aforementioned issues (3). These recommendations were developed as a consensus from an international panel of MR experts and were intended for use as a standard of care at all MR centers (Fig. 9-1; the entire document may be found in Appendix III). Elster et al. (6) also published a screening recommendation in 1994. This information was somewhat similar to the content of the recommendations provided by the Safety Committee, which is not surprising, because many of the same MR clinicians and scientists were involved in the development of both documents.

With the use of any form of written questionnaire, limitations exist related to incomplete or incorrect answers provided by the patient, guardian, or other individual preparing to enter the MR setting (6). For example, there may be difficulties associated with individuals who have impaired vision, fluency, or literacy level (6). Therefore, it may be useful or necessary to have a version of the screening questionnaire in the native language of the individual and/or to have a direct verbal interaction with individuals who may have problems with a written questionnaire.

In addition to reviewing the information provided on the questionnaire, it is recommended that an oral interview be conducted by the MR technologist or other trained staff member to ensure further the safety of the individual entering the MR environment or undergoing an MR procedure. This will allow a mechanism for clarification or confirmation of the answers to the questions posed to the individual so that there is no miscommunication (6). The "oral phase" of MR screening is believed to be especially vital for establishing the reliability of the individual's answers (6).

SCREENING PROCEDURES AND BIOMEDICAL IMPLANTS, MATERIALS, AND DEVICES

Numerous studies have assessed the relative safety of performing MR procedures in patients with biomedical implants, materials, or devices (1,2,7,9–18).

This information has served as the basis for determining what objects an individual may have and be permitted or excluded from exposure to the MR system.

With respect to the ferromagnetic qualities of metallic implants, materials, and devices, investigations have generally demonstrated that an MR procedure may be performed safely in a patient with a metallic object if it is nonferromagnetic or if it is attracted only minimally by the static magnetic field in relation to the in vivo application of the object (i.e., the associated deflection force or attraction to the magnetic field is insufficient to move or dislodge the metallic object in situ) (7–17).

In consideration of the above, MR users should note that manufacturers of biomedical implants, materials, and devices may alter the composition of these objects without being required to notify the FDA or the end-users as long as the modification does not substantially alter the effectiveness of the device (19–21). Therefore, MR sites may elect to follow certain policies and procedures, such as contacting the company that manufactured the device in question to determine if any alterations in component materials occurred since the date it was manufactured. This is particularly important when the metallic implant, material, or device is such that, if it were moved or dislodged, may result in serious injury to the patient.

With specific regard to performing MR procedures in patients with aneurysm clips, each individual aneurysm clip, regardless of its type and known or suspected ferromagnetic qualities, should undergo ex vivo testing before implantation in a patient who may subsequently undergo an MR procedure (with the exception of clips that have always been made out of Elgiloy) (20,21). This ex vivo testing would comprise subjecting the aneurysm clip to a static magnetic field of the strength that would subsequently be used to perform the MR procedure on the patient. If no motion or torque of the aneurysm clip is identified, the specific manufacturer, lot number, and model number of the clip should be recorded in the operative note, including the results of the evaluation of ferromagnetism (20,21). Additional information regarding performing MR procedures in patients with aneurysm clips may be found in Chapter 10.

The presence of an electrically, magnetically, or mechanically activated device is usually considered to be a contraindication for an MR procedure (1–21). Therefore, any individual with this type of object must be excluded from the area of the MR system unless, of course, the particular device has been previously shown to be unaffected by the electromagnetic fields generated by the MR system and there is an acceptably low possibility of injuring the individual who has the device (1–3,8–17). MR users should predominantly rely on the peer-reviewed literature regarding the information related to safety with respect to performing MR procedures in patients with potentially hazardous electrically, magnetically, or mechanically activated objects.

SCREENING INDIVIDUALS WITH METALLIC FOREIGN BODIES

All patients or other individuals with a history of being injured by a metallic foreign body such as a bullet, shrapnel, or other type of metallic fragment should be thoroughly evaluated before admission to the area of the MR system (1–3). This is particularly important with respect to the static magnetic field of the MR system because the exposure may cause serious injury as a result of movement or dislodgement of the metallic foreign body.

The relative risk of injury depends on the ferromagnetic properties of the foreign body, the geometry and dimensions of the object, and the strength of the static magnetic field of the MR system. Additionally, the potential for injury is related to the amount of force with which the object is fixed within the tissue and whether or not it is positioned in or adjacent to a particularly sensitive site of the body such as a vital neural, vascular, or soft tissue structure (1,2,9–17).

A patient or other individual who encounters the static magnetic field of an MR system with an intraocular metallic foreign body is at a particular risk for significant eye injury (1,2,28–32). The single reported case of a patient who experienced a vitreous hemorrhage resulting in blindness occurred during an MR imaging procedure that was performed using a 0.35-T MR system (28). The patient had a 2.0 × 3.5 mm intraocular metal fragment that became dislodged while exiting the MR system (28). This incident emphasizes the importance of adequately screening patients and other individuals with suspected intraocular metallic foreign bodies before performing MR procedures or allowing them to enter into the area of the MR system.

Research has demonstrated that small intraocular metallic fragments as small as 0.1 × 0.1 × 0.1 mm may be detected using standard plain film radiographs (29,30). Although thin slice (i.e., <3 mm) computed tomography (CT) has been shown to identify metallic foreign bodies as small as approximately 0.15 mm (29), it is unlikely that a metallic fragment of this size would be dislodged by static magnetic field strengths of up to 2.0 T (29–31).

Metallic fragments of various sizes and dimensions ranging from 0.1 mm × 0.1 mm × 0.1 mm to 3.0 mm × 1.0 mm × 1.0 mm in size have been examined to determine if they were moved or dislodged from the eyes of laboratory animals during exposure to a 2.0-T MR system (30). The largest fragment, 3.0 mm × 1.0 × 1.0 mm in size, rotated but did not move as a result of attraction by this powerful static magnetic field. Furthermore, there was no discernible damage to the ocular tissue (30).

Therefore, it appears that plain film radiography is an acceptable technique for identifying or excluding an intraocular metallic foreign body that represents a potential hazard to the individual entering the area of the MR system or about to undergo an MR procedure (1,5,6,15,26,30). Any individual with a high suspicion of having an intraocular metallic foreign body (e.g., a metal worker exposed to metallic slivers with a history of an eye injury requiring medical attention) should have plain film radiographs of the orbits to rule out the presence of a metallic fragment before exposure to the static magnetic field of the MR system (1,5,6,15,26,30). If an individual with a suspected ferromagnetic intraocular foreign body has no history of a prior injury, no previous or present symptoms, and a plain film series of the orbits does not demonstrate a radiopaque foreign body, the risk of injury associated with exposure to the MR system is considered to be minimal (1,3,5,6,26). Of note is that detection of a high-density focus associated with a metal in the ocular region is not always easy (26). For example, using CT, it is possible to mistake a calcification for a metallic foreign body in the orbit (26,28).

A recent case report illustrates that special precautions are needed for screening adolescent patients before MR procedures (32). This article described an incident in which a 12-year-old patient accompanied by his parent completed all routine procedures before preparation for MR imaging of the lumbar spine. The pre-MR examination screening process included the recommendations and questionnaire developed by the Safety Committee of the Society for Magnetic Resonance (3). The patient and parent provided negative answers to questions regarding prior injury by metallic objects or the presence of a metallic foreign body.

While entering the MR system room, the adolescent patient appeared to be anxious about the examination (32). He was placed in a feet-first, supine position on the scanner table and prepared for MR imaging. The patient became more anxious and restless, shifting his position several times on the table. As the patient was moved slowly toward the bore of a 1.5-T MR system, he complained of pressure in the left eye. The MR technologist immediately removed him from the MR system and out of the room.

Once again, the patient was questioned regarding any previous eye injuries, and again he denied any history of injury or problems (32). Despite this, an intraocular foreign body was suspected to be present in the patient. To be prudent, plain film x-ray Waters views were obtained, with upward and downward fixed glazes. These plain films revealed a metallic foreign body in the left orbit, curvilinear in shape and approximately 5 mm in size. Fortunately, the patient did not appear to have sustained an injury to the eye during this incident. The patient and parent were counseled regarding the implications of future MR procedures with respect to the possibility of significant eye injury related to movement or dislodgement of the metallic foreign body.

This case clearly demonstrates that routine guidelines and safety protocols may not always be sufficient for evaluation of potential hazardous situations that may be present, particularly in adolescents referred for MR procedures. There are possible additional risks involved whenever parents or guardians fill out MR screening forms because children may not be willing to disclose previous injuries or accidents.

To avoid unfortunate accidents related to the electromagnetic fields used for MR procedures, it is recommended that adolescents be provided additional screening that includes private counseling about the hazards associated with the MR environment (32). Furthermore, the technical staff should be educated about these similarly related issues (32).

In addition to being used to detect metallic objects in the ocular region, plain film radiography should be used as the standard of care when screening a patient for the presence of a metallic object located in other potentially hazardous sites of the body (1,5,6,15). Each MR site must establish a standardized policy for screening individuals with suspected metallic foreign bodies. The policy should include guidelines concerning which individuals or patients require work-up by radiographic procedures and the specific procedure to be performed (i.e., number and type of views, position of the anatomy, etc.) and each case should be considered on an individual basis. These precautions must be taken with respect to any type of MR system regardless of field strength, magnet type, and presence or absence of magnetic shielding (1,2,5).

METAL DETECTORS AND MAGNETOMETERS

Metal detectors and magnetometers are devices that may be used by some MR users as a component of the screening protocol for MR procedures (1,2,6,26). Metal detectors have a tuned electronic circuit with a resonance frequency selected to identify specific types of metals (6). Magnetometers measure magnetic fields and can identify materials with magnetic properties (26). Unfortunately, MR sites may rely excessively on these devices as part of their screening process, placing substantial emphasis on the use of a metal detector or magnetometer to identify metallic objects that could present a problem to an individual or patient in association with the MR environment. This is believed to be an unwise practice because of the frequent occurrences of false-positive and false-negative results (1,2).

The ability of a metal detector or magnetometer to identify metal depends on several factors, including the rate of motion of the device relative to the metal, the size and mass of the metallic object, the sensitivity setting of the device (this is generally user selected), the proximity of the device to the metallic object, and the technique and skill of the operator (1). Small or deeply embedded metallic objects in biologically delicate locations of the body (e.g., the eye) might easily escape detection, even by an expert examiner using a metal detector or magnetometer. Therefore, the use of these devices as the primary or only means of finding a metallic object is considered to be inadequate for screening individuals or patients before entering the MR environment (26).

The only acceptable application of an externally applied screening device is the use of a powerful hand-held magnet for assessment of objects that are attached to or found in association with the individual or patient entering the MR environment (i.e., excluding all internal metallic objects). For example, a hand-held magnet is useful as a simple means of evaluating a traction device, wheel chair, or gurney (see next section). It should be noted that this will identify only ferromagnetic components and will not provide any information related to the conductive qualities of the object, which is another potential source of hazard to an individual in the MR setting (1,2,4,8,11,15,16).

SCREENING INDIVIDUALS TO PROTECT FROM THE "MISSILE EFFECT"

The "missile effect" refers to the capability of the fringe field component of the static magnetic field to attract ferromagnetic objects (e.g., oxygen tanks, tools, etc.) that may be subsequently drawn into the MR system by considerable force (1). The missile effect can pose a significant risk to the patient inside the MR system and/or anyone who is in the path of the ferromagnetic object attracted by the magnetic fringe field. In extreme cases, the magnet may need to be "quenched" for MR systems with superconducting magnets or turned off to extract sizable ferromagnetic objects from the MR systems, resulting in substantial financial loss because of down-time, replacement of cryogens, etc. Therefore, a protocol should be established by every MR site for detection of metallic objects before allowing individuals to enter into the area of the MR system in order to avoid injuries or other problems related to missile effects.

To guard against these catastrophes, the immediate area around the MR system should be clearly demarcated, labeled with appropriate warning signs, and secured by trained staff who are cognizant of MR-related safety procedures. In addition, patients and other individuals who must enter the MR system area should be carefully screened for objects that may be involved in the missile effect.

For patients preparing to undergo an MR procedure, all metallic personal belongings (i.e., analog watches, jewelry, etc.) and devices must be removed as well as clothing items that have metallic fasteners, loose metallic components, or metallic threads. One of the more effective means of preventing a ferromagnetic object from inadvertently becoming a missile is to require that patients be placed in a gown and that accompanying individuals be required to remove all objects from their pockets and hair before entering the MR area. Furthermore, patients and other individuals should be educated about the potential hazards and problems associated with the magnetic fringe field before entering the area of the MR system.

Any patient who is nonambulatory must enter the area of the MR system only in a nonferromagnetic wheel chair or on a nonferromagnetic gurney. Wheel chairs and gurneys should also be inspected for the presence of a ferromagnetic oxygen tank before allowing the patient into the MR setting. Fortunately, there are several commercially available, MR-compatible devices that may be used to transport and support nonambulatory patients to and from the MR system room.

MR PROCEDURES AND PREGNANCY

Pregnant patients or those who suspect that they are pregnant must be identified before exposure to the electromagnetic fields used for MR procedures so that the risks versus the benefits of the examination may be assessed (see Chapter 4 for additional discussion related to this issue). According to the recommendations provided by the Safety Committee of the Society for Magnetic Resonance Imaging, MR procedures may be used in pregnant patients if other non-ionizing forms of diagnostic imaging are inadequate or if the examination provides important information that would otherwise require exposure to a diagnostic procedure that requires ionizing radiation (e.g., CT, fluoroscopy, etc.) (5).

The guidelines issued by the FDA indicate that the safety of MR when used to image the fetus has not been established or proved (24,25). Therefore, patients should be provided this information and should also be informed that there are no known deleterious effects related to the use of MR procedures during pregnancy (1,2,4,15).

With regard to screening other pregnant women who may encounter the electromagnetic fields of the MR system, it should be realized that these individuals are not subjected to the same type of exposure levels used to examine patients during MR procedures. Epidemiologic data obtained from a study pertaining to this issue indicate that there is no evidence of an increase in adverse reproductive outcomes for pregnant technologists or other health care providers associated with limited or no exposure to the time-varying electromagnetic fields produced during the operation of MR systems (33). Therefore, MR sites can develop a screening policy concerning these individuals, accordingly (see Chapter 4 for additional information on this topic).

PERMANENT COLORING TECHNIQUES AND COSMETICS

Before undergoing an MR procedure, the patient should be asked if he or she has ever had any type of permanent coloring technique (i.e., tattooing) applied to any part of the body. This includes cosmetic applications such as eye liner, lip-liner, and decorative designs. This question is necessary because of the associated imaging artifacts and, more importantly, because a small number of patients (fewer than 10) who have experienced transient skin irritation or cutaneous swelling at the site of the application of the permanent coloring in association with MR procedures (34–36). More recently, there has been one anecdotal report of a patient undergoing MR imaging who complained of a burning sensation at the site where a large tattoo had been applied on the arm using a black pigment.

Investigation of the incidents related to patients experiencing adverse effects in relation to the presence of tattoos revealed that there was a tendency for the problem to occur whenever pigments that contained iron oxide or other ferromagnetic substance(s) were used (8,29–30). This includes those pigments that are especially black or blue in color. Supposedly, certain ferrous pigments used for the tattooing process can interact with the electromagnetic fields used for MR procedures, producing the reported problems (8,28).

When one considers the many millions of MR procedures that have been conducted in patients over the past 12 years, and that only a few individuals have had a minor, short-term difficulty related to the presence of permanent coloring techniques, it is apparent that this problem occurs rarely. Therefore, the risk associated with the use of permanent coloring techniques in patients during MR procedures is considered to be relatively minor. Any difficulty performing an MR procedure in a patient who has a tattoo is unlikely to prevent the examination because the important diagnostic information provided by this imaging modality is typically critical to the care of the patient.

If a patient with a tattoo requires an MR procedure, the individual should be informed of the relative minor risk associated with the site of the permanent coloring application. In addition, the patient should be requested to advise the MR operator regarding any unusual sensations felt at the site of the tattoo during the MR examination. Patients with tattoos located on extremities or peripheral sites should be positioned in the MR system to avoid direct contact with the body coil or surface coils (e.g., foam rubber pads may be placed in between the site of the tattoo and the coil) to minimize the potential problem. Similar to other patients undergoing MR procedures, patients with tattoos must be closely monitored throughout the entire operation of the MR system to ensure their safety.

With respect to eye make-up, there has been a report of a patient who developed eye irritation when her make-up, which contained ferromagnetic particles, became displaced from her eyelid into her eye during exposure to the MR system (8). Therefore, it is necessary to inform individuals about the potential problems related to the presence of eye make-up and request that they remove it (if appropriate) before undergoing the MR procedure.

REFERENCES

1. Kanal E, Shellock FG. Safety considerations in MR imaging. *Radiology* 1990;176:593–606.
2. Shellock FG. Biological effects and safety aspects of magnetic resonance imaging. *Magn Reson Q* 1989;5:243–261.
3. Shellock FG, Kanal E. SMRI Report. Policies, guidelines and recommendations for MR imaging safety and patient management. Questionnaire for screening patients before MR procedures. *J Magn Reson Imag* 1994;4:749–751.
4. Persson BRR, Stahlberg F. *Health and safety of clinical NMR examinations.* Boca Raton, Fla: CRC Press; 1989.
5. Shellock FG, Kanal E. Policies, guidelines, and recommendations for MR imaging safety and patient management. *J Magn Reson Imag* 1991;1:97–101.
6. Elster AD, Link KM, Carr JJ. Patient screening prior to MR imaging: a practical approach synthesized from protocols at 15 U.S. medical centers. *AJR Am J Roentgenol* 1994;162:195–199.
7. Hayes DL, Holmes DR, Gray JE. Effect of a 1.5 Tesla nuclear magnetic resonance imaging scanner on implanted permanent pacemakers. *J Am Coll Cardiol* 1987;10:782–786.
8. Gangarosa RE, Minnis JE, Nobbe J, Praschan D, Genberg RW. Operational safety issues in MRI. *Magn Reson Imag* 1987;5:287–292.
9. Shellock FG, Crues JV. High-field MR imaging of metallic biomedical implants: an ex vivo evaluation of deflection forces. *AJR Am J Roentgenol* 1988;151:389–392.

10. Shellock FG, Curtis JS. MR imaging and biomedical implants, materials, and devices. An updated review. *Radiology* 1991;180:541–550.
11. Pohost GM, Blackwell GG, Shellock FG. Safety of patients with medical devices during application of magnetic resonance methods. In: *Biological effects and safety aspects of nuclear magnetic resonance imaging and spectroscopy.* New York: New York Academy of Sciences; 1992: 302–312.
12. Shellock FG. MR imaging of metallic implants and materials: a compilation of the literature. *AJR Am J Roentgenol* 1988;151:811–814.
13. Shellock FG, Crues JV. MRI: safety considerations in magnetic resonance imaging. *MRI Decisions* 1988;2:25–30.
14. Shellock FG. Safety Considerations in MR Imaging of Biomedical Implants and Devices. In: Thrall J, ed. *Current practice in radiology.* Philadelphia: BC Decker/Mosby–Year Book; 1992.
15. Shellock FG, Litwer C, Kanal E. MRI bioeffects, safety, and patient management: a review. *Rev Magn Reson Imag* 1992;4:21–63.
16. Shellock FG, Crues JV. Safety aspects of MRI in patients with metallic implants or foreign bodies: absolute and relative contraindications. *Appl Radiol* 1992;Nov:44–47.
17. Shellock FG. *Pocket guide to MR procedures and metallic objects: update 1996.* New York: Lippincott–Raven Press; 1996.
18. Klucznik RP, Carrier DA, Pyka R, Haid RW. Placement of a ferromagnetic intracerebral clip in a magnetic field with a fatal outcome. *Radiology* 1993;187:855–856.
19. FDA stresses need for caution during MR scanning of patients with aneurysm clips. In: *Medical devices bulletin.* Center for Devices and Radiological Health; March, 1993;11:1–2.
20. Kanal E, Shellock FG. MR imaging of patients with intracranial aneurysm clips. *Radiology* 1993;187:612–614.
21. Kanal E, Shellock FG. The value of published data on MR compatibility of metallic implants. *AJNR Am J Neuroradiol* 1994;15:1394–1396.
22. Bellon EM, Haacke EM, Coleman PE, Sacco DC, Steiger DA, Gangarosa RE. MR artifacts: a review. *Magn Reson Imag* 1984;2:41–52.
23. Pusey E, Lufkin RB, Brown RKJ, et al. Magnetic resonance imaging artifacts: mechanisms and clinical significance. *RadioGraphics* 1986;6:891–911.
24. Premarket notification: 510(k) regulatory requirements for medical devices. In: US Department of Health and Human Services, Public Health Service, Food and Drug Administration; 1988.
25. F.D.A. Magnetic resonance diagnostic device; Panel recommendation and report on petitions for MR reclassification. *Fed Reg* 1988;53:7575–7579.
26. Boutin RD, Briggs JE, Williamson MR. Injuries associated with MR imaging: survey of safety records and methods used to screen patients for metallic foreign bodies before imaging. *AJR Am J Roentgenol* 1994;162:189–194.
27. Dupuy DE, Hartnell GC, Lipsky M. MR imaging of a patient with a ferromagnetic foreign body. *AJR Am J Roentgenol* 1993;160:893.
28. Kelly WM, Pagle PG, Pearson A, San Diego AG, Soloman MA. Ferromagnetism of intraocular foreign body causes unilateral blindness after MR study. *AJNR Am J Neuroradiol* 1986;7:243–245.
29. Mani RL. In search of an effective screening system for intraocular metallic foreign bodies prior to MR–an important issue of patient safety. *AJNR Am J Neuroradiol* 1988;9:1032.
30. Williams S, Char DH, Dillon WP, Lincoff N, Moseley M. Ferrous intraocular foreign bodies and magnetic resonance imaging. *Am J Opthalolmol* 1988;105:398–401.
31. Shellock FG, Kanal E. Re: Metallic foreign bodies in the orbits of patients undergoing MR imaging: prevalence and value of pre-MR radiography and CT. *AJR Am J Roentgenol* 1994;162:985–986.
32. Elmquist C, Shellock FG, Stoller D. Screening adolescents for metallic foreign bodies before MR procedures. *J Magn Reson Imag* 1996;5:784–785.
33. Kanal E, Gillen J, Evans JA, Savitz DA, Shellock FG. Survey of reproductive health among female workers. *Radiology* 1993; 187:395–399.
34. Jackson JG, Acker JD. Permanent eyeliner and MR imaging. *AJR Am J Roentgenol* 1987;49: 1080.
35. Lund G, Nelson JD, Wirtschafter JD, Williams PA. Tatooing of eyelids: Magnetic resonance imaging artifacts. *Ophthalmic Surg* 1986;17:550–553.
36. Sacco D, Steiger DA, Bellon EM, Coleman PE, Haacke EM. Artifacts caused by cosmetics in MR imaging of the head. *AJR Am J Roentgenol* 1987;148:1001–1004.

10

Magnetic Resonance Procedures and Patients with Biomedical Implants, Materials, and Devices

Magnetic resonance (MR) procedures may be contraindicated for a patient because of the risks associated with movement or dislodgement of a ferromagnetic biomedical implant, material, device, or object (1–89). There are other possible hazards related to the presence of a bioimplant, including induction of electric current, excessive heating, and the misinterpretation of an imaging artifact as an abnormality (21,48,49,55,57,58,90–109).

The potential for MR procedures to injure patients by inducing electric currents in conductive materials or devices such as gating leads, unused surface coils, halo vests, or improperly used physiologic monitors has been previously reported (21,48,49,55,57,58). Recommendations concerning techniques to protect patients from injuries related to induced current that may develop during an MR procedure, especially those associated with the use of monitoring devices, have been presented (21,49,55,58) (see Chapter 7 for additional information).

Temperature elevations produced during MR procedures have been studied using ex vivo testing techniques to evaluate several metallic implants, materials, devices, and objects of various sizes and metallic composition (9,45,55,58). These data indicate that only minor temperature changes occur in association with MR procedures involving metallic objects (11,40,50,54). Therefore, heating generated during MR procedures involving patients with bioimplants does not appear to be a substantial hazard. Of additional note is that there has never been a report of a patient being seriously injured as a result of excessive heat developing in a biomedical implant or device (with the exception of burns that have occurred as a result of induced current in electrically conductive devices).

The type and extent of various artifacts caused by metallic implants, materials, and devices have also been described and are well recognized on MR images (81,82,90–92,100–106). The distortion of the image by a metallic object is caused by a disruption of the local magnetic field that perturbs the relationship between position and frequency crucial for accurate image reconstruction. For this reason, biomedical implants, materials, devices, or objects that incorporate magnets can produce artifacts on MR images that are especially profound (29,50,58).

The degree of image distortion depends on the magnetic susceptibility, quantity, shape, orientation, and position of the object in the body as well as the techniques used for imaging (i.e., the specific pulse sequence parameters) and image processing (i.e., 2D Fourier transform reconstruction, back projection, etc.) (81,82). Artifacts caused by the presence of metallic objects in patients during MR imaging are seen typically as local or regional distortions of the image and/or as signal void. However, the extent, configuration, and characteristics of the artifacts may be unpredictable.

Nonferromagnetic objects tend to produce artifacts that are less severe than ferromagnetic objects. Artifacts caused by nonferromagnetic bioimplants result from eddy currents that can be generated in the objects by gradient magnetic fields used for MR imaging that, in turn, disrupt the local magnetic field and distort the image (81,82).

Numerous studies have assessed the ferromagnetic qualities of various biomedical implants, materials, devices, and objects by measuring deflection forces, attraction, or other aspects of interaction associated with the static and/or gradient magnetic fields generated by MR systems. With respect to the evaluation of ferromagnetism, these investigations have demonstrated that MR procedures may be performed safely in patients if the metallic object is nonferromagnetic or is only minimally attracted by the magnetic field in relation to its in vivo application (i.e., the associated attractive force is insufficient to move or dislodge the object in situ or affect its intended function) (46,47,56,57,63,64,67,74,95,96).

Each implant, material, device, or object (particularly those made from unknown materials) should be evaluated using ex vivo techniques before performing an MR procedure in a patient that possesses it (46,47,56,67). By following this procedure, the presence and relative degree of ferromagnetism may be determined so that a competent decision can be made concerning any associated risks caused by possible adverse interactions with the magnetic fields of the MR systems.

Various factors influence the risk of performing an MR procedure in a patient with a ferromagnetic implant, material, or device, including the strength of the static and gradient magnetic fields, the degree of ferromagnetism of the object, the mass of the object, the geometry of the object, the location and orientation of the object in situ, and the length of time the object has been in place. These factors should be carefully considered before subjecting a patient with a ferromagnetic object to an MR procedure, particularly if it is located in a potentially dangerous area of the body such as near a vital neural, vascular, or soft tissue structure where movement or dislodgement could injure the patient. Furthermore, there is a possibility of changing the operational or functional aspects of the implant, material, or device as a result of exposure to the electromagnetic fields used by the MR systems.

USING THE INFORMATION CONCERNING IMPLANTS, MATERIALS, DEVICES, AND OBJECTS EVALUATED FOR COMPATIBILITY WITH MR PROCEDURES

Although lists of implants, materials, devices, and objects tested for ferromagnetism have been published and updated on several occasions, words of advice and caution on how to use them are in order (83). The data presented in any list of this nature represents a "snapshot in time" for the period indicated and for the specific implants, materials, devices, and objects that have been evaluated using the particular technique described in the published report (83).

Manufacturers may change the composition of the implant, material, device, or object without being required to notify or seek new approval from the FDA as long the function of the device remains the same (83,85). Therefore, MR sites may elect to follow guidelines, such as contacting the company that manufactured the device to determine if any alterations in component materials occurred since it was tested previously (83). This is particularly important for those devices that would present a serious hazard to the patient if it were moved or dislodged (e.g., aneurysm clips, otologic implants, etc.).

Additionally, it is important to note that there is now a proliferation of MR systems with static magnetic field strengths that exceed 2.0 T. Very few of the implants, materials, devices, or objects have been evaluated for attraction to these higher static magnetic fields. It is conceivable that there may be an instance in which a device that exhibited only "mild" or "slight" ferromagnetism in association with a static magnetic field strength of 1.5 T or lower may now be attracted with sufficient force to pose a hazard to a patient undergoing an MR procedure on an MR system that has a static magnetic field strength of 2.0 T or higher.

The following is a summary of information related to the interaction of magnetic fields of MR systems with various implants, materials, devices, and objects that have been evaluated usually by ex vivo testing methods. The reader is advised to refer to Appendix I for the specific sited references and for additional information.

ANEURYSM AND HEMOSTATIC CLIPS

According to test results, several aneurysm clips display ferromagnetic qualities and, therefore, are considered to be a contraindication for patients undergoing MR procedures (6,11,46,47,56,62) (Fig. 10-1). Unfortunately, one patient mortality has occurred as a result of a ferromagnetic aneurysm clip being displaced from its position during an MR procedure (78). In this incident, a 74-year-old patient with an intracranial aneurysm clip was permitted to undergo MR imaging in a 1.5-T MR system. The personnel at the site were aware that the patient had an aneurysm clip in place but it was thought to be a type that is nonferromagnetic. Only after the patient experienced a fatal intracranial hemorrhage from what appears to have been the result of dislodgement of this aneurysm clip in the static field of the MR system was it revealed that the history provided during pre-MR screening was incorrect and that the clip was actually a ferromagnetic type (22,78).

Because of the profound safety implications related to performing an MR procedure in a patient with an aneurysm clip, each aneurysm clip, regardless of its type and known or suspected ferromagnetic qualities, should undergo ex vivo testing before implantation in a patient who may subsequently undergo an MR procedure (22). This ex vivo testing can take the form of subjecting the aneurysm clip to a magnetic field similar to that that will subsequently be used to perform the MR procedure in the patient. If no motion or torque of the aneurysm clip is identified, the specific manufacturer, lot number, and model number of the clip should be recorded in the operative note, including the results of the evaluation of ferromagnetism (22). In the future, it would thus be

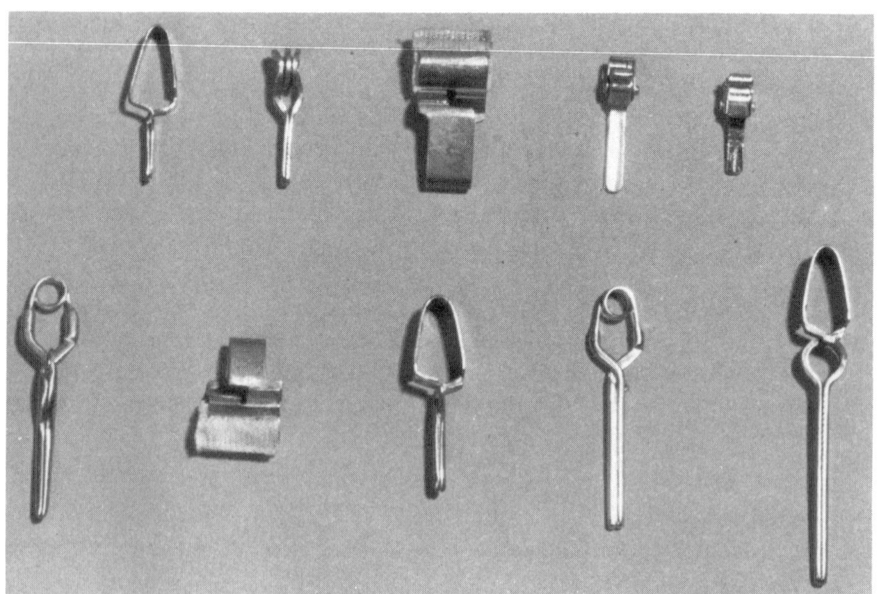

FIG. 10-1. Examples of cerebral vascular aneurysm clips. Some of these implants are composed of ferromagnetic materials and are considered to be contraindicated for patients undergoing MR procedures.

easy to verify precisely what was implanted and that the aneurysm clip had been tested.

If the aneurysm clip is found to be ferromagnetic, it is strongly advised that it not be used for surgery (22). If the aneurysm clip needs to be implanted, the patient should be educated in the postoperative period and a note should be placed in the patient's chart, similar to that used to indicate a severe allergy. This will provide a warning for all further health care practitioners as well as the patient him- or herself as to the possible hazards of MR imaging of this patient. Additional recommendations are discussed in the article by Kanal and Shellock (22).

Gordon C. Johnson of the Center for Devices and Radiological Health, Food and Drug Administration, in response to the need for caution during MR imaging of patients with aneurysm clips, has suggested the following (85):

> To minimize the possibility of inadvertently imaging a patient with a magnetically active metallic implant, implanting physicians should provide patients with information about the type and identity of their particular implants and suggest, where appropriate, that patients carry an alert card or wear a medical alert bracelet or necklace identifying them as having such an implant. In addition, physicians who order MR procedures should carefully screen patients and inform the MR imaging facility of any metallic implants the patient may have. MR imaging facilities should review their procedures to be sure that all patients are adequately screened for the presence of metallic implants before MR imaging.

None of the various hemostatic vascular clips that have been evaluated were attracted by static magnetic fields up to 1.5 T (46,47,56,62). These hemostatic clips are made from nonferromagnetic materials such as tantalum and nonferromagnetic forms of stainless steel (Fig. 10-2). Therefore, patients who have any

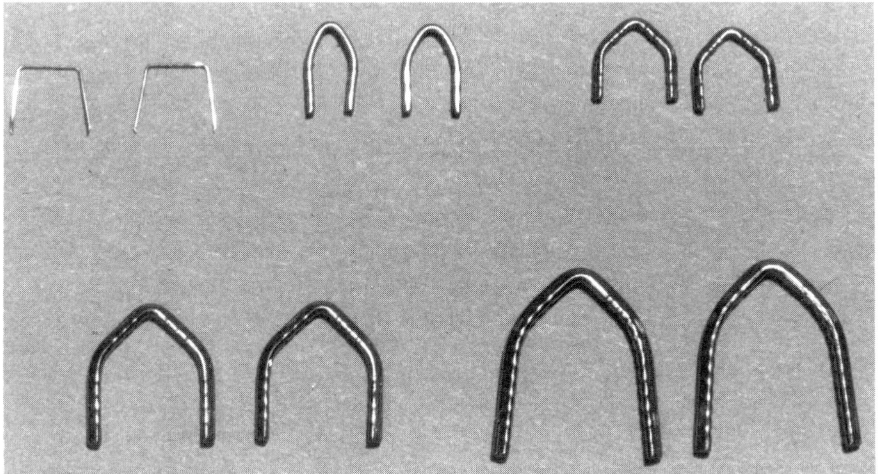

FIG. 10-2. Examples of vascular clips. Each of the vascular clips tested was found to be nonferromagnetic materials and are safe for patients undergoing MR procedures.

of the hemostatic vascular clips listed in Appendix I are not at risk for injury during MR procedures.

BIOPSY NEEDLES AND DEVICES

Recently, MR imaging has been used, with encouraging results, to guide tissue biopsy. The performance of these specialized procedures requires tools that are compatible with MR systems. Commercially available biopsy needles and devices (i.e., guide wires, stylets, marking wires, biopsy guns, etc.) have been evaluated with respect to compatibility with MR procedures, not only to determine ferromagnetic qualities but to also characterize imaging artifacts (100,101). The results have indicated that most of the commercially available biopsy needles and devices are not useful for MR-guided biopsy procedures because of the presence of ferromagnetism and the associated imaging artifacts.

The presence of these ferromagnetic biopsy needles and lesion marking wires in a tissue phantom used for testing produced such substantial artifacts that they would not be useful for MR-guided procedures (100,101). Indeed, needles or devices containing any type of ferromagnetic material may have too much associated magnetic susceptibility to cause their use for MR-guided procedures to be limited. Fortunately, several needles and devices have been constructed out of nonferromagnetic materials specifically for use in MR-guided procedures (100,101).

Although most of the biopsy guns tested for attraction to the static magnetic fields of MR systems were found to be ferromagnetic, because they are not used in the immediate area of the tissue that is to be sampled, the artifact associated with these devices is unlikely to affect the resulting image during an MR-guided biopsy procedure. Nevertheless, the presence of ferromagnetism is likely to preclude the optimal use of most biopsy guns in the MR environment. Currently, there is at least one commercially available biopsy gun that has been developed specifically for use in MR-guided procedures (101).

BREAST TISSUE EXPANDERS AND IMPLANTS

Breast tissue expanders and mammary implants are used for breast reconstruction following mastectomy, for the correction of breast and chest-wall deformities and underdevelopment, for tissue defect procedures, and for cosmetic augmentation. These devices are equipped with either an integral injection site or a remote injection dome that is used to accept a needle for placement of saline for expansion of the prosthesis intraoperatively and/or postoperatively.

The Becker and Siltex prostheses are additionally equipped with a choice of a standard injection dome or a microinjection dome. The Radovan expander is indicated for temporary implantation only (102). The injection ports contain 316 L stainless steel to guard against piercing the injection port by the needle. There are two breast tissue expanders that are constructed with magnetic ports to allow for a more accurate detection of the injection site. These devices are substantially attracted to the static magnetic field of MR systems and, therefore, may be injurious to a patient undergoing an MR procedure (29).

The relative amount of image distortion caused by the metallic components of these devices should not greatly affect the diagnostic quality of an MR examination, unless the imaging area of interest is at the same location as the metallic portion of the breast tissue expander (102). For example, there may be a situation during which a patient is referred for MR imaging for the determination of breast cancer or a breast implant rupture such that the presence of the metallic artifact could obscure the precise location of the abnormality. In view of this possibility, it is recommended that patients be identified with breast tissue expanders that have metallic components so that the individual interpreting the MR images is aware of the potential problems related to the generation of artifacts.

CAROTID ARTERY VASCULAR CLAMPS

Each of the different carotid artery vascular clamps tested for ferromagnetism displayed attraction to a 1.5-T static magnetic field (68). However, only the Poppen-Blaylock carotid artery vascular clamp was felt to be contraindicated for patients undergoing MR procedures because of the existence of substantial attractive force (68). The other carotid artery clamps were considered to be safe for patients exposed to the magnetic fields of MR systems because they were only "slightly" ferromagnetic (68). With the exception of the Poppen-Blaylock clamp, patients with metallic carotid artery vascular clamps have been imaged by MR systems with static magnetic fields ranging up to 1.5 T without experiencing any discomfort or neurologic sequelae (68).

DENTAL IMPLANTS, DEVICES, AND MATERIALS

Many of the dental implants, devices, materials, and objects evaluated for ferromagnetic qualities exhibited measurable deflection forces, but only the ones that have a magnetically activated component present a potential problem for patients during MR procedures (see section on Magnetically Activated Implants and Devices) (46,47,56,62) (Fig. 10-3). The other dental implants, devices, and materials are held in place with sufficient counter-forces to prevent them from being moved or dislodged by magnetic fields of the MR system.

HALO VESTS AND CERVICAL FIXATION DEVICES

Halo vests or cervical fixation devices may be constructed from either ferromagnetic, nonferromagnetic, or a combination of metallic components (4,8,51,62,103) (Fig. 10-4). Although some commercially available halo vests or

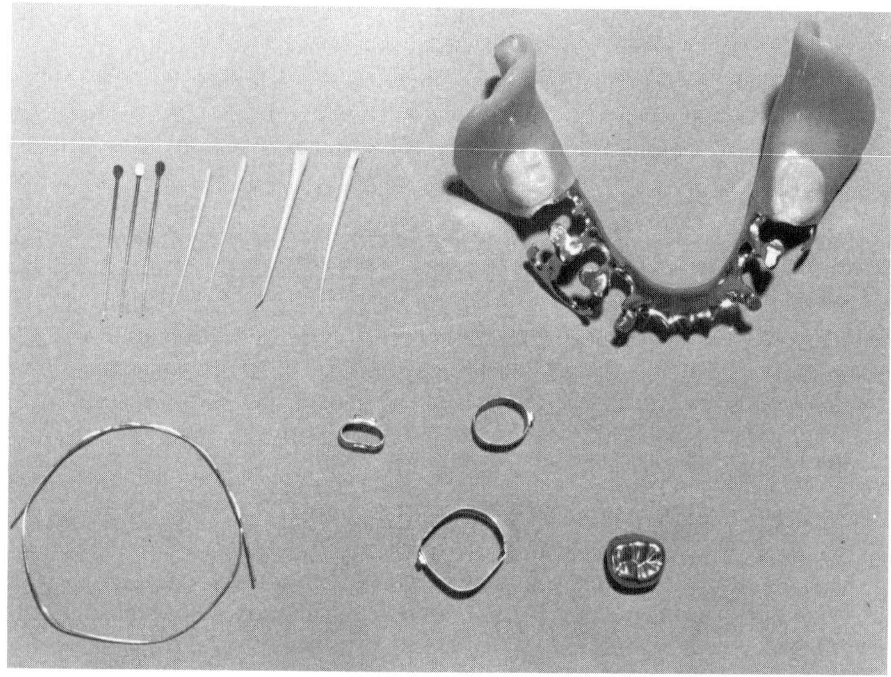

FIG. 10-3. Examples of various dental implants and materials tested for MR compatibility.

cervical fixation devices are composed entirely of nonferromagnetic materials, there is a theoretical hazard of inducing electric current in the ring portion of any halo device made from electrically conductive materials according to Faraday's law of electromagnetic induction (51). Additionally, there is a potential for the patient's tissue to be involved in part of this current loop, so that there would be the concern of a possible burn or electrical injury to the patient. The induced current within such a ring or conductive loop is of additional concern because of eddy current induction and potential image degradation effects.

Currently, there are no reports of injuries associated with MR procedures performed in patients with halo devices. However, one incident of "electrical arcing" without injury was reported in the 1988 Society for Magnetic Resonance Imaging Safety Survey (Phase I Study; E. Kanal, personal communication, 1988).

Because of safety and image quality issues, MR procedures should be performed only on patients with specially designed halo vests or cervical fixation devices made from nonferromagnetic and nonconductive materials that have little or no interaction with the electromagnetic fields generated by MR systems (56,62,103).

Recently, there have been anecdotal reports of patients experiencing a sensation of heat during MR imaging. Therefore, a study was conducted to assess the

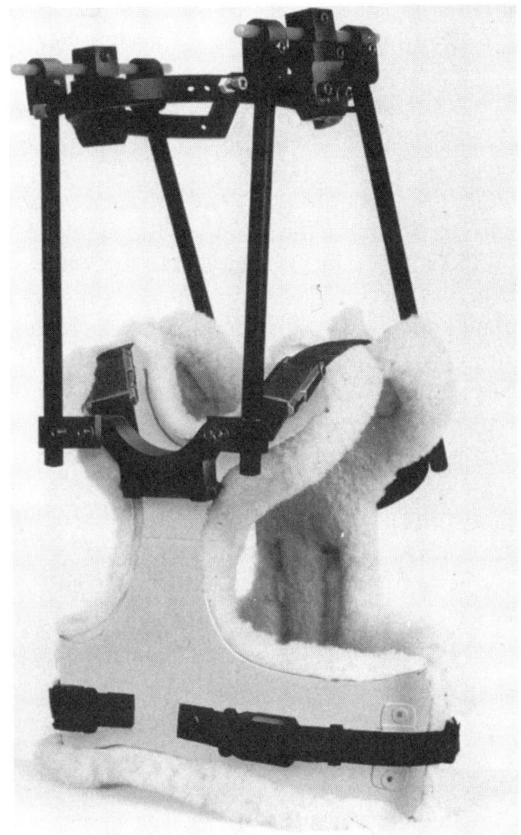
A

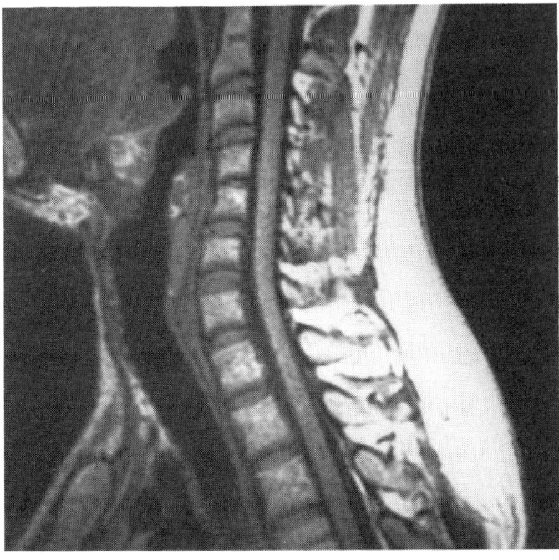
B

FIG. 10-4. A: Example of nonconductive, nonferromagnetic halo vest designed for use during MR procedures. **B:** T1-weighted, sagittal plane image of the cervical spine obtained from a patient wearing an MR-compatible halo vest.

possible heating of halo vests and cervical fixation devices during MR imaging performed using a 1.5-T MR system and various pulse sequences typically used to image the cervical spine (103). Of interest is that there appeared to be subtle motions of the halo ring associated with the use of a magnetization transfer contrast (MTC) pulse sequence, as shown by recordings obtained using a motion-sensitive, laser-Doppler flow monitor (103). Apparently, the specific imaging parameters used for the MTC pulse sequence produced sufficient vibration of the halo ring to create the sensation of heating. These vibrations may have been felt by the subject and interpreted as a "heating" sensation. This is likely to occur when the frequency and/or amount of vibration is at a certain level that stimulates nerve receptors located in the subcutaneous region that detect sensations of pain and temperature changes. The aforementioned is merely a hypothesis based on the available data and requires further investigation to substantiate this theory.

In consideration of the above, it may be inadvisable to permit patients with certain cervical fixation devices to undergo MR procedures using an MTC pulse sequence until this problem can be further characterized in order to avoid other similar patient responses, regardless of the lack of safety concern related to excessive heating. Other comparable pulse sequences should likewise be avoided when performing MR imaging of patients with halo vests until the precise cause of this problem is determined (103).

HEART VALVE PROSTHESES

Many heart valve prostheses have been evaluated for the presence of attraction to static magnetic fields of MR systems at field strengths of as high as 2.35 T (41,56,62,63,95) (Fig. 10-5). Of these, most displayed measurable attraction to the static magnetic field of the MR system used for testing. However, because the actual deflection forces of these heart valves were minimal compared with the force exerted by the beating heart (i.e., approximately 7.2 N) (64), an MR procedure is not considered to be hazardous for a patient who has any of the heart valve prostheses listed in Appendix I. This includes the Starr-Edwards Model Pre-6000 heart valve prosthesis, which was previously suggested to be a potential hazard for a patient undergoing an MR procedure. With respect to clinical MR procedures, there has never been a report of a patient incident or injury related to the presence of a heart valve prosthesis.

INTRAVASCULAR COILS, FILTERS, AND STENTS

Various types of intravascular coils, filters, and stents have been evaluated for compatibility with MR systems (62,65–67) (Figs. 10-6 and 10-7). Eight of these exhibited ferromagnetism. Fortunately, these devices typically become incorporated securely into the vessel wall primarily because of tissue ingrowth within approximately 6 weeks from their introduction. Therefore, it is unlikely that

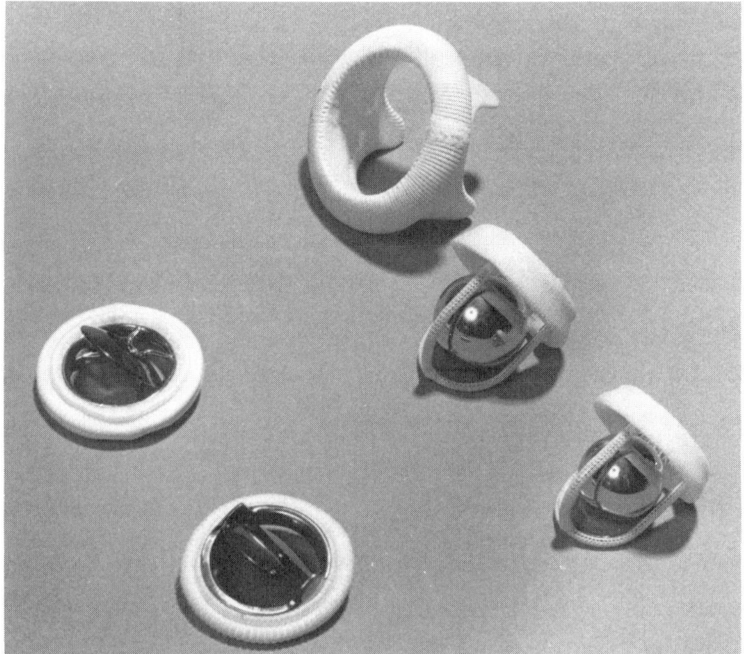

FIG. 10-5. Examples of prosthetic heart valves. Each of these heart valves has a metallic component. Some of these valves are made from materials that are "mildly" ferromagnetic. However, all these prosthetic heart valves are considered to be safe for patients undergoing MR procedures because the associated deflection forces are less than the in vivo forces.

any of them would become moved or dislodged as a result of being attracted by static magnetic fields up to 1.5 T (65). Patients with the intravascular coils, filters, and stents listed in Appendix I have undergone procedures using MR systems with static magnetic fields of up to 1.5 T without incident. An MR procedure should not be performed if there is any possibility or suspicion that the intravascular coil, filter, or stent is not positioned properly or firmly in place.

OCULAR IMPLANTS AND DEVICES

Of the different ocular implants and devices tested (Figs. 10-8 and 10-9), the Fatio eyelid spring, the retinal tack made from martensitic (i.e., ferromagnetic) stainless steel (Western European), the Troutman magnetic ocular implant, and the Unitek round wire eyelid spring were attracted by a 1.5-T static magnetic field (62,96). A patient with a Fatio eyelid spring or round wire eyelid spring may experience discomfort but probably would not be injured severely as a result of exposure to the magnetic fields of an MR system. Patients have un-

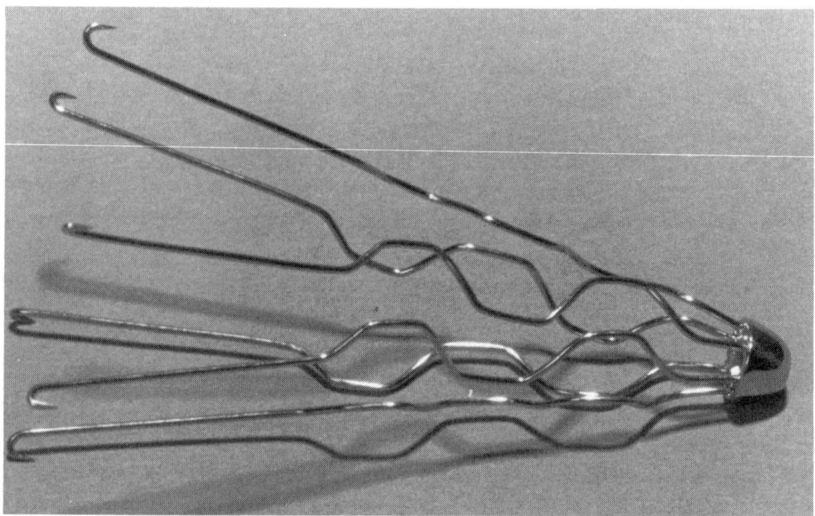

FIG. 10-6. Greenfield filter, stainless steel version. This intravascular filter is considered to be safe for patients undergoing MR procedures after 6 weeks of implantation because the associated deflection force is minimal compared with the in vivo force.

dergone MR procedures with eyelid wires after having a protective plastic covering placed around the globe along with a firmly applied eye patch.

The retinal tack made from martensitic stainless steel and the Troutman magnetic ocular implant may injure a patient undergoing an MR procedure (see also section on Magnetically Activated Implants and Devices for additional information pertaining to the Troutman magnetic ocular implant).

ORTHOPEDIC IMPLANTS, MATERIALS, AND DEVICES

Most of the orthopedic implants, materials, and devices evaluated for ferromagnetism are made from nonferromagnetic materials and, therefore, are safe for patients undergoing MR procedures (62) (Fig. 10-10). Only the Perfix interference screw used for reconstruction of the anterior cruciate ligament was found to be highly ferromagnetic (60). Because this interference screw is embedded in bone for its application, it is held in place with sufficient force to prevent movement or dislodgement (60).

Of note is that the presence of the Perfix interference screw causes extensive image distortion during MR imaging of the knee (60) (Fig. 10-11). Therefore, one of the nonferromagnetic interference screws available should be used for reconstruction of the anterior cruciate ligament if MR imaging is to be utilized for subsequent evaluation of the knee (60). Patients with each of the orthopedic implants, materials, and devices listed in Appendix I have undergone MR pro-

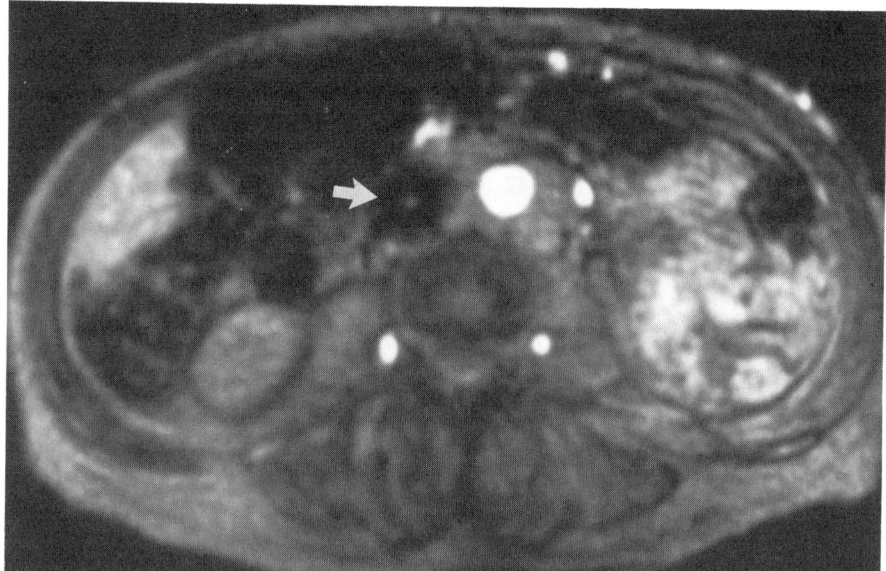

A

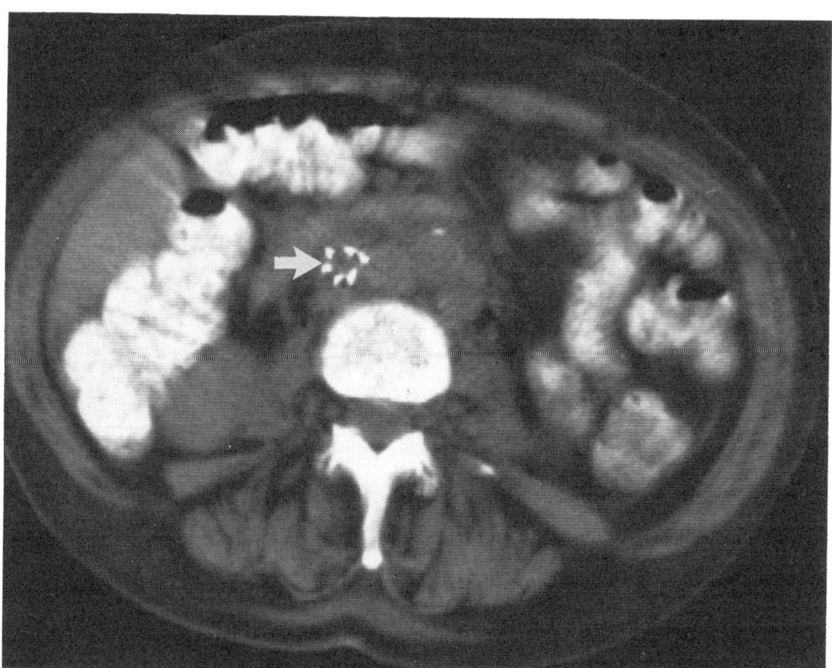

B

FIG. 10-7. A: Gradient echo, axial plane image of a patient with a Greenfield filter in place. Note the unusual artifact in the vena cava (*arrow*). **B:** CT of same patient as in A showing metallic artifact produced by presence of Greenfield filter (*arrow*).

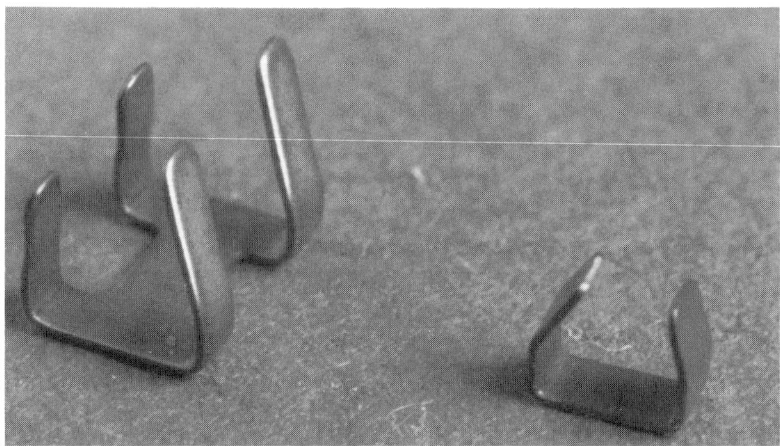

FIG. 10-8. Example of clips used for scleral buckling. These clips are made from nonferromagnetic materials and, are safe for patients undergoing MR procedures.

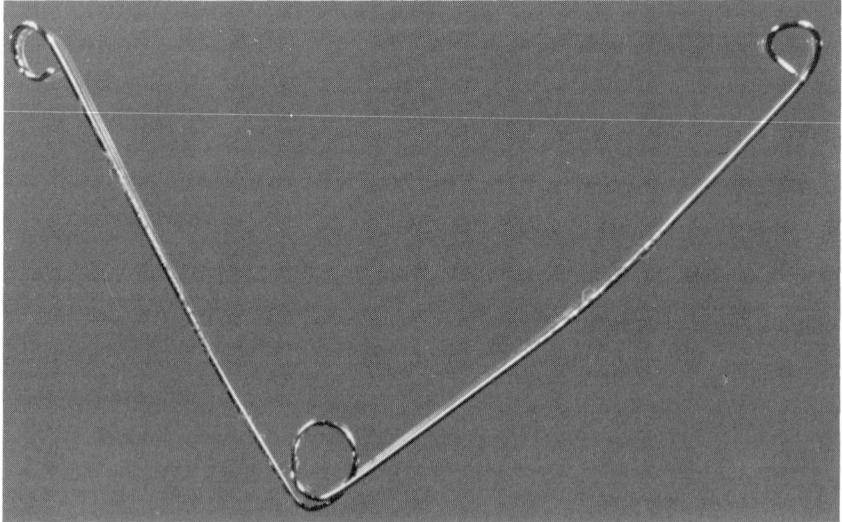

FIG. 10-9. Fatio eyelid wire. This implant may be composed of either gold or a ferromagnetic material.

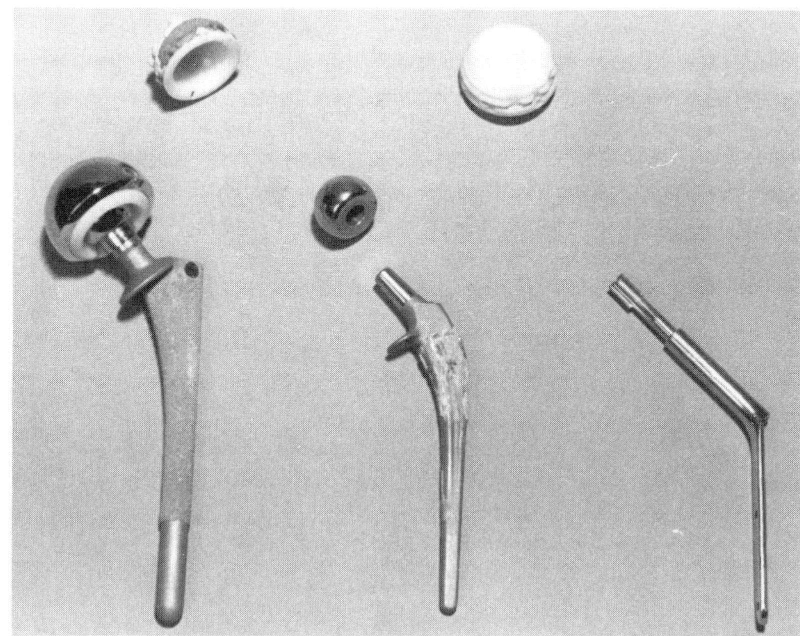

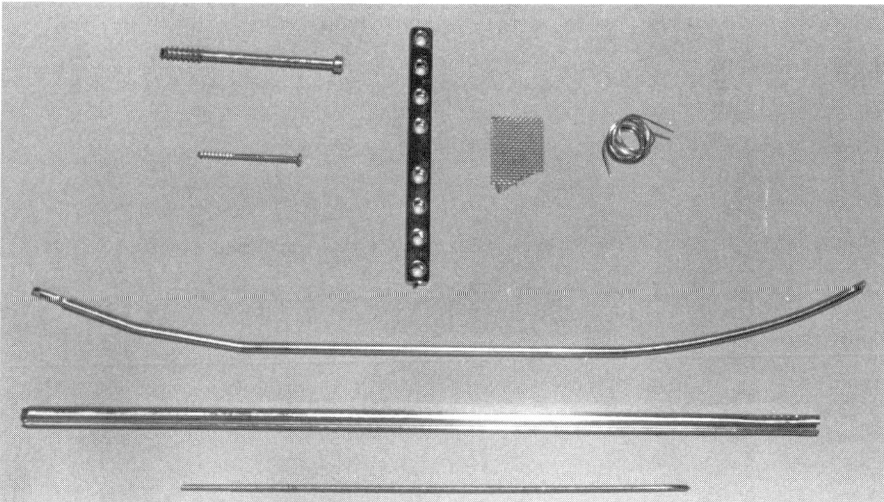

FIG. 10-10. Examples of various metallic orthopedic implants and materials tested for MR compatibility. All these implants are considered safe for patients undergoing MR procedures because they are composed of nonferromagnetic materials.

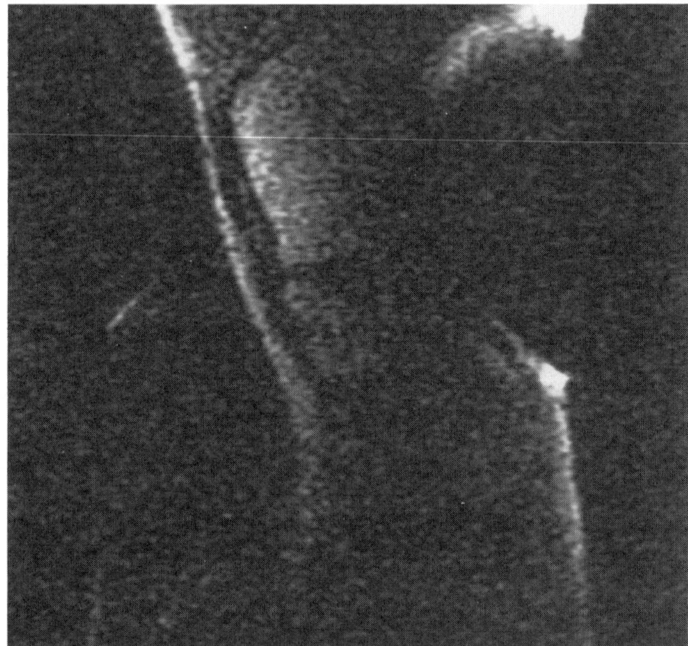

A

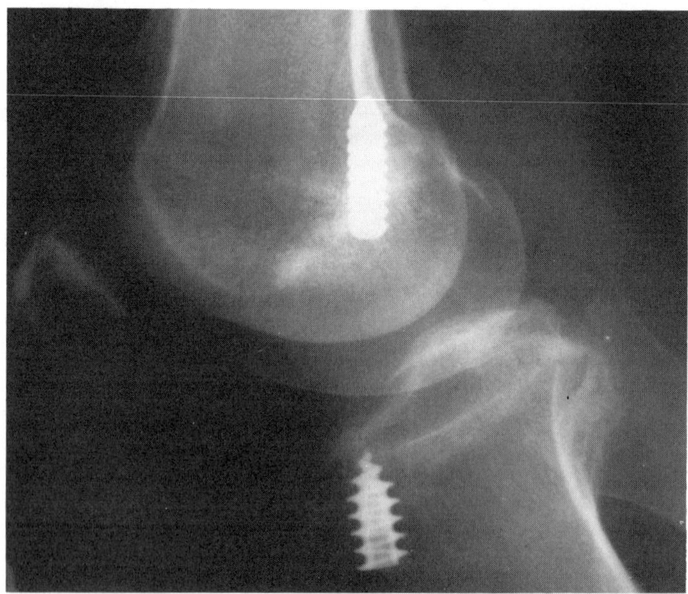

B

FIG. 10-11. A: T1-weighted, sagittal plane image of the knee obtained in a patient with two Perfix interference screws in place for reconstruction of the anterior cruciate ligament. Note the substantial artifact caused by the presence of these ferromagnetic implants. **B:** Plain film radiograph of the knee obtained in the patient as A showing the positions of the two Perfix interference screws.

cedures using MR systems with static magnetic fields of up to 1.5 T without incident.

OTOLOGIC IMPLANTS

A patient who has any of the three different cochlear implants listed in Appendix I should not be exposed to the magnetic fields of the MR system because these devices are ferromagnetic (2,3,62). Furthermore, they are activated by electronic and/or magnetic mechanisms (see also section on Magnetically Activated Implants and Devices for additional information) (2,3,62,104).

Of the remaining otologic implants that have been evaluated for the presence of ferromagnetism, only the McGee stapedectomy piston prosthesis, made from platinum and $Cr_{17}Ni_4$ stainless steel, is ferromagnetic (2,3,62). This type of otologic implant has been recalled by the manufacturer and patients who received these devices have been issued warnings to avoid MR procedures (3). The specific item and lot numbers of the McGee implants that were recalled and considered to be contraindicated for MR procedures are as follows (personal communication, Winston Geer, Smith & Nephew Richards Inc., Barlett, TN, 1995):

Item No.	*Lot No:*
14-0330	1W91100, 4UO9690
14-0331	4U09700
14-0332	1W91110, 4U58540, 4U86300
14-0333	4U09710, 1W91120
14-0334	4U09720, 1W34390, 2WR4073
14-0335	1W34400, 4U09730
14-0336	3U18350, 3U50470, 4UR2889
14-0337	3U18370, 4UR2889
14-0338	3UI8390, 4U02900, 4UR1453
14-0339	3U18400, 3U50480
14-0340	3U18410, 3U50500
14-0341	3U41200, 4UR2889

PATENT DUCTUS ARTERIOSUS, ATRIAL SEPTAL DEFECT, AND VENTRICULAR SEPTAL DEFECT OCCLUDERS

Metallic cardiac occluders are implants used to treat patients with patent ductus arteriosus (PDA), atrial septal defect (ASD), or ventricular septal defect (VSD) congenital heart conditions. As long as the proper size of occluder is used, the amount of retention provided by the folded-back, hinged arms of the device is sufficient to keep it in place, acutely. Eventually, tissue growth covers the cardiac occluder (86–88).

The metallic PDA, ASD, VSD occluders tested for ferromagnetism were made from either 304V stainless steel or MP35n. The occluders made from

304V stainless steel displayed relatively minor ferromagnetism whereas those made from MP35n were nonferromagnetic (86). Patients with cardiac occluders made from 304V stainless steel may undergo MR procedures approximately 6 weeks after placement of these devices, in order to allow tissue growth to provide additional retentive force, unless there is a concern about the retention of one of these implants. Patients with cardiac occluders made from MP35n may undergo MR procedures any time after placement of these implants (86).

PELLETS AND BULLETS

Most pellets and bullets tested for MR compatibility are composed of nonferromagnetic materials (69,70). Ammunition that proved to be ferromagnetic tended to be manufactured in foreign countries and/or used for military applications (69,70). Because pellets, bullets, and shrapnel may be contaminated with ferromagnetic materials, the risk versus benefit of performing an MR procedure in a patient should be carefully considered as well as whether or not the metallic object is located near a vital anatomic structure. Of note is that shrapnel typically contains steel and, therefore, presents a potential hazard for patients undergoing MR procedures (69,70). In one case, a small metallic foreign body located in a subcutaneous site caused painful symptoms in a patient exposed to the magnetic field of the MR system (55).

To reduce lead poisoning in "puddling"-type ducks, the federal government requires many of the eastern United States to use steel shotgun pellets instead of lead (70). The presence of steel shotgun pellets would present a potential hazard to patients undergoing MR procedures and cause severe imaging artifacts (70).

PENILE IMPLANTS

Two of the penile implants evaluated for ferromagnetic qualities had substantial deflection forces measured when exposed to a 1.5-T static magnetic field (44) (Fig. 10-12). Although it is unlikely that a penile implant would severely injure a patient undergoing an MR procedure because of the manner in which it is used, it would undoubtedly be uncomfortable. For this reason, subjecting a patient with one of these implants to an MR procedure is inadvisable.

VASCULAR ACCESS PORTS AND CATHETERS

Vascular access ports and catheters are bioimplants commonly used to provide long-term vascular administration of chemotherapeutic agents, antibiotics, and analgesics (105,106). These devices are implanted typically in a subcutaneous pocket over the upper chest wall with the catheters inserted either in

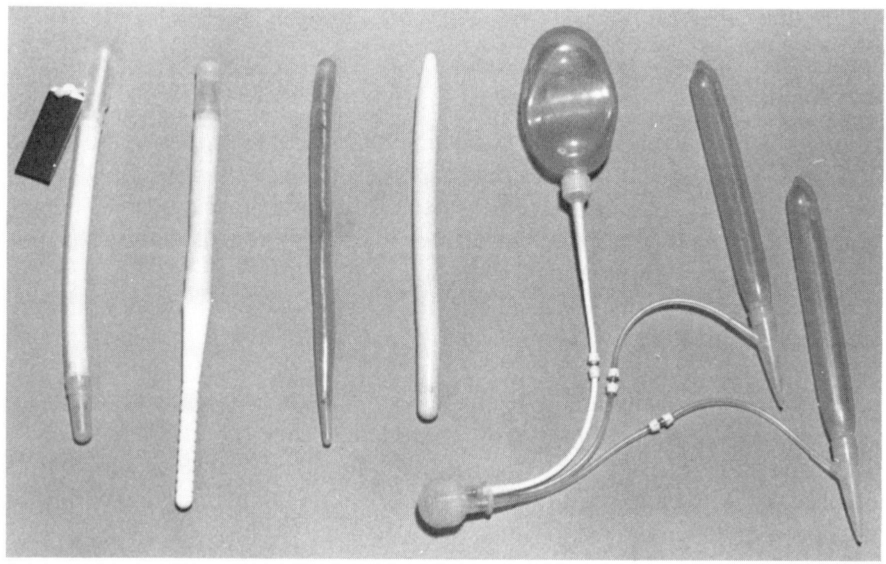

FIG. 10-12. Examples of penile implants tested for MR compatibility.

the jugular, subclavian, or cephalic vein. Smaller ports, which are less obtrusive and tend to be tolerated better, have also been designed for implantation in the arms of children or adults, with vascular access via an antecubital vein.

Vascular access ports have a variety of inherent features (e.g., a reservoir, central septum, and catheter) and are constructed from various types of materials including stainless steel, titanium, silicone, and various forms of plastic. Because of the widespread use of vascular access ports and associated catheters and the high probability that patients with these devices may require MR procedures, it was important to determine the MR compatibility of these implants.

Three of the implantable vascular access ports and catheters evaluated for compatibility with MR procedures showed measurable attraction to the static magnetic fields of the MR systems used for testing, but the forces were considered to be minor relative to the in vivo application of these implants (53,105,106). Therefore, MR procedures are safe to perform in a patient who may have one of the vascular access ports or catheters listed in Appendix I.

With respect to MR imaging and artifacts in general, the vascular access ports that will produce the least amount of artifact in association with MR imaging are made entirely from nonmetal materials whereas the ones that produce the greatest amount of artifact are composed of metal(s) or have metal that was in an unusual shape (e.g., the OmegaPort Access devices) (105). Various manufacturers of vascular access ports have decided to make devices entirely from nonmetallic materials under the assumption that this is required for the device to be "MRI compatible." In fact, several manufacturers have produced brochures that state that their devices allow "distortion-free imaging" or "will not obscure important structures" during MR imaging.

In one marketing brochure, an MR image is shown that is color enhanced so that the artifact caused by a "competitor's" metallic vascular access port appears to be inordinately large, whereas the manufacturer's plastic vascular access port caused essentially no distortion of the image (unpublished observation, F. Shellock, 1994). This misrepresents the actual MR imaging compatibility issue and promotes a marketing claim that is without support from a diagnostic MR imaging standpoint.

Of note is that even the so-called MRI compatible or MRI ports made entirely from nonmetal materials were, in fact, seen on the MR images in this study because they contain silicone (105). The septum portion of each of the vascular access ports is typically made from silicone. Using MR imaging, the Larmor precessional frequency of fat is close to that of silicone (i.e., 100 Hz at 1.5 T). Therefore, silicone used in the construction of vascular access ports may be observed on MR images with varying degrees of signal intensity depending on the pulse sequence selected for imaging (105,106).

Manufacturers of plastic vascular access ports have not addressed this finding during advertising and marketing of their products. On the contrary, vascular access ports made from nonmetallic materials are claimed to be MRI compatible and be invisible on MR images. However, if a radiologist did not know that a vascular access port was present in a patient, the MR signal produced by the silicone component of the device could be considered an abnormality, or at the very least, present a confusing image. For example, this may present a diagnostic problem in a patient being evaluated for a rupture of a silicone breast implant because silicone from the vascular access port may be misread as an extracapsular silicone implant rupture.

In more general terms, it is improbable that an artifact produced by the presence of any of the vascular access ports or catheters that have been tested will detract from the diagnostic capabilities of MR imaging because the extent of the artifact is relatively minor and, as such, is unlikely to obscure any important anatomical structures by their presence. Of note is that MR imaging examinations of the chest, where most vascular access ports are typically implanted in a subcutaneous pocket, account for less than 5% of diagnostic studies performed using this imaging modality.

Finally, an important issue related to the construction of vascular access ports should be discussed. Metal is used typically to make these devices to guard against piercing of the injection site by repetitive insertions of needles used to refill the reservoir. Additionally, repeated needle access of a plastic reservoir compared with a metal reservoir may perturb the functional integrity and long-term durability of the vascular access port, as suggested by recent evidence (unpublished findings, 1994). This could result in embolization by fragmented plastic pieces or a reduced ability to properly flush the vascular access port. Therefore, vascular access ports with reservoirs made from metallic or other similar hard material may be more acceptable for use in a patient compared with those made from plastic (105).

Future developments in vascular access port technology will produce devices that are activated and regulated electronically. The presence of this type of vascular access port would likely be contraindicated for a patient undergoing an MR procedure.

MISCELLANEOUS

Of the many different miscellaneous implants, materials, devices, and objects tested for ferromagnetic qualities, the cerebral ventricular shunt tube connector (type unknown) and Sophy adjustable pressure valve are the only devices that have substantial attraction to the static magnetic field of the MR system and, therefore, may present a hazard to a patient. Another metallic implant, the O-ring washer vascular marker, displayed only slight ferromagnetic qualities and, therefore, does not pose a risk to any patient examined by an MR system.

Contraceptive diaphragms were attracted strongly by the 1.5-T static magnetic field used for testing these devices (62) (Figs. 10-13 and 10-14). However, MR imaging has been performed in patients with these devices and they did not complain of any sensation related to movement of the diaphragms. Therefore,

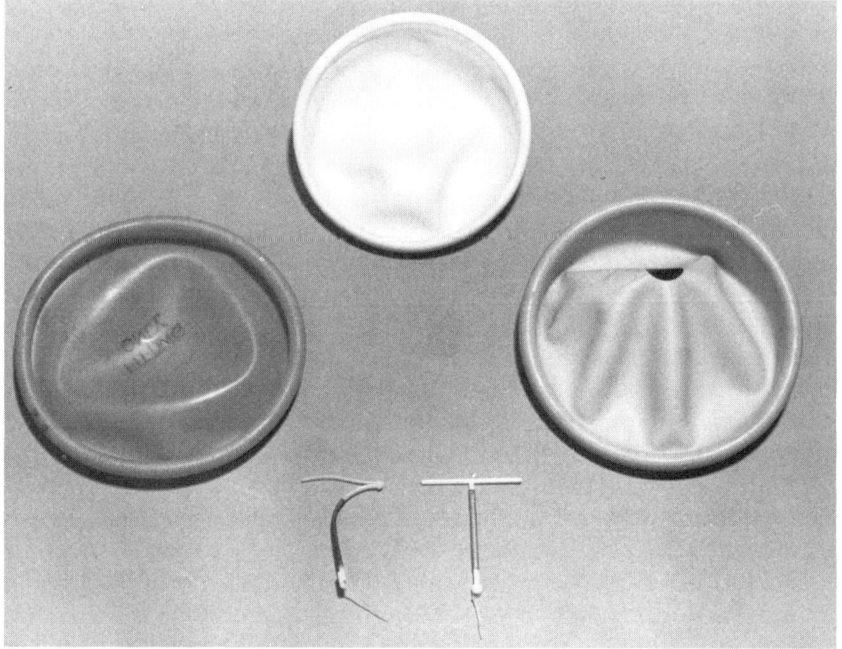

FIG. 10-13. Examples of IUDs and contraceptive diaphragms tested for MR compatibility.

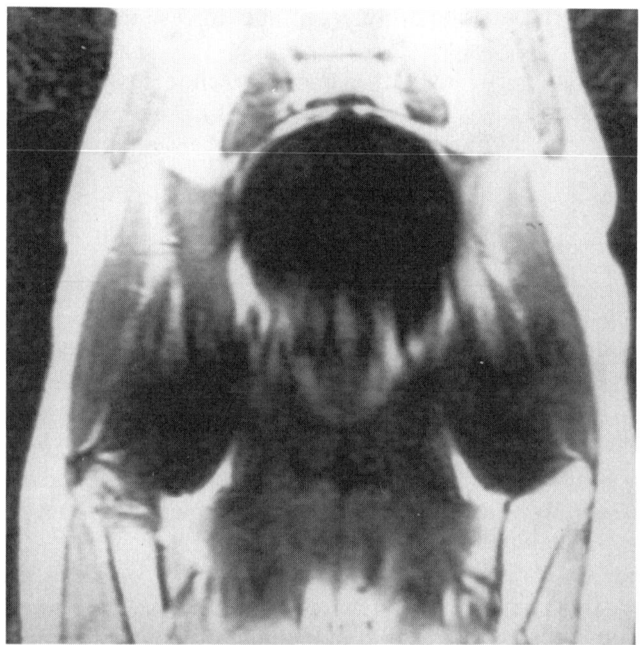

FIG. 10-14. T1-weighted, coronal plane image of the hips and pelvis obtained from a patient with a contraceptive diaphragm in place. Note the presence of the substantial artifact.

the presence of a diaphragm is not believed to be a contraindication for a patient undergoing an MR procedure. There is a remote possibility, however, that the contraceptive properties of the diaphragm may be hindered if it is inadvertently moved during an MR procedure (62).

The Deponit, nitroglycerin transdermal delivery system, contains aluminum, which is nonferromagnetic and, therefore, not attracted to the static magnetic field of an MR system. However, a patient wearing one of these patches received a second degree burn during MR imaging (R. E. Mucha, personal communication, 1995) Therefore, it is recommended that any patient using this or a similar transdermal delivery system with a metallic component should have the patch removed before an MR procedure and have a new patch applied after the examination is completed (R. E. Mucha, personal communication, 1995).

Although a triple-lumen, thermodilution Swan-Ganz catheter is constructed of nonferromagnetic materials, the presence of this device may be injurious to the patient during an MR procedure (13). A report indicated that a portion of a thermodilution Swan-Ganz catheter that was outside the patient melted during MR imaging (13). It was postulated that the high-frequency electromagnetic fields generated by the MR system caused eddy current–induced heating of either the wires within the thermodilution catheter or the radiopaque material used in the construction of the catheter (13). This incident suggests that patients with triple-lumen, thermodilution Swan-Ganz catheters or other similar devices could be potentially injured during an MR procedure.

Recently, there has been a need for specially designed devices and instruments for use during MR-guided therapy and surgical procedures. At least one manufacturer has used ceramic material as a means of constructing MR-compatible devices including scalpels, drill bits, scissors, and tweezers (Fig. 10-15).

MAGNETICALLY ACTIVATED IMPLANTS AND DEVICES

Various ferromagnetic implants and devices such as cochlear implants, certain breast tissue expanders and implants, ocular prostheses, and dental implants are activated by magnetic mechanisms (62) (see Chapter 11). Many of these may be hazardous to patients undergoing MR procedures (62). Besides moving or dislodging the magnetically activated implants and devices, exposure to the electromagnetic fields used for MR procedures may alter or damage the operation of the magnetic component (62,75), possibly requiring surgery for replacement.

Furthermore, if the portion of the prosthesis that the magnet attracts is implanted in soft tissue (e.g., with certain ocular prostheses, the magnet is contained in the prosthesis and a ferromagnetic "keeper" is implanted in the subcutaneous tissue), it is inadvisable to perform an MR procedure in a patient

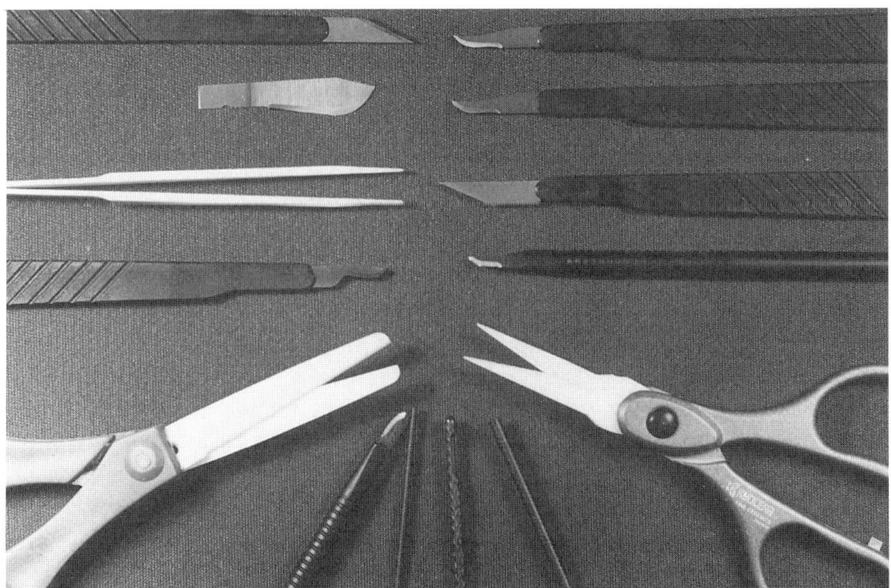

A

FIG. 10-15. A: Scissors, tweezers, scalpels, and drill bits made from MR-compatible ceramic material.

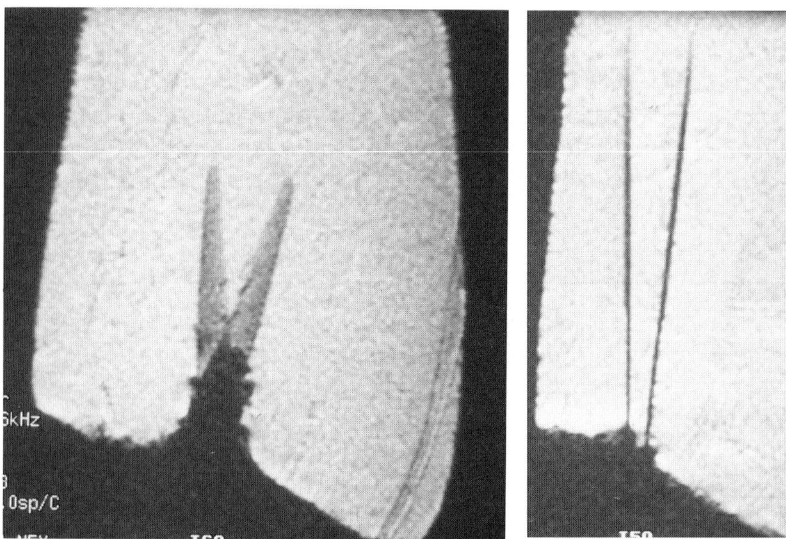

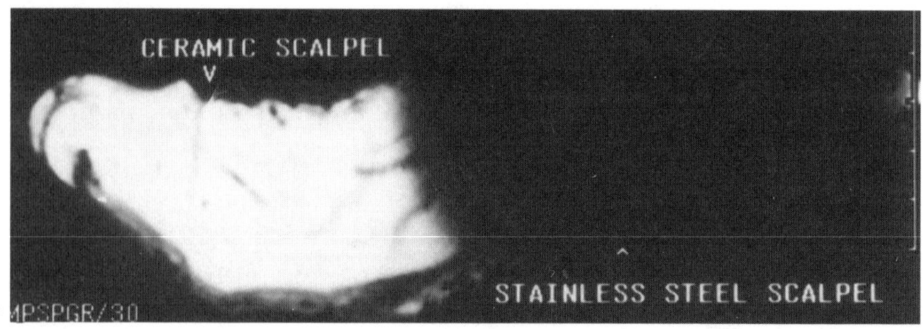

FIG. 10-15. B: MR image of ceramic scissors inserted into a beef phantom and scanned with a gradient echo pulse sequence (TR/TE 34/4.4 ms, flip angle 30°). Note that the imaging artifact is confined to the extent of the size of the ceramic scissors. **C:** MR image of ceramic tweezers inserted into a beef phantom and scanned with a gradient echo pulse sequence (TR/TE 34/4.4 ms, flip angle 30°). Note that the imaging artifact is confined to the extent of the size of the ceramic tweezers. **D:** MR image of ceramic scalpel and conventional stainless steel scalpel inserted into a beef phantom and scanned with a fast spoiled gradient echo pulse sequence (TR/TE 100/7.4 ms, flip angle 30°). Note that the imaging artifact is confined to the extent of the size of the ceramic scalpel, whereas the stainless steel scalpel produces extensive signal loss.

with this device because of potential adverse effects associated with displacement of the "keeper" (62,75). MR procedures may be performed safely in patients with dental magnet appliances that are properly attached to supporting structures after the magnet-containing portion of the device is removed.

CONCLUSIONS

In general, a patient with any electrically, magnetically, or mechanically activated implant, device, material, or object should be excluded from examination by MR techniques unless it has been demonstrated to be unaffected by the electromagnetic fields of the MR system. Certain electrically, magnetically, or mechanically activated implants or devices may be specially designed to be compatible with the MR environment. However, the federal government agencies responsible for the safe operation of MR systems must designate whether the implant or device is acceptable before subjecting a patient with such a device to an MR procedure. This information is typically indicated in the product insert for the object. In lieu of this, MR users may rely on the peer-reviewed literature to guide them with respect to the safety of performing MR procedures when a patient has an implant or device.

REFERENCES

1. Albert DW, Olson KR, Parel JM, et al. Magnetic resonance imaging and retinal tacks. *Arch Ophthalamol* 1990;108:320–321.
2. Applebaum EL, Valvassori GE. Effects of magnetic resonance imaging fields on stapedectomy prostheses. *Arch Orolaryngol* 1985;11:820–821.
3. Applebaum EL, Valvassori GE. Further studies on the effects of magnetic resonance fields on middle ear implants. *Ann Otol Rhinol Laryngol* 1990;99:801–804.
4. Ballock RT, Hajed PC, Byrne TP, et al. The quality of magnetic resonance imaging, as affected by the composition of the halo orthosis. *J Bone Joint Surg* 1989;71-A:431–434.
5. Barrafato D, Henkelman RM. Magnetic resonance imaging and surgical clips. *Can J Surg* 1984;27:509–512.
6. Becker RL, Norfray JF, Teitelbaum GP, et al. MR imaging in patients with intracranial aneurysm clips. *AJR Am J Roentgenol* 1988;9:885–889.
7. Brown MA, Carden JA, Coleman RE, et al. Magnetic field effects on surgical ligation clips. *Magn Reson Imag* 1987;5:443–453.
8. Clayman DA, Murakami ME, Vines FS. Compatibility of cervical spine braces with MR imaging: a study of nine nonferrous devices. *AJNR Am J Neuroradiol* 1990;11:385–390.
9. Davis PL, Crooks L, Arakawa M, et al. Potential hazards in NMR imaging: heating effects of changing magnetic fields and RF fields on small metallic implants. *AJR Am J Roentgenol* 1981;137:857–860.
10. de Keizer RJ, Te Strake L. Intraocular lens implants (pseudophakoi) and steelwire sutures: a contraindication for MRI? *Doc Opthalmol* 1984;61:281–284.
11. Dujovny M, Kossovsky N, Kossowsky R, et al. Aneurysm clip motion during magnetic resonance imaging: in vivo experimental study with metallurgical factor analysis. *Neurosurgery* 1985;17:543–548.
12. Dupuy DE, Hartnell GC, Lipsky M. MR imaging of a patient with a ferromagnetic foreign body. *AJR Am J Roentgenol* 1993;160:893.
13. ECRI, Health devices alert. A new MRI complication? May 27, 1988.
14. Gegauff A, Laurell KA, Thavendrarajah A, et al. A potential MRI hazard: forces on dental magnet keepers. *J Oral Rehabil* 1990;17:403–410.
15. Go KG, Kamman RL, Mooyaart EL. Interaction of metallic neurosurgical implants with magnetic resonance imaging at 1.5 Tesla as a cause of image distortion and of hazardous movement of the implant. *Clin Neurosurg* 1989;91:109–115.
16. Gold JP, Pulsinelli W, Winchester P, et al. Safety of metallic surgical clips in patients undergoing high-field-strength magnetic resonance imaging. *Ann Thorac Surg* 1989;48:643–645.
17. Hassler M, Le Bas JF, Wolf JE, et al. Effects of magnetic fields used in MRI on 15 prosthetic heart valves. *J Radiol* 1986;67:661–666.
18. Hathout G, Lufkin RB, Jabour B, et al. MR-guided aspiration cytology in the head and neck at high-field strength. *J Magn Reson Imag* 1992;2:93–94.
19. Joondeph BC, Peyman GA, Mafee MF, et al. Magnetic resonance imaging and retinal tacks. *Arch Ophthalmol* 1987;105:1479–1480.

20. Kagetsu NJ, Litt AW. Important considerations in measurement of attractive force on metallic implants in MR imagers. *Radiology* 1991;179:505–508.
21. Kanal E, Shellock FG, Talagala L. Safety considerations in MR imaging. *Radiology* 1990;176: 593–606.
22. Kanal E, Shellock FG. MR imaging of patients with intracranial aneurysm clips. *Radiology* 1993;187:612–614.
23. Kelly WM, Paglan PF, Pearson JA, et al. Ferromagnetism of intraocular foreign body causes unilateral blindness after MR study. *AJNR Am J Neuroradiol* 1986;7:243–245.
24. Kuethe DO, Small KW, Blinder RA. Nonferromagnetic retinal tacks are a tolerable risk in magnetic resonance imaging. *Invest Radiol* 1991;26:1–7.
25. Laakman RW, Kaufman B, Hans JS, et al. MR imaging in patients with metallic implants. *AJR Am J Roentgenol* 1985;8:837–840.
26. Leibman CE, Messersmith RN, Levin DN, et al. MR imaging of inferior vena caval filter: safety and artifacts. *AJR Am J Roentgenol* 1988;150:1174–1176.
27. Lemmens JAM, van Horn R, den Boer, et al. MR imaging of 22 Charnley-Muller total hip prostheses. *Fortschr Rontgenstr* 1986;33:311–315.
28. Leon JA, Gabriele OF. Middle ear prothesis: significance in magnetic resonance imaging. *Magn Reson Imag* 1987;5:405–406.
29. Liang MD, Narayanan K, Kanal E. Magnetic ports in tissue expanders: a caution for MRI. *Magn Reson Imag* 1989;7:541–542.
30. Lissac MI, Metrop D, Brugigrad, et al. Dental materials and magnetic resonance imaging. *Invest Radiol* 1991;26:40–45.
31. Lufkin R, Jordan S, Lylyck P, et al. MR imaging with topographic EEG electrodes in place. *AJNR Am J Neuroradiol* 1988;9:953–954.
32. Lyons CJ, Betz RR, Mesgarzadeh M, et al. The effect of magnetic resonance imaging on metal spine implants. *Spine* 1989;14:670–672.
33. Mark AS, Hricak H. Intrauterine contraceptive devices: MR imaging. *Radiology* 1987;162: 311–314.
34. Marshall MW, Teitelbaum GP, Kim HS, et al. Ferromagnetism and magnetic resonance artifacts of platinum embolization microcoils. *Cardiovasc Intervent Radiol* 1991;14:163–166.
35. Matsumoto AH, Teitelbaum GP, Barth KH, et al. Tantalum vascular stents: in vivo evaluation with MR imaging. *Radiology* 1989;170:753–755.
36. Mattucci KF, Setzen M, Hyman R, et al. The effect of nuclear magnetic resonance imaging on metallic middle ear protheses. *Otolaryngnol Head Neck Surg* 1986;94:441–443.
37. Mechlin M, Thickman D, Kressel HY, et al. Magnetic resonance imaging of postoperative patients with metallic implants. *AJR Am J Roentgenol* 1984;143:1281–1284.
38. Mesgarzadeh M, Revesz G, Bonakdarpour A, et al. The effect on medical metal implants by magnetic fields of magnetic resonance imaging. *Skeletal Radiol* 1985;14:205–206.
39. New PFJ, Rosen BR, Brady TJ, et al. Potential hazards and artifacts of ferromagnetic and nonferromagnetic surgical and dental materials and devices in nuclear magnetic resonance imaging. *Radiology* 1983;147:139–148.
40. Power W, Collum LMT. Magnetic resonance imaging and magnetic eye implants. *Lancet* 1988;2:227.
41. Randall PA, Kohman LJ, Scalzetti EM, et al. Magnetic resonance imaging of prosthestic cardiac valves in vitro and in vivo. *Am J Cardiol* 1988;62:973–976.
42. Roberts CW, Haik BG, Cahill P. Magnetic resonance imaging of metal loop intraocular lenses. *Arch Opthalmol* 1990:108:320–321.
43. Seiff SR, Vestel KP, Truwit CL. Eyelid palpebral springs in patients undergoing magnetic resonance imaging: an area of possible concern. *Arch Opthalmol* 1991;109:319.
44. Shellock FG, Crues JV, Sacks SA. High-field magnetic resonance imaging of penile protheses: in vitro evaluation of deflection forces and imaging artifacts. In: *Book of Abstracts, Society of Magnetic Resonance in Medicine.* Berkeley, CA: Society of Magnetic Resonance in Medicine; 1987:915.
45. Shellock FG, Crues JV. High-field-strength MR imaging and metallic bioimplants: an in vitro evaluation of deflection forces and temperature changes induced in large prostheses. *Radiology* 1987;165(P):150.
46. Shellock FG, Crues JV. High-field strength MR imaging and metallic biomedical implants: an ex vivo evaluation of deflection forces. *AJR Am J Roentgenol* 1988;151:389–392.
47. Shellock FG. MR imaging of metallic implants and materials: a compilation of the literature. *AJR Am J Roentgenol* 1988;151:811–814.

48. Shellock FG, Crues JV. MRI: safety considerations in magnetic resonance imaging. *MRI Decisions* 1988;2:25–30.
49. Shellock FG. Biological effects and safety aspects of magnetic resonance imaging. *Magn Reson Q* 1989;5:243–261.
50. Shellock FG. Ex vivo assessment of deflection forces and artifacts associated with high-field strength MRI of "mini-magnet" dental prostheses. *Magn Reson Imag* 1989;7(suppl 1):P38.
51. Shellock FG, Slimp G. Halo vest for cervical spine fixation during MR imaging. *AJR Am J Roentgenol* 1990;154:631–632.
52. Shellock FG, Schatz CJ, Shelton C, et al. Ex vivo evaluation of 9 different ocular and middle ear implants exposed to a 1.5 Tesla MR scanner. *Radiology* 1990;177(P):271.
53. Shellock FG, Meeks T. Ex vivo evaluation of ferromagnetism and artifacts for implantable vascular access ports exposed to a 1.5 T MR scanner. *J Magn Reson Imag* 1991;1:243.
54. Shellock FG, Schatz CJ. High-field strength MR imaging and metallic otologic implants. *AJNR Am J Neuroradiol* 1991;12:279–281.
55. Shellock FG, Kanal E, SMRI Safety Committee. Policies, guidelines, and recommendations for MR imaging safety and patient management. *J Magn Reson Imag* 1991;1:97–101.
56. Shellock FG, Swengros-Curtis J. MR imaging and biomedical implants, materials, and devices: an updated review. *Radiology* 1991;180:541–550.
57. Shellock FG. Safety Considerations in MR Imaging of Biomedical Implants and Devices. In: Thrall J, ed. *Current practice in radiology*. Philadelphia: BC Decker/Mosby–Year Book; 1992.
58. Shellock FG, Litwer C, Kanal E. MRI bioeffects, safety, and patient management: a review. *Rev Magn Reson Imag* 1992;4:21–63.
59. Shellock FG, Crues JV. Safety aspects of MRI in patients with metallic implants or foreign bodies: absolute and relative contraindications. *Appl Radiol* 1992;Nov:44–47.
60. Shellock FG, Mink JH, Curtin S, et al. MRI and orthopedic implants used for anterior cruciate ligament reconstruction: assessment of ferromagnetism and artifacts. *J Magn Reson Imag* 1992;2:225–228.
61. Shellock FG, Myers SM, Schatz CJ. Ex vivo evaluation of ferromagnetism determined for metallic scleral "buckles" exposed to a 1.5 T MR scanner. *Radiology* 1992;185(P):288–289.
62. Shellock FG, Morisoli S, Kanal E. MR procedures and biomedical implants, materials, and devices: 1993 update. *Radiology* 1993;189:587–599.
63. Soulen RL, Budinger TF, Higgins CB. Magnetic resonance imaging of prosthetic heart valves. *Radiology* 1985;154:705–707.
64. Soulen RL. Magnetic resonance imaging of prosthetic heart valves. *Radiology* 1986;158:279.
65. Teitelbaum GP, Bradley WG, Klein BD. MR imaging artifacts, ferromagnetism, and magnetic torque of intravascular filters, stents, and coils. *Radiology* 1988;166:657–664.
66. Teitelbaum GP, Ortega HV, Vinitski S, et al. Low artifact intravascular devices: MR imaging evaluation. *Radiology* 1988;168:713–719.
67. Teitelbaum GP, Raney M, Carvlin MJ, et al. Evaluation of ferromagnetism and magnetic resonance imaging artifacts of the Strecker tantalum vascular stent. *Cardiovasc Intervent Radiol* 1989;12:125–127.
68. Teitelbaum GP, Lin MCW, Watanabe AT, et al. Ferromagnetism and MR imaging: safety of cartoid vascular clamps. *AJNR Am J Neuroradiol* 1990;11:267–272.
69. Teitelbaum GP, Yee CA, Van Horn DD, et al. Metallic ballistic fragments: MR imaging safety and artifacts. *Radiology* 1990;175:855–859.
70. Teitelbaum GP. Metallic ballistic fragments: MR imaging safety and artifacts. *Radiology* 1990;177:883.
71. To SYC, Lufkin RB, Chiu L. MR-compatible winged infusion set. *Comput Med Imag Graphics* 1989;13:469–472.
72. Watanabe AT, Teitelbaum GP, Gomes AS, et al. MR imaging of the bird's nest filter. *Radiology* 1990;177:578–579.
73. White DW. Interation between magnetic fields and metallic ossicular prostheses. *Am J Otolaryngol* 1987;8:290–292.
74. Williamson MR, McCowan TC, Walker CW, et al. Effect of a 1.5 Tesla magnetic field on Greenfield filters in vitro and in dogs. *Angiology* 1988;12:1022–1024.
75. Yuh WTC, Hanigan MT, Nerad JA, et al. Extrusion of an eye socket magnetic implant after MR imaging examination: potential hazard to a patient with eye prosthesis. *J Magn Reson Imag* 1991;1:711–713.
76. Zheutlin JD, Thompson JT, Shofner RS. The safety of magnetic resonance imaging with

intraorbital metallic objects after retinal reattachment or trauma [Letter]. *Am J Ophthalmol* 1987;103:831.
77. FDA stresses the need for caution during MR scanning of patients with aneurysm clips. In: *Medical devices bulletin,* Center for Devices and Radiological Health, March, 1993;11:1–2.
78. Klucznik RP, Carrier DA, Pyka R, Haid RW. Placement of a ferromagnetic intracerebral aneurysm clip in a magnetic field with a fatal outcome. *Radiology* 1993;187:855–856.
79. Lufkin R, Layfield L. Coaxial needle system of MR- and CT-guided aspiration cytology. *J Comput Assist Tomogr* 1989;13:1105–1107.
80. Lufkin R, Teresi L, Hanafee W. New needle for MR-guided aspiration cytology of the head and neck. *AJR Am J Roentgenol* 1987;149:380–382.
81. Bellon EM, Haacke EM, Coleman PE, et al. MR artifacts: a review. *Magn Reson Imag* 1984;2: 41–52.
82. Pusey E, Lufkin RB, Brown RKJ, et al. Magnetic resonance imaging artifacts: mechanism and clinical significance. *RadioGraphics* 1986;6:891–911.
83. Kanal E, Shellock FG. The value of published data regarding MR compatibility of metallic implants and devices. *AJNR Am J Neuroradiol* 1994;15:1394–1396.
84. Food and Drug Administration. Magnetic resonance diagnostic device: panel recommendation and report on petitions for MR reclassification. *Fed Reg* 1988;53:7575–7579.
85. Johnson GC. Need for caution during MR imaging of patients with aneurysm clips. *Radiology* 1993;188:287.
86. Shellock FG, Morisoli SM. Ex vivo evaluation of ferromagnetism and artifacts for cardiac occluders exposed to a 1.5 Tesla MR system. *J Magn Reson Imag* 1994;4:213–215.
87. Dupuy DE, Hartnell GC, Lipsky M. MR imaging of a patient with a ferromagnetic foreign body. *AJR Am J Roentgenol* 1993;160:893.
88. Mani RL. In search of an effective screening system for intraocular metallic foreign bodies prior to MR—an important issue of patient safety. *AJNR Am J Neuroradiol* 1988;9:1032.
89. Williams S, Char DH, Dillon WP, Lincoff N, Moseley M. Ferrous intraocular foreign bodies and magnetic resonance imaging. *Am J Opthalolmol* 1988;105:398–401.
90. Jackson JG, Acker JD. Permanent eyeliner and MR imaging. *AJR Am J Roentgenol* 1987;49: 1080.
91. Lund G, Nelson JD, Wirtschafter JD, Williams PA. Tatooing of eyelids: Magnetic resonance imaging artifacts. *Opthalmic Surg* 1986;17:550–553.
92. Sacco, Steiger DA, Bellon EM, Coleman PE, Haacke EM. Artifacts caused by cosmetics in MR imaging of the head. *AJR Am J Roentgenol* 1987;148:1001–1004.
93. Erlebacher JA, Cahill PT, Pannizzo F, et al. Effect of magnetic resonance imaging on DDD pacemakers. *Am J Cardiol* 1986;57:437–440.
94. Fetter J, Aram G, Holmes DR, et al. The effects of nuclear magnetic resonance imagers on external and implantable pulse generators. *PACE* 1984;7:720–727.
95. Shellock FG, Morisoli SM. Ex vivo evaluation of ferromagnetism, heating, and artifacts for heart valve prostheses exposed to a 1.5 Tesla MR system. *J Magn Reson Imag* 1994;4:756–758.
96. Bakshandeh H, Shellock FG, Schatz CJ, Morisoli SM. Metallic clips used for scleral buckling: ex vivo evaluation of ferromagnetism determined at 1.5 T. *J Magn Reson Imag* 1993;3:559.
97. Hayes DL, Holmes DR, Gray JE. Effect of a 1.5 Tesla magnetic resonance imaging scanner on implanted permanent pacemakers. *J Am Coll Cardiol* 1987;10:782–786.
98. Holmes DR, Hayes DL, Gray JE, et al. The effects of magnetic resonance imaging on implantable pulse generators. *PACE* 1986;9:360–370.
99. Shellock FG, Kanal E. Burns associated with the use of monitoring equipment during MR procedures. *J Magn Reson Imag* 1996;4:271–272.
100. Moscatel M, Shellock FG, Morisoli S. Biopsy needles and devices: assessment of ferromagnetism and artifacts during exposure to a 1.5 Tesla MR system. *J Magn Reson Imag* 1995;5: 369–372.
101. Shellock FG, Shellock VJ. Additional information pertaining to the MR-compatibility of biopsy needles and devices. *J Magn Reson Imag* 1996;6:441.
102. Fagan LL, Shellock FG, Brenner RJ, Rothman B. Ex vivo evaluation of ferromagnetism, heating, and artifacts of breast tissue expanders exposed to a 1.5 T MR system. *J Magn Reson Imag* 1995;5:614–616.

103. Shellock FG. MR imaging and cervical fixation devices: assessment of ferromagnetism, heating, and artifacts. *Magn Reson Imag* 1996 (in press).
104. Nogueira M, Shellock FG. Otologic bioimplants: Ex vivo assessment of ferromagnetism and artifacts at 1.5 Tesla. *AJR Am J Roentgenol* 1995;63:1472–1473.
105. Shellock FG, Nogueira M, Morisoli M. MRI and vascular access ports: ex vivo evaluation of ferromagnetism, heating, and artifacts at 1.5 T. *J Magn Reson Imag* 1995;4:481–484.
106. Shellock FG, Shellock VJ. Vascular access ports and catheters tested for ferromagnetism, heating, and artifacts associated with MR imaging. *Magn Reson Imag* 1996 (in press).

11

Magnetic Resonance Procedures and Patients with Electrically, Magnetically, and Mechanically Activated Implants and Devices

The FDA requires labeling of MR systems to indicate that a patient with any electrically, magnetically, or mechanically activated implant or device should not undergo an MR procedure because the electromagnetic fields used by the MR system may interfere with the operation of the implant or device and there is a possibility that the patient could be injured (1–6). Examples of electrically, magnetically, and mechanically activated implants and devices include cardiac pacemakers, implantable cardiac defibrillators, external hearing aids, magnetic dental implants, cochlear implants, neurostimulators, bone-growth stimulators, and implantable electronic drug infusion pumps. In addition, there are several experimental implants and devices currently undergoing clinical trials that incorporate electrically, magnetically, or mechanically activated mechanisms (also see Chapter 10). This chapter discusses the safety aspects of performing MR procedures in patients with the preceding implants and devices.

CARDIAC PACEMAKERS, IMPLANTABLE CARDIAC DEFIBRILLATORS, AND EXTERNAL HEARING AIDS

Cardiac Pacemakers

Cardiac pacemakers are the most common electrically activated implants found in patients who may be referred for MR procedures. In fact, approximately 80,000 cardiac pacemakers are implanted yearly in patients in the United States alone. Unfortunately, the presence of a cardiac pacemaker is considered to be a strict contraindication for patients referred for MR procedures (1). The effects of MR systems on the function of a cardiac pacemaker are variable and depend on several factors, including the type of cardiac pacemaker, the static magnetic field strength of the MR system, and the specific type of imaging conditions being used (i.e., the anatomic region imaged, the type of surface coil used, the pulse sequence, etc.) (2–12).

A commonly asked question is whether or not MR procedures may be safely performed under any conditions on patients with implanted cardiac pacemakers. Pacemakers present potential problems to patients undergoing MR procedures from several mechanisms (2–12):

1. motion of the pacemaker in strong static magnetic fields;
2. modification of the function of the pacemaker, temporarily and/or permanently, by the static magnetic field of the MR system;
3. heating induced in/of the pacemaker leads because of the time-varying RF magnetic fields of the imaging system during the MR imaging process; and
4. voltages and currents induced in the pacemaker leads and/or myocardium during the MR procedure process by the time-varying RF and possibly the gradient magnetic fields.

Recent work has been performed in this area (R. Gimble, personal communication, 1996). A survey has revealed that there have been numerous patients (at least two dozen) who have been placed in MR systems (either intentionally or inadvertently). There appears to be documentation that at least six of these patients have died. (It should be stressed that, in the opinion of the investigator, the cause of death is unknown.)

Much has been written, especially in the radiologic literature, about the static field of the MR system closing the reed switches of many pacemakers. Indeed, these switches close in static fields as low as 15 gauss, with the newest pacemakers having reed switch activation occur in static magnetic fields as low as 5 to 7 gauss. Nevertheless, all that reed switch closure accomplishes is placing the pacemaker into asynchronous mode. A predetermined fixed pacing rate takes over during the time period that the reed switch is activated. However, this does not explain why patients would experience cardiac distress or death in MR systems. In fact, thousands of patients are placed into asynchronous mode each day in outpatient visits to cardiologists' offices as their pacemakers are interrogated as part of their routine pacemaker maintenance program. Thus, it would appear that this often quoted reed switch activation by the static magnetic field of the MR system may not be the causative factor for adverse patient outcomes in the MR environment.

However, there is an interesting potential complication in this discussion. At least one study demonstrated that one pacemaker (Cordis 415A) appeared to have a malfunction of the reed switch after the cessation of RF pulsing during the MR procedure, such that the device neither switched into asynchronous mode nor generated its programmed pulses (6). Thus, the device appeared to have been entirely inhibited by exposure to MR imaging.

Another study was performed on pacemakers from Pacesetter (Model 283),

Intermedics (Model 283-01), and Medtronics (Model 7000A) (3). This study reported no apparent electrocardiographically detectable output from these pacemakers when studied in a 0.5-T MR scanner (using 10 kW RF pulses at a 20.91 MHz carrier frequency). The apparent total pacemaker inhibition in one study and pacemaker malfunction in the other have serious safety implications for studying pacemaker-dependent patients using MR procedures.

There have been several studies in which laboratory dogs as well as human subjects have been tachyarrhythmic and/or hypotensive during MR imaging. It is possible that the cause may be the induction of voltages or currents within the pacemaker-lead-myocardial loop that is sufficient to induce action potentials or contraction of the myocardium and an electrical, as well as physiologic, systole. In fact, some cardiologists have reported that they observed cardiac pacing at the selected repetition time (TR). The accuracy of this statement is unclear in light of multislice and/or multiecho and/or spin echo MR imaging protocols, etc. (e.g., RF cycling rates in spin echo imaging sequences are greater than that determined by the selected TR even in single slice acquisitions). Nevertheless, such rapid pacing at rates that yield cardiac outputs that are not compatible with sustaining life seems to be responsible for the death in some of the pacemaker patients who underwent MR procedures.

Interestingly, with the RF field turned on and the gradients turned off, rapid pacing was still observed. However, with the RF fields inactivated and the gradients left on, this rapid pacing was no longer observed in this experiment (6).

Heating of the pacemaker/pacing leads during MR imaging is also potentially problematic, and thermal injury to the endocardium or myocardium must be considered a potential adverse outcome if RF power is transmitted near the pacemaker and/or its leads.

In consideration of all of the above, it is fair to conclude that, without an integrated and coordinated approach together with Cardiology and knowledgeable personnel from Radiology (and perhaps Institutional Review Board and/or Human Rights Committee), involvement and informed consent from the patient, which includes possible arrhythmias, pacemaker malfunction, and death, and without exceptionally strong indications that there is clinical need for performance of the MR procedure, it should still be considered contraindicated to permit any patient with a cardiac pacemaker to enter the MR environment.

However, it is possible that this will change as more knowledge is acquired about this issue and as more information becomes available defining which patients may be safely imaged with MR systems and under what specific conditions. Various theories do suggest that it may be possible to perform MR procedures safely in certain patients (such as patients who are not pacemaker dependent) with certain pacemakers, for studies in which the body RF coil is not used for RF excitation, where continuous physiologic monitoring is being performed throughout the examination, etc.

How should the above response to the pacemaker question be modified if cardiac pacemaker leads are present but the pulse generator itself has been removed from the body? There are several potential concerns regarding pacemaker wires, just as there are for pacemakers themselves. These include ferromagnetic interactions, wire or lead heating as a result of interactions between the transmitted radiofrequency oscillating magnetic field (RF) pulses and the implanted leads, and induced arrhythmias. However, we are unaware of pacemaker leads that have demonstrated significant ferromagnetic properties. As such, it is unlikely that wire or lead motion in the static field of the MR system is a significant safety concern.

Heating of the wire or lead of the pacemaker is at least a theoretical concern for any wire in the bore, especially an MR system operating with a high static magnetic field (e.g., 1.5 T). Cardiac pacemaker leads, however, are typically intravascular for most of their length. Heat transfer and dissipation from the leads into the blood may likely prevent dangerous levels of lead heating to be reached or maintained for the intravascular segments of pacemaker leads. For the extravascular segments of these leads, however, it is at least theoretically possible that sufficient power deposition or heating may be induced within these leads to result in local tissue injury or burn.

The amount of power deposited into these leads depends on many factors, including the transmitted RF power and the distance of the leads from the RF transmitter. In the case where the transmitting coil is, for example, a transmit-receive extremity coil around the ankle, the expected power deposition into a normally positioned pacemaker lead would approach zero. It is anticipated that a body coil would be used to transmit the RF pulses for other types of studies, where there may well be significant power deposition in the anatomic distribution of the pacemaker's leads. Thus, the possibility for tissue injury or burn cannot be dismissed in the case presented in the question.

Of note is that there has been a report of a Swan-Ganz thermodilution catheter that melted in a patient during an MR imaging procedure (13). This was believed to occur because of electromagnetic fields produced by the MR system that generated eddy current inductive heating of the nonferromagnetic, electrically conductive material contained within the catheter (13). Because of this obvious deleterious and unpredictable effect, patients referred for MR procedures with residual external pacing wires, temporary pacing wires, Swan-Ganz thermodilution catheters, and/or any other type of internally or externally positioned conductive wire or similar device should not undergo MR procedures because of the possible associated risks (4,7,10,11).

Finally, as noted above, there is a possibility of inducing cardiac arrhythmias, presumably as a result of induced voltages/currents in the leads themselves. A study was performed with laboratory dogs in which arrhythmias were induced in the test animals when they were exposed to trains of RF pulses in the presence of cardiac pacemakers and intact pacemaker leads (3). When the RF pulses were turned off and the gradient fields were turned on (superimposed on the static magnetic field), no such arrhythmias were induced or noted, and there was no effect observed on pacing (3). This suggests that it is the RF time-varying magnetic field and not the gradient magnetic field (at least of the magnitude used in that study) that is active in inducing the abnormal pacing observed.

Another study demonstrated that, during RF stimulation, rapid cardiac pacing was seen in the presence of a Cordis 415A pacemaker while both leads were connected (6). Yet, when the ventricular lead was disconnected, rapid ventricular pacing was no longer observed (6). This suggests that rapid pacing required an intact ventricular lead. In other words, it might well be that, with isolated pacemaker leads and without an intact pacemaker, it may be more difficult to induce arrhythmias. Nevertheless, arrhythmias may be induced even without the pacemaker in the circuit. It may simply be that it is more difficult to do so (e.g., may require higher induced voltages or currents).

Most of these prior studies were performed with older MR systems (i.e., virtually a decade ago) using weaker RF transmitter and gradient subsystems. Therefore, there may be reason to hesitate regarding the substantially stronger RF transmitters and gradient magnetic fields more commonly used in many present-day MR systems. This is especially so for the echo planar imaging MR systems that have gradient fields that may be 5 to 10 times more powerful than the ones available 10 years ago. Perhaps at these gradient magnetic field levels the issue of induced arrhythmias secondary to changing gradient magnetic fields needs to be re-examined.

Therefore, although there do not appear to be any studies to date that demonstrate arrhythmias specifically in the presence of pacemaker leads alone (i.e., without an attached cardiac pacemaker), it is prudent to prevent a patient to undergo an MR procedure if the patient has retained intracardiac pacemaker leads alone (i.e., no pacemaker) and if the examination requires exposure to the RF fields in the region of the retained pacemaker leads. Perhaps one might consider relaxing this hesitation regarding permitting an MR examination if the bulk of the transmitted RF power is not in the anatomic vicinity of the retained pacemaker leads (e.g., a knee study with a transmit/receive knee coil).

A Letter to the Editor indicated that a patient who was not pacemaker-dependent was examined by MR imaging after having his cardiac pacemaker "disabled" during the procedure (14). Although this patient did not experience any apparent discomfort and the cardiac pacemaker was not damaged (14), it is inadvisable to routinely perform this type of maneuver on patients with cardiac pacemakers because of the potential of encountering the various aforementioned hazards.

In the event of exposure (inadvertent or intentional) of a patient with an implanted pacemaker to the static and/or time-varying magnetic fields of an MR imaging system, it would be prudent to have the functionality of the pacemaker checked and verified by a cardiologist and, if possible, have the functionality verification affirmed by the manufacturer of the particular pacing device. Although it is entirely possible that no permanent modification of sensing or pacing function(s) may result from such an exposure, the marked variety of past and currently available types, designs, and even size, age, and construction of the various pacing devices virtually requires that the device's manufacturer reinspect to ensure continued safe and proper operation.

Another commonly asked question involving pacemakers deals with the issue of distribution of liability related to MR procedures. Specifically, whose responsibility is it to screen for the presence of a pacemaker? What, if any, is the role and therefore the liability of the referring physician, primary care physician, and others involved in the patient's management?

As per discussion with legal counsel (personal communication, Craig Frischman, plaintiff's medical malpractice attorney, Pittsburgh, PA), a general answer to such a general question is that the referring and/or primary care physician(s) would typically not be held liable for an adverse outcome of performing an MR procedure in a patient with a pacemaker, unless they had knowledge of the hazard and failed to act. Therefore, the radiologist and MR facility would certainly be prime candidates for a malpractice attorney to pursue, as it is their responsibility to ensure that only patients on whom an MR procedure can be performed with a reasonable level of safety be permitted into the environment of the MR system. The referring and/or primary care physician(s) rely on the radiologist and personnel at the MR site to know how the test is performed—and on whom it may be safely applied.

Implantable Cardiac Defibrillators

Implantable cardiac defibrillators are used to treat patients with sustained ventricular arrhythmias that are refractory to antiarrhythmic pharmacologic treatment (15). These devices use an external magnet to test the battery charger and to activate and deactivate the system (15). Deactivation of an implantable cardiac defibrillator is accomplished by holding a magnet over the device for approximately 30 s (15) and has occurred accidentally as a result of patients encountering the magnetic fields in the home and workplace environments. For example, deactivation of implantable defibrillators has occurred in patients from exposure to the magnetic fields found in stereo speakers, bingo wands, and 12-volt starters (15).

Obviously, magnetic fields of MR systems would have a similar effect on implantable cardiac defibrillators and, therefore, patients with these devices should avoid exposure to MR systems. In addition, because implantable cardiac defibrillators also have electrodes that are placed in the myocardium, patients should not undergo MR procedures because of the previously mentioned risks related to the presence of these conductive materials (10,11).

External Hearing Aids

External hearing aids are included in the category of electrically activated implants that may be found in patients referred for MR procedures. The magnetic fields used for MR procedures can easily damage these devices. Fortunately, external hearing aids can be readily identified and may simply be removed from patients to allow them to safely undergo MR procedures.

Magnetic Fringe Field–Related Issues

Cardiac pacemakers, implantable defibrillators, or other similar magnetically activated devices may also be affected by the magnetic fringe field associated with the static magnetic field of the MR systems. Therefore, patients or other individuals should avoid areas that may affect these devices within the fringe field. As a person with a cardiac pacemaker or implantable cardiac defibrillator approaches the MR system, the magnetic fringe field may be strong enough to throw the reed relay switch of the cardiac pacemaker or to deactivate the implantable defibrillator (2–4,8,9). The acceptable safe levels for exposure to magnetic fringe fields with respect to patients who have cardiac pacemakers have been reported to be between 5 and 15 gauss (8,9).

Special precautions should be taken to establish a security zone in the vicinity of the MR system to alert individuals with cardiac pacemakers or implantable defibrillators (and other similar implants or devices that may be adversely affected by the magnetic fringe fields) of the potential risks of the magnetic fringe fields (12). Additionally, appropriate barriers and warning signs should be used to control access to this area.

MAGNETICALLY ACTIVATED IMPLANTS AND DEVICES

Various types of implants and devices incorporate magnets as a means of activating the implant, retaining the implant in place, guiding an external component to change the operation of the implant, or to program the device (see Chapter 10 for additional information). Because there is a high likelihood of perturbing the function of magnetically activated implants, demagnetizing the implants, or displacing the implants, MR procedures should not be performed in patients with magnetically activated implants or devices (10,11,16).

Implants and devices that use magnets (e.g., certain types of dental implants, magnetic sphincters, magnetic stoma plugs, magnetic ocular implants, and other similar prosthetic devices) may be damaged by the magnetic fields of the MR systems which, in turn, may necessitate surgery to replace or reposition the damaged implant or device. Whenever possible, a magnetically activated implant or device (i.e., such as an externally applied prosthesis or magnetic stoma plug) should be removed from the patient before the MR procedure. This will permit the examination to be performed safely (16–19). Knowledge of the specific aspects of the magnetically activated implant or device is essential to recognize potential problems and to guarantee that an MR procedure may be performed on a patient without risk.

Extrusion of an eye socket magnetic implant in a patient imaged with a 0.5-T MR system has been described (20). This type of magnetic prosthesis is used in patients after enucleation. A removable eye prosthesis adheres with a magnet of opposite polarity to a permanent implant sutured to the rectus muscles and conjunctiva by magnetic attraction through the conjunctiva (20). This "magnetic linkage" enables the eye prosthesis to move in a coordinated fashion with that of normal eye movement. In the reported incident, the static magnetic field of the MR system produced sufficient attraction of the ferromagnetic portion of the magnetic prosthesis to cause it to extrude through the tissue, thus injuring the patient (20) (Fig. 11-1).

Inflatable tissue expanders may also pose a hazard to patients undergoing MR procedures. One version of this device has a magnetic port that is used to enable the surgeon to accurately find the site for injection of fluid such as saline, so that the size of the expander may be altered (21). The intrinsic magnetic field of the tissue expander with a magnetic port presents a relative contraindication for patients undergoing MR procedures because of the significant torque and movement of the implant by the strong static magnetic fields of MR systems (21).

Cochlear Implants

Some types of cochlear implants employ a relatively strong cobalt samarium magnet used in conjunction with an external magnet to align and retain a radiofrequency transmitter coil (22,23). Other types of cochlear implants are electronically activated (22,23). Consequently, MR procedures are strictly contraindicated in patients with these types of implants because of the possibility of injuring the patient and/or damaging or altering the function of the cochlear implant (22,23).

IMPLANTED NEUROSTIMULATORS AND BONE GROWTH STIMULATORS

The incidence of patients receiving implanted neurostimulators for treatment of various forms of neurological disorders is increasing. There are two types of neurostimulators (24):

1. *Passive receivers*: neurostimulators that receive RF energy that is magnetically coupled from an external device by means of a coil placed over the implanted device
2. *Hermetically encased pulsed generators:* neurostimulators that contain a battery and are programmed by an external device to produce the various stimulus parameters.

Because of the specific design and intended function of neurostimulators

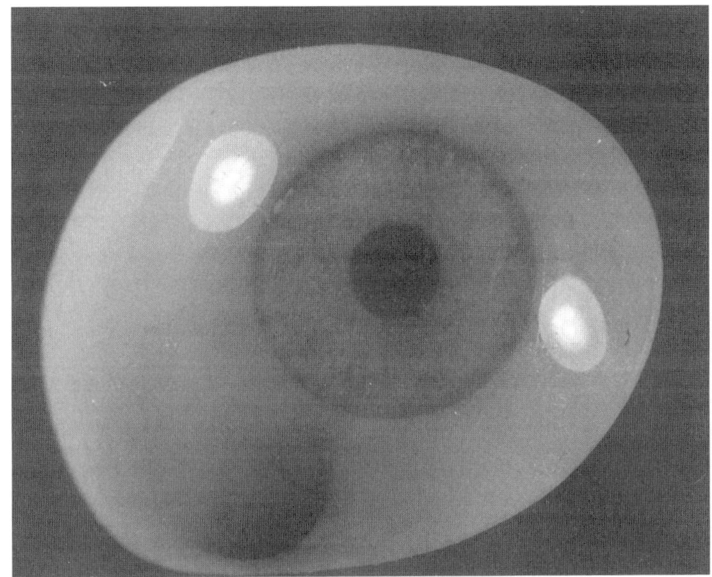

A

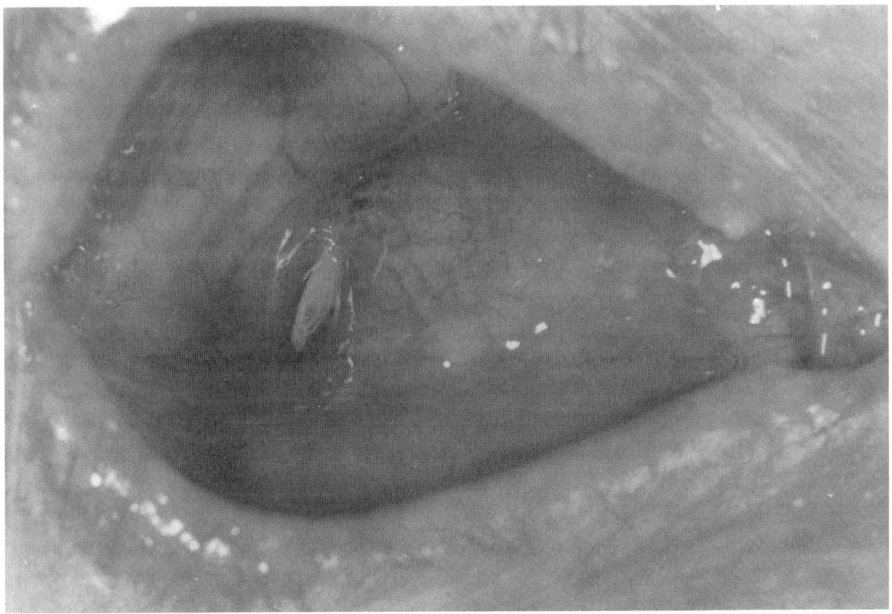

B

FIG. 11-1. A: Magnetically activated ocular prosthesis. **B:** Injured ocular tissue resulting from extrusion of metallic portion of ocular prosthesis due to attraction by magnetic field of MR system (see ref. 20 for additional details).

(Fig. 11-2), the electromagnetic fields used for MR procedures may produce problems with the operation of these devices. Malfunction of a neurostimulator that results from exposure to the electromagnetic fields of an MR system may cause discomfort or pain to the patient (24). In extreme cases, damage to the nerve fibers at the site of the implanted electrodes of the neurostimulator may also occur (24). Therefore, the present policy regarding patients with neurostimulators is that patients with these devices should not undergo MR procedures for reasons similar to those indicated for patients with cardiac pacemakers (4,7,10,11).

Six implantable neurostimulators models have been evaluated in an ex vivo manner in conjunction with 0.35- and 1.5-T MR systems (24). The authors of this study reported that "patients with certain types of implanted neurostimulators can be scanned safely under certain conditions" (24). It should be noted that this investigation had several limitations, including the fact that it did not assess the effects of the variety of pulse sequences used for MR imaging that may substantially alter the function of an implantable neurostimulator, nor was an in vivo evaluation performed (24).

Furthermore, the FDA indicates that the presence of an implantable neurostimulator is a contraindication for patients undergoing MR procedures (1). Therefore, MR procedures should not be performed in patents with implantable neurostimulators until the FDA reviews the available safety data and provides the proper approval or recommendations.

The clinical use of bone growth stimulators is also increasing. These devices usually have an external electronic component that attaches to electrodes implanted in areas of fractured bones and are used to enhance and facilitate the rate of bone healing. Similar to neurostimulators, patients with bone growth stimulators should not undergo MR procedures until data are available to support that there are no hazards associated with the presence of these devices in patients during the operation of MR systems. Currently, there is no neurostimulator or bone growth stimulator that has received from the FDA the designation of being "MR-compatible."

ELECTRONICALLY ACTIVATED, IMPLANTABLE DRUG INFUSION PUMP

There is a programmable, implantable drug infusion pump (SynchroMed, Medtronic) used for automatic delivery of antineoplastic agents, morphine, or antispasticity drugs. The implantable drug infusion pump has ferromagnetic components, a magnetic switch, and is programmed by telemetry (25). The presence of these features in a device are usually considered reasons for the device being designated as contraindicated for patients undergoing MR procedures (1,10,11). Nevertheless, the function and integrity of this implantable drug infusion pump was evaluated for compatibility with a 1.5-T MR system

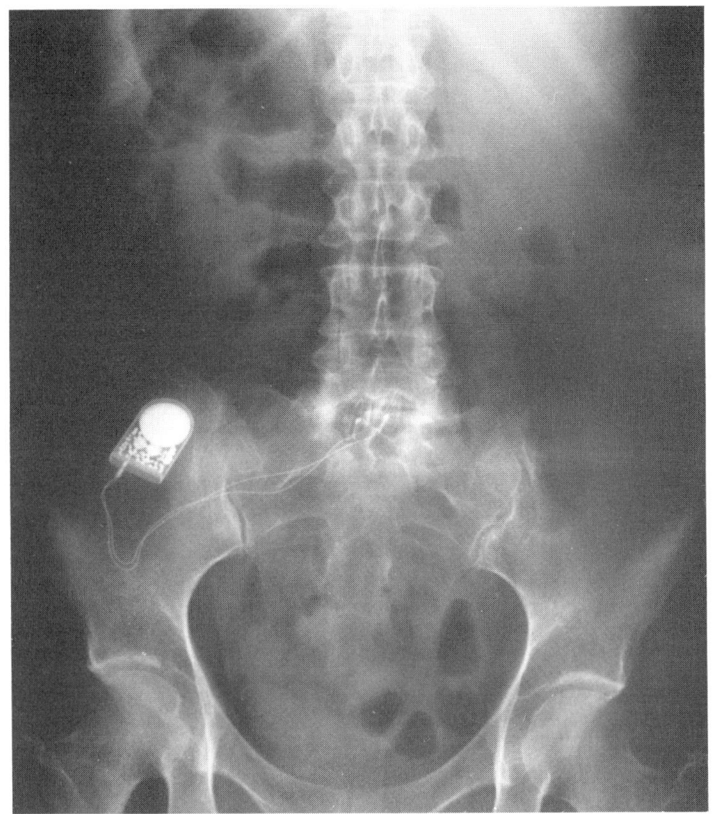

A

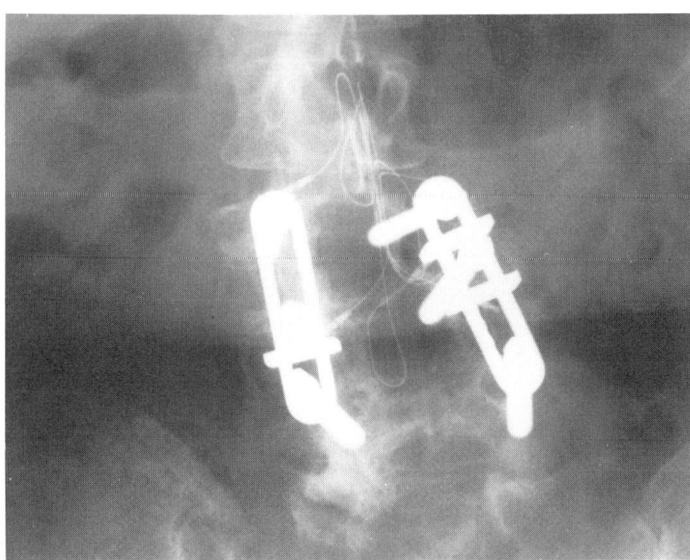

B

FIG. 11-2. Plain films showing implantable bone growth stimulators. **A:** Bone growth stimulator with electronic component attached to wires and implanted in vertebra. **B:** Residual wires from bone growth stimulator. Note coiled configuration of wires and metal from bone fixation devices.

(25). The authors concluded that MR imaging was accurate and safe so long as it was understood that the area of interest must be at least 10 cm from the pump and that there was an awareness that a temporary cessation of infusion (i.e., the roller pump rotor appeared to be frozen when the infusion pump was inside the MR system) occurs during the MR procedure (25).

There were several limitations of the assessment performed to determine compatibility of the SynchroMed drug infusion pump with MR systems. For example, only a single volunteer was examined by MR imaging and the infusion pump was placed externally on this subject (25). It is possible that substantially different test results would have been obtained with an implanted infusion pump. Additionally, only conventional T1-, proton density, and T2-weighted pulse sequences were used by a single type of MR system during the evaluation (25). Different MR systems operating with different static magnetic field strengths and frequencies using pulse sequences that require higher levels of RF energy (i.e., fast spin echo) or very rapid gradient magnetic fields (i.e., fast gradient echo or echo planar techniques) were not assessed. Therefore, it is probably premature, considering the limited testing procedures conducted on this device, to recommend that MR procedures may be performed safely on patients with the SynchroMed infusion pump.

FUTURE CONSIDERATIONS

There are several types of investigational implants and devices undergoing clinical trials that incorporate electrically, magnetically, or mechanically activated mechanisms. MR users should be aware of these experimental implants and devices because they may be encountered in patients referred for MR procedures in the near future.

For example, an electromagnetically controlled heart valve has been described that can be activated so that it stays open or closed depending on the requirements of the cardiovascular system (26). This implant uses a small electromagnet that surrounds a ferromagnetic disk within the valve mechanism. Movement of the valve is controlled by the field created by the electromagnet and its force on the disk (26). Obviously, the operation of this electromagnetically controlled heart valve would be seriously compromised if a patient with this implant were exposed to the electromagnetic fields of an MR system.

An endovascular catheter used for aneurysm embolization has been described that uses an external magnetic field for guidance of the device (27). Because this catheter must be retained in the aneurysm, this device would likely be a contraindication for patients undergoing MR procedures because of the possibility of inadvertent movement or dislodgement by the magnetic fields of the MR system.

Another experimental technique used for embolization of blood vessels has been described, whereby ferrous particles are introduced into the vascular system and guided by an external magnet to the site of the vascular abnormality (27). If this technique of embolization is used in the clinical setting, patients who have undergone this procedure will need to be identified because of potential risks associated with displacement of the ferrous particles during exposure to MR systems.

The clinical applications of magnetic microspheres used for the targeted and controlled release of medications or diagnostic agents to single or multiple organs are currently being evaluated (28). The magnetic microspheres are usually injected into the arterial system near the targeted organ and subjected to an extracorporal gradient magnetic field gradient ranging from 0.55 to 0.8 T to position them properly in the tissue (28). The magnetic fields associated with MR systems would probably cause disruption of the magnetic microspheres and dislodge them from the intended organ. MR procedures should not be performed in patients with magnetic microspheres until the safety implications have been assessed further.

The remote magnetic manipulation of a small ferromagnetic "seed" used for delivery of drugs, focal hyperthermia, or other therapies to brain tissues has been reported (29). Initial experiments evaluating the use of this magnetic stereotaxic system in laboratory animals have yielded encouraging results. The ferromagnetic seed used for this treatment is typically maneuvered to a precise location within the brain using static magnetic fields at field strengths less than those used for clinical MR procedures (29). Iatrogenic displacement of the ferromagnetic seed is likely to occur if a patient with one of these implants is subjected to an MR procedure. Therefore, the risks related to having a patient with a ferromagnetic seed exposed to the static magnetic fields of the MR system must be thoroughly evaluated before allowing the patient to undergo MR imaging or spectroscopy.

CONCLUSIONS

In general, a patient with any other electrically, magnetically, or mechanically activated implant or device should be excluded from examination by MR techniques unless the particular implant or device has been previously demonstrated to be unaffected by the magnetic and electromagnetic fields used for MR procedures. Certain electrically, magnetically, or mechanically activated implants and devices may be designed so that they are compatible with the MR environment. However, it should be noted that the respective federal government agencies responsible for the safety aspects of MR systems must designate whether or not the implant or device is acceptable and compatible with MR procedures before MR users routinely perform examinations on patients.

REFERENCES

1. Food and Drug Administration. Magnetic resonance diagnostic device: panel recommendation and report on petitions for MR reclassification. *Fed Reg* 1988;53:7575–7579.

2. Erlebacher JA, Cahill PT, Pannizzo F, et al. Effect of magnetic resonance imaging on DDD pacemakers. *Am J Cardiol* 1986;57:437–440.
3. Fetter J, Aram G, Holmes DR, et al. The effects of nuclear magnetic resonance imagers on external and implantable pulse generators. *PACE* 1984;7:720–727.
4. Gangarosa RE, Minnis JE, Nobbe J, et al. Operational safety issues in MRI. *Magn Reson Imag* 1987;5:287–292.
5. Hayes DL, Holmes DR, Gray JE. Effect of a 1.5 Tesla magnetic resonance imaging scanner on implanted permanent pacemakers. *J Am Coll Cardiol* 1987;10:782–786.
6. Holmes DR, Hayes DL, Gray JE, et al. The effects of magnetic resonance imaging on implantable pulse generators. *PACE* 1986;9:360–370.
7. Kanal E, Shellock FG, Talagala L. Safety considerations in MR imaging. *Radiology* 1990;176: 593–606.
8. Pavlicek W, Geisinger M, Castle L, et al. The effects of nuclear magnetic resonance on patients with cardiac pacemakers. *Radiology* 1983;147:149–153.
9. Persson BRR, Stahlberg F. *Health and safety of clinical NMR examinations.* Boca Raton, Fla: CRC Press; 1989.
10. Shellock FG, Kanal E. Policies, guidelines, and recommendations for MR imaging safety and patient management. *J Magn Reson Imag* 1991;1:97–101.
11. Shellock FG, Litwer CA, Kanal E. Magnetic resonance imaging: Bioeffects, safety, and patient management. *Rev Magn Reson Med* 1992;4:21–63.
12. Zimmermann BH, Faul DD. Artifacts and hazards in NMR imaging due to metal implants and cardiac pacemakers. *Diagn Imag Clin Med* 1984;53:53–56.
13. ECRI. A new MRI complication? *Health Devices Alert* 1988;F5:1.
14. Alagona P, Toole JC, Maniscalco BS, et al. Nuclear magnetic resonance imaging in a patient with a DDD pacemaker. *PACE* 1989;12:619.
15. Bonnet CA, Elson JJ, Fogoros RN. Accidental deactivation of the automatic implantable cardioverter defibrillator. *Am Heart J* 1990;3:696–697.
16. Shellock FG, Curtis JS. MR imaging and biomedical implants, materials, and devices: an updated review. *Radiology* 1991;180:541–550.
17. Gegauff AG, Laurell KA, Thavendrarajah A, et al. A potential MRI hazard: forces on dental magnet keepers. *J Oral Rehab* 1990;17:403–410.
18. Gillings BRD, Samant A. Overdentures with magnetic attachments. *Dent Clin North Am* 1990;34:683–709.
19. Shellock FG. Ex vivo assessment of deflection forces and artifacts associated with high-field MRI of 'mini-magnet' dental prostheses. *Magn Reson Imag* 1989;7(S1):P38.
20. Yuh WTC, Hanigan MT, Nerad JA, et al. Extrusion of eye socket magnetic implant after MR imaging: potential hazard to patient with eye prosthesis. *J Magn Reson Imag* 1991;1:711–713.
21. Liang MD, Narayanan K, Kanal E. Magnetic ports in tissue expanders—a caution for MRI. *Magn Reson Imag* 1989;7:541–542.
22. Mattucci KF, Setzen M, Hyman R, et al. The effect of nuclear magnetic resonance imaging on metallic middle ear protheses. *Otolaryngol Head Neck Surg* 1986;94:441–443.
23. Dormer KJ, Richard GL, Hough JVD, et al. The use of rare-earth magnet couplers in cochlear implants. *Laryngoscope* 1981;91:1812–1820.
24. Gleason CA, Kaula NF, Hricak H, et al. The effect of magnetic resonance imagers on implanted neurostimulators. *PACE* 1992;15:81–94.
25. Von Roemeling R, Lanning RM, Eames FA. MR imaging of patients with implanted drug infusion pumps. *J Magn Reson Imag* 1991;1:77–81.
26. Young DB, Pawlak AM. An electromagnetically controllable heart valve suitable for chronic implantation. *ASAIO Trans* 1990;36:M421–M425.
27. Gaston A, Marsault C, Lacaze A, et al. External magnetic guidance of endovascular catheters with a superconducting magnet: preliminary trials. *J Neuroradiol* 1988;15:137–147.
28. Ranney DF, Huffaker HH. Magnetic microspheres for the targeted controlled release of drugs and diagnostic agents. *Ann NY Acad Sci* 1987;507:104–119.
29. Grady MS, Howard MA, Molloy JA, et al. Nonlinear magnetic stereotaxis: three-dimensional, in vivo remote magnetic manipulation of a small object in canine brain. *Med Phys* 1990;17: 405–415.

12

Cryogen and Quench Considerations of Magnetic Resonance Systems

QUENCH AND CRYOGEN CONSIDERATIONS OF MR SYSTEMS WITH SUPERCONDUCTING MAGNETS

There are some hazards that apply to certain MR systems and not to others. A prime example of this is the potential safety issue associated with the use of cryogenic liquids. Such cryogens are used only in sites with MR systems that incorporate a superconductive-type magnet to produce their static magnetic fields. These constitute the majority of MR systems currently in use throughout the United States for both mobile and fixed MR sites.

Even within this category, not all superconductive magnets used for MR systems are the same. Some older magnets use both liquid nitrogen and liquid helium to cool the static field coils, whereas the newer models tend to use just helium—but all superconductive MR systems in clinical use today use liquid helium. Nevertheless, the safety issues and appropriate practices for MR sites using cryogens are essentially identical, regardless of whether one or both these cryogenic liquids are used.

The cryogens are used to cool the static-field–producing coils to a temperature that is so low that they are able to conduct electricity with essentially no resistance to electrical current (i.e., they become superconductive) (1; J. E. Gray, personal communications, 1989; A. Aisen, personal communication, 1989).

For the types of materials used in these coils (e.g., niobium-titanium alloys embedded in copper), a superconductive state is reached only at exceedingly low temperatures. Liquid helium is able to reach low temperatures. In fact, for helium to be maintained as a liquid it must be kept at or below temperatures of approximately −269°C (4.17°K) because above this temperature helium will achieve the gaseous state, or "boil off" (1). Thus, if for whatever reason the temperature of the liquid helium should exceed this level, the liquid helium will enter the gaseous state. If this occurs, helium (and/or nitrogen) would undergo a marked increase in volume as it transforms into a gaseous state, because the gas/liquid volume ratio for helium is approximately 760 to 1. For nitrogen the ratio is approximately 695 to 1. This will result in a marked increase in the pressure within the cryostat of the MR system that contains these cryogenic liquids. In this instance, a pressure-sensitive valve within the cryostat will release with a rather loud popping noise, followed by the rapid egress of gaseous helium (and/or nitrogen) as it escapes from the cryostat. In a manner similar to the sound created by steam escaping rapidly past the narrow opening of a teapot, the escaping cryogenic gases may produce a loud roaring sound as they leave the cryostat and exit the MR system past the orifice of the burst pressure pop-up valve (2).

Ordinarily, with appropriate site and MR system design, venting gases can be guided through a "stack," or conduit, out of the MR system room and into the outside environment if an incident occurs. It is possible, however, that venting may accidentally release some cryogenic gases into the ambient atmosphere of the MR system room. The rate of egress of these gases, the ventilation capacity of the room, the total amount of gas released into the scan room, and the dimensions of the scan room will determine how much of the air (and, more importantly, oxygen) within the MR system room will be displaced.

Assuming that the escaped gas is predominantly helium, there is the fortuitous benefit of having the helium gas substantially lighter than air. Thus, the helium will preferentially rise toward the ceiling and away from the occupant(s) (such as the patient and/or health practitioners) in the lower aspect of the room. Helium vapor may be exceedingly cold (yet looks like steam) and is entirely odorless and tasteless. Vented nitrogen would, of course, be much closer in density to that of the ambient air, and may remain more readily near the level of the patient at the bottom third level of the MR system room.

Prolonged inhalation of helium gas may lead to an increase in the pitch of the voice, asphyxiation, and/or frostbite. In addition, the loss of superconductivity (i.e., quench) of an MR system may be associated with the release of a considerable quantity of helium gas into the MR system room. There are several reports of this resulting in increased pressure within the MR system room and damage to the MR facility. For doors to these rooms that are designed to open into the rooms, the pressure increase associated with the escaping gas might secondarily result in difficulty in opening the doors because of the substantial pressure differential produced. In these cases, it may be necessary to enter the MR system room through a window. If one attempts to enter the room to reach the patient via a sealed window by throwing an object through the window to break it, it is important to be careful not to injure oneself or others by flying glass shards that might result from the pressure differential between the scan room and the control room on the other side of the window. Today, the MR system room should be designed with these considerations in mind, with sliding windows or windows and doors that open outward.

Figure 12-1 illustrates an example of a case in which the stack was unable to handle the amount of venting gases that occurred during a quench while a patient was undergoing an MR imaging procedure. This resulted in physical disruption of the stack from the MR system and rapid venting of the cryogenic gases into the room. The MR system room filled with a "cloud" of condensed and frozen water vapors, accompanied by a sound that was described as a "freight train" or "tornado tearing through the room." Pressure in the room increased to a point at which the door could not be opened. After breaking the

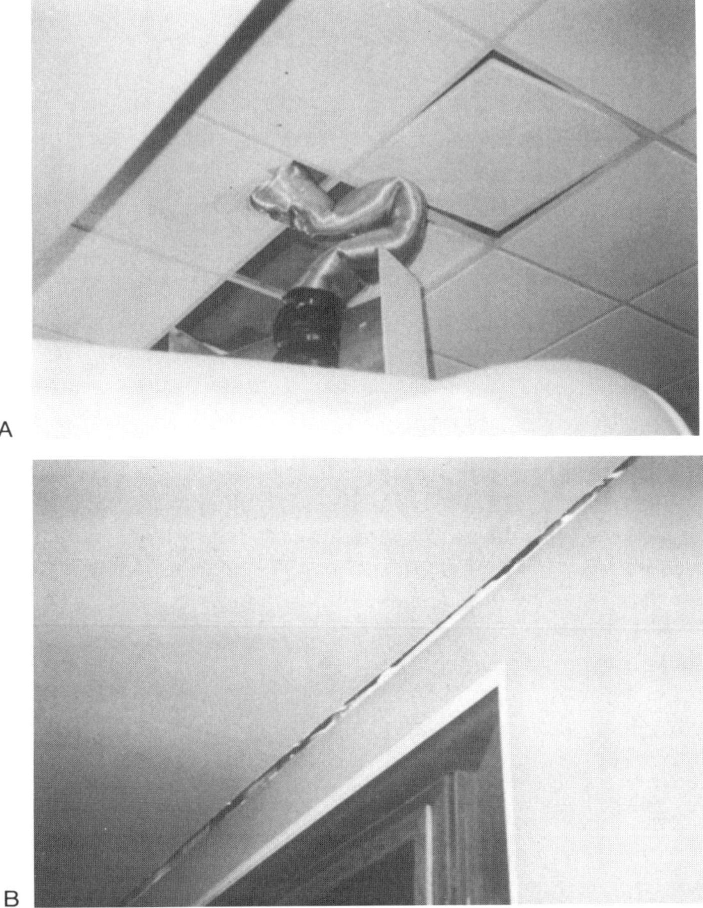

FIG. 12-1. Views of MR system room after quench of superconducting magnet. Note the damage to the stack of the MR system (**A**) and the separated ceiling and walls (**B,C**) that occurred as a result of the rapid increase in pressure from the quench.

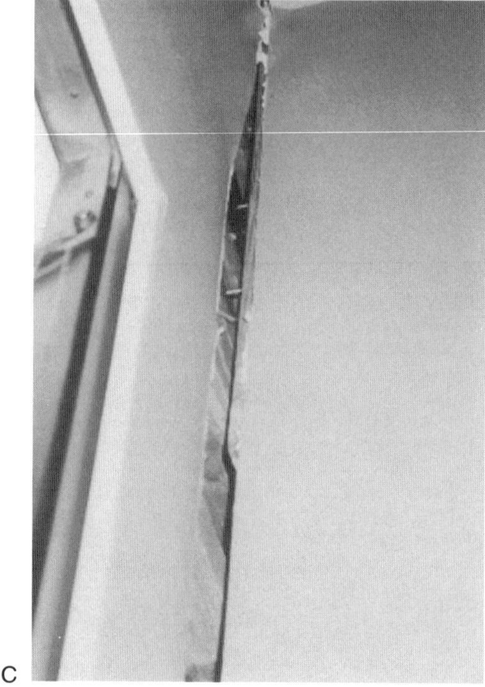

C

FIG. 12-1. *Continued.*

glass between the operator's console and the MR system room, the pressure decreased sufficiently to permit personnel to enter the area and remove the patient from the environment of the quench. This incident was handled in a most appropriate manner, with the number one priority being to evacuate the patient from the area during the quench. Unfortunately, extensive damage was caused to the MR system room by the excessive build-up of pressure from the escaping gases (Fig. 12-1).

In the unlikely event of a superconductive magnet quench, the major efforts should be directed toward immediately evacuating the area of the MR system room and anywhere the helium vapor may reach. The MR system manufacturer and other appropriate personnel who are responsible for clearing the site from escaped gas(es) should be advised regarding the incident, and all personnel should be kept away from the area of the quench until there has been an opportunity for the helium and/or nitrogen gases to be vented and cleared from the area.

Because of considerable improvements in the design of cryostats, use of insulation, and the incorporation of refrigerant systems in many superconducting MR systems, most (if not all) of the newer superconducting magnets use only liquid helium. Nevertheless, a considerable number of clinical MR systems that also use liquid nitrogen are still in use today.

Liquid nitrogen serves as a buffer between the liquid helium and the outside atmosphere, as its boiling point is 77.3°K (1). In the event of an accidental release of liquid nitrogen into the atmosphere of the MR system room, there is again the potential for frostbite, as with the release of gaseous helium. With gaseous nitrogen release, however, because nitrogen has roughly the same density as air, there is the additional concern that the nitrogen gas could more easily settle near the floor level, where patients, attendant family members, and health care personnel may be located.

Once again, the total amount of nitrogen gas that would be contained within the MR system room would be determined by the total amount of gas released into the room, the rate at which it was released, the dimensions of the scan room, and the room's ventilation capacity (the existence and size of other routes of egress, such as doors, windows, ventilation ducts, and fans, available for the nitrogen gas). A pure nitrogen environment is especially hazardous, and unconsciousness generally results in humans as rapidly as within 5 or 10 seconds after exposure. To quote one source (J. E. Gray, personal communication, 1989),

> "Acute asphyxia, such as from breathing pure inert gases, produces immediate unconsciousness without warning and so quickly that the individual cannot help or protect himself. The worker may fall as if struck down by a blow on the head and will die within a few minutes if not resuscitated."

Therefore, it is imperative that all patients and health care personnel be evacuated from the area as soon as it is recognized that nitrogen gas is being released into the MR system room. They should not return until appropriate corrective measures have been taken to assure that the gas has been cleared from the room and the oxygen environment has been restored to normal.

In humans, when the oxygen concentration falls between 21% and 14%, there initially will be a compensatory increase in the respired volume and heart rate. There may even be subtle decreases in muscle coordination, the ability to maintain attention, and to think clearly. Breathing air containing between 10% and 14% oxygen concentration results in further impairment of judgment and coordination and possible signs of somnolence or fatigue. Respiring air with between 6% and 10% oxygen concentration may result in nausea and vomiting and complete loss of coordination, yet, paradoxically, may occur with the individual now completely unaware that anything is even amiss.

With oxygen concentrations below 6%, breathing may come to a complete halt and convulsions may occur. If prolonged over 10 to 15 seconds, complete unconsciousness will rapidly occur. If prolonged over 6 minutes, 50% of these individuals will die. If prolonged over 8 or more minutes, it is inevitably fatal. Finally, breathing a pure inert gas such as helium or nitrogen produces immediate unconsciousness, not permitting the exposed individual to have the opportunity to recognize that anything is wrong or take any steps to attempt to correct or escape the situation.

Dewar (cryogen storage containers) storage should also be within a well ventilated area, lest normal boil-off rates increase the concentration of inert gas within the storage room to a dangerous level (J. E. Gray, personal communication, 1989). At least one reported death has occurred in an industrial setting during the shipment of cryogens (J. E. Gray, personal communication, 1989), although no such fatality has occurred to our knowledge in the medical community.

There is one report of a loss of consciousness of unexplained etiology by a technologist passing through a cryogen storage area (A. Aisen, personal communication, 1989). Although there is no verification of ambient atmospheric oxygen concentration available in that instance to confirm any relationship to the cryogens per se, the history is strongly suggestive of such a relationship.

For these reasons, an oxygen monitor, with an audible alarm, should be situated at an appropriate height (less than 6 feet from the ground) within each room that contains a superconductive MR system. This should be considered a mandatory minimum safety precaution for all MR sites. Automatic linking to the MR system room ventilation system, in case the oxygen monitor detects oxygen levels that fall below 18% or 19%, should also be considered at each MR facility.

In designing MR sites, one should be aware that the exit port(s) for cryogenic gas venting must be verified to be directed in such a way as to release the gases harmlessly into the outside atmosphere and not into an area that can threaten patients, pedestrians, delicate and temperature-sensitive materials, or other structures.

It is also important to stress that collections of liquids around MR systems or cryogenic dewars should be treated with the utmost respect and caution because they may represent super-cold collections of liquid cryogens that may have spilled or leaked from their containers. Only those individuals specially trained in the appropriate and safe handling of such liquids should be permitted to "clean up" a spill once it is identified as a cryogenic substance.

Of note is that there is a small, but finite, possibility of damage to the static-field--producing coils themselves from any quench. The MR system should thus undergo a complete "check-up" by the manufacturer to ensure its acceptable status for patient imaging or spectroscopy subsequent to a magnet quench.

From the above discussion it should be evident that, despite an overwhelmingly safe record over the more than 10 years of clinical use, the use of cryogens in superconductive MR systems does present several unique safety considerations for MR sites. The proper handling and storage of these cryogens as well as appropriate behavior in the presence of possible leaks should be taught and stressed at each facility. Appropriate steps to be taken in the event of a quench or a sounding of the oxygen monitoring alarm should be outlined and rehearsed at recurring intervals to ensure the safety of patients and health care practitioners around MR systems that have superconducting magnets.

ELECTRICAL CONSIDERATIONS OF A QUENCH

Until now, we have been concerned directly with the cryogens themselves. However, there are other considerations of a quench that should be addressed. Faraday's Law of Induction states that a changing magnetic field induces an electrical current voltage; therefore, there is also a concern about electrical currents that may be induced in electrical conductors, such as biologic tissues, in the vicinity of the rapidly changing magnetic field associated with a quench (2).

In a study where physiologic monitoring of a pig was performed and environmental measurements were obtained during an intentional quench of a 1.76-T MR system, there did not appear to be any significant effects on the blood pressure, heart rate, temperature, electrocardiogram, or electroencephalogram measurements of the pig during or immediately after the quench (2). Although such a single observation does not, of course, prove safety for humans undergoing exposure to a quench, the data do suggest that there is good reason to presume that the experience in humans would be similar. Furthermore, it is reasonable to assume that no serious or deleterious effects would likely be experienced by humans undergoing a similar experience and exposure.

REFERENCES

1. Williamson KW, Eduskuty FJ, eds. *Liquid cryogens, vol 1, theory and equipment.* Boca Raton, Fla: CRC Press; 1983.
2. Bore PJ, Galloway GJ, Styles P, Radda GK, Flynn G, Pitts PR. Are quenches dangerous? *Magn Reson Med* 1986;3:112–117.

Appendix I

List of Items Tested

LIST OF IMPLANTS, MATERIALS, DEVICES, AND OBJECTS TESTED FOR ATTRACTION/DEFLECTION FORCES DURING EXPOSURE TO STATIC MAGNETIC FIELDS

Implant, material, device, or object	Attraction/ deflection	Highest field strength (T)	Reference
Aneurysm and hemostatic clips			
Downs multi-positional (15-7PH)	Yes	1.39	1
Drake (DR 14, DR 21) Edward Weck Triangle Park, NJ	Yes	1.39	1, 2
Drake (DR 16) Edward Weck Triangle Park, NJ	Yes	0.147	1
Drake (301 SS) Edward Weck Triangle Park, NJ	Yes	1.5	2, 3
Gastrointestinal anastomosis clip Auto Suture SGIA, (SS) United States Surgical Corp. Norwalk, CT	No	1.5	3
Heifetz (17-7PH) Edward Weck Triangle Park, NJ	Yes	1.89	4, 5
Heifetz (Elgiloy) Edward Weck Triangle Park, NJ	No	1.89	2, 4, 5
Hemoclip, #10, (316L SS) Edward Weck Triangle Park, NJ	No	1.5	3

APPENDIX I. *Continued.*

Implant, material, device, or object	Attraction/ deflection	Highest field strength (T)	Reference
Hemoclip (tantalum) Edward Weck Triangle Park, NJ	No	1.5	3
Housepian	Yes	0.147	1
Kapp (405 SS) V. Mueller	Yes	1.89	2, 5
Kapp, curved (404 SS) V. Mueller	Yes	1.39	1
Kapp, straight (404 SS) V. Mueller	Yes	1.39	1
Ligaclip, #6, (316L SS) Ethicon, Inc. Sommerville, NJ	No	1.5	3
Ligaclip (tantalum) Ethicon, Inc. Sommerville, NJ	No	1.5	3
Mayfield (301 SS) Codman Randolf, MA	Yes	1.5	3
Mayfield (304 SS) Codman Randolf, MA	Yes	1.89	5
McFadden (301 SS) Codman Randolf, MA	Yes	1.5	2, 3
Olivecrona	No	1.39	1
Pivot (17-7PH)	Yes	1.89	5
Scoville (EN58J) Downs Surgical, Inc. Decatur, GA	Yes	1.89	2, 5
Stevens (50-4190, silver alloy)	No	0.15	6
Sugita (Elgiloy) Downs Surgical, Inc. Decatur, GA	No	1.89	2, 5
Sundt-Kees (301 SS) Downs Surgical, Inc. Decatur, GA	Yes	1.5	2, 3
Sundt-Kees Multi-Angle (17-7PH) Downs Surgical, Inc. Decatur, GA	Yes	1.89	2, 5
Surgiclip, Auto Suture M-9.5 (SS) United States Surgical Corp. Norwalk, CT	No	1.5	3
Vari-Angle (17-7PH) Codman Randolf, MA	Yes	1.89	5
Vari-Angle McFadden (MP35N) Codman Randolf, MA	No	1.89	2, 5
Vari-Angle Micro (17-7PM SS) Codman Randolf, MA	Yes	0.15	2, 6

APPENDIX I. *Continued.*

Implant, material, device, or object	Attraction/ deflection	Highest field strength (T)	Reference
Vari-Angle Spring (17-7PM SS) Codman Randolf, MA	Yes	0.15	2, 6
Yasargil (316 SS) Aesculap	No	1.89	5
Yasargil (Phynox) Aesculap	No	1.89	2
Biopsy needles and devices			
Adjustable, Automated Biopsy Gun 6, 13, and 19 mm (304 SS) MD Tech Watertown, MA	Yes	1.5	7
Adjustable, Automated Aspiration Biopsy Gun 10, 15, and 20 mm (304 SS) MD Tech Watertown, MA	Yes	1.5	7
ASAP 16, Automatic 16 G Core Biopsy System 19 cm length (304 SS)	Yes	1.5	7
Automatic Cutting Needle with Depth Markings 14 G, 10 cm length (304 SS) Manan Northbrook, IL	Yes	1.5	7
Automatic Cutting Needle with Ultrasound Tip & Depth Markings 18 G, 16 cm length (304 SS) Manan Northbrook, IL	Yes	1.5	7
Automatic Cutting Needle with Ultrasound Tip & Depth Markings 18 G, 20 cm length (304 SS) Manan Northbrook, IL	Yes	1.5	7
Basic II Hookwire Breast Localization Needle (304 SS) MD Tech Watertown, MA	Yes	1.5	7
Beaded Breast Localization Wire Set 20 G, 2 inch needle with 5-7/8 inch wire (304 SS) Inrad Grand Rapids, MI	Yes	1.5	7
Beaded Breast Localization Wire Set 19 G, 3-1/2 inch needle with 7-7/8 inch wire (304 SS) Inrad Grand Rapids, MI	Yes	1.5	7

APPENDIX I. *Continued.*

Implant, material, device, or object	Attraction/ deflection	Highest field strength (T)	Reference
Biopsy Gun 13 mm Meadox Oakland, NJ	Yes	1.5	7
Biopsy Gun 25 mm Meadox Oakland, NJ	Yes	1.5	7
Biopsy Needle 17 G, 10 cm length Meadox Oakland, NJ	Yes	1.5	7
Biopsy Needle 20 G, 15 cm length Meadox Oakland, NJ	Yes	1.5	7
Biopsy Needle 22 G, 15 cm length Meadox Oakland, NJ	Yes	1.5	7
Biopsy Needle 22 G, 15 cm length Cook, Inc. Bloomington, IN	Yes	1.5	7
Biopty-Cut Biopsy Needle 14 G, 10 cm length (304 SS) C.R. Bard, Inc. Covington, GA	Yes	1.5	7
Biopty-Cut Biopsy Needle 16 G, 16 cm length (304 SS) C.R. Bard, Inc. Covington, GA	Yes	1.5	7
Biopty-Cut Biopsy Needle 18 G, 18 cm length (304 SS) C.R. Bard, Inc. Covington, GA	Yes	1.5	7
Biopty-Cut Biopsy Needle with centimeter markings 18 G, 20 cm length (304 SS) C.R. Bard, Inc. Covington, GA	Yes	1.5	7
Breast Localization Needle 20 G, 5 cm length (304 SS) Manan Northbrook, IL	Yes	1.5	7
Breast Localization Needle 20 G, 7 cm length (304 SS) Manan Northbrook, IL	Yes	1.5	7
Chiba Needle with HiLiter Ultrasound Enhancement 22 G, 3-7/8 inch needle (304 SS) Inrad Grand Rapids, MI	Yes	1.5	7

APPENDIX I. *Continued.*

Implant, material, device, or object	Attraction/ deflection	Highest field strength (T)	Reference
Coaxial Needle Set Chiba-type needle 22 G, 5-7/8 inch needle (304 SS) Inrad Grand Rapids, MI	Yes	1.5	7
Coaxial Needle Set Introducer Needle 19G, 2-15/16 inch needle (304 SS) Inrad Grand Rapids, MI	Yes	1.5	7
Cutting Needle 14 G, 9 cm length West Coast Medical Laguna Beach, CA	Yes	1.5	7
Cutting Needle 16 G, 17 mm length (304 SS) BIP USA, Inc. Niagara Falls, NY	Yes	1.5	7
Cutting Needle 16 G, 19 mm length (304 SS) BIP USA, Inc. Niagara Falls, NY	Yes	1.5	7
Cutting Needle 18 G, 100 mm length Meadox Oakland, NJ	Yes	1.5	7
Cutting Needle 18 G, 150 mm length Meadox Oakland, NJ	Yes	1.5	7
Cutting Needle 18 G, 9 cm length West Coast Medical Laguna Beach, CA	Yes	1.5	7
Cutting Needle 18 G, 15 cm length West Coast Medical Laguna Beach, CA	Yes	1.5	7
Cutting Needle 19 G, 6 cm length West Coast Medical Laguna Beach, CA	Yes	1.5	7
Cutting Needle 19 G, 9 cm length West Coast Medical Laguna Beach, CA	Yes	1.5	7
Cutting Needle 19 G, 15 cm length West Coast Medical Laguna Beach, CA	Yes	1.5	7
Cutting Needle 20 G, 9 cm length West Coast Medical Laguna Beach, CA	Yes	1.5	7

APPENDIX I. *Continued.*

Implant, material, device, or object	Attraction/ deflection	Highest field strength (T)	Reference
Cutting Needle 20 G, 15 cm length West Coast Medical Laguna Beach, CA	Yes	1.5	7
Cutting Needle 20 G, 20 cm length West Coast Medical Laguna Beach, CA	Yes	1.5	7
Cutting Needle & Gun 18 G, 155 mm length Meadox Oakland, NJ	Yes	1.5	7
Hawkins Blunt Needle (304 SS) MD Tech Watertown, MA	Yes	1.5	7
Hawkins III Breast Localization Needle MD Tech Watertown, MA	Yes	1.5	7
Lufkin Aspiration Cytology Needle 20 G, 5 cm length (high nickel alloy) E-Z-Em, Inc. Westbury, NY	No	1.5	9
Lufkin Biopsy Needle 18 G, 5 cm length (high nickel alloy) E-Z-Em, Inc. Westbury, NY	No	1.5	8
Lufkin Biopsy Needle 18 G, 15 cm length (high nickel alloy) E-Z-Em, Inc. Westbury, NY	No	1.5	8
Lufkin Biopsy Needle 22 G, 5 cm length (high nickel alloy) E-Z-Em, Inc. Westbury, NY	No	1.5	8
Lufkin Biopsy Needle 22 G, 10 cm length (high nickel alloy) E-Z-Em, Inc. Westbury, NY	No	1.5	8
Lufkin Biopsy Needle 22 G, 15 cm length (high nickel alloy) E-Z-Em, Inc. Westbury, NY	No	1.5	8
MReye Chiba Biopsy Needle William Cook Europe A/S Bjaeverskov, Denmark	No	1.5	N/A
MReye Embolization Coil William Cook Europe A/S Bjaeverskov, Denmark	No	1.5	N/A

APPENDIX I. *Continued.*

Implant, material, device, or object	Attraction/ deflection	Highest field strength (T)	Reference
MReye Franseen Lung Biopsy Needle William Cook Europe A/S Bjaeverskov, Denmark	No	1.5	N/A
MReye Interventional Needle William Cook Europe A/S Bjaeverskov, Denmark	No	1.5	N/A
MReye Kopans Breast Lesion Localization Needles (21, 20, 19 gauge; 5.0, 9.0, 15.0 length) William Cook Europe A/S Bjaeverskov, Denmark	No	1.5	N/A
MRI BioGun 18 G, 10 cm length (high nickel alloy) E-Z-Em, Inc. Westbury, NY	No	1.5	8
MRI Histology Needle 18 G, 5 cm length (high nickel alloy) E-Z-Em, Inc. Westbury, NY	No	1.5	8
MRI Histology Needle 18 G, 15 cm length (high nickel alloy) E-Z-Em, Inc. Westbury, NY	No	1.5	7
MRI Histology Needle 20 G, 5 cm length (high nickel alloy) E-Z-Em, Inc. Westbury, NY	No	1.5	7
MRI Histology Needle 20 G, 7.5 cm length (high nickel alloy) E-Z-Em, Inc. Westbury, NY	No	1.5	8
MRI Histology Needle 20 G, 10 cm length (high nickel alloy) E-Z-Em, Inc. Westbury, NY	No	1.5	8
MRI Histology Needle 20 G, 15 cm length (high nickel alloy) E-Z-Em, Inc. Westbury, NY	No	1.5	8
MRI Lesion Marking System 20 G, 7.5 cm length (high nickel alloy) E-Z-Em, Inc. Westbury, NY	No	1.5	8
MRI Needle (surgical grade SS) Cook, Inc. Bloomington, IN	No	1.5	7

APPENDIX I. *Continued.*

Implant, material, device, or object	Attraction/ deflection	Highest field strength (T)	Reference
Percucut Biopsy Needle and Stylet 19.5 gauge 3 10 cm (316L SS) E-Z-Em, Inc. Westbury, NY	Yes	1.5	7
Percucut Biopsy Needle and Stylet 21 gauge 3 10 cm (316L SS) E-Z-Em, Inc. Westbury, NY	Yes	1.5	7
Sadowsky Breast Marking System 20 G, 5 cm length needle and 7 inch hook wire (316 L SS) Ranfac Corporation Avon, MA	Yes	1.5	7
Soft Tissue Biopsy Needle Gun & Needle, (304 SS) Anchor Products Co. Addison, IL	Yes	1.5	7
Trocar Needle (304 SS) BIP USA, Inc. Niagara Falls, NY	Yes	1.5	7
Trocar Needle, Disposable (SS) Cook, Inc. Bloomington, IN	Yes	1.5	7
Ultra-Core, biopsy needle 16 G, 16 cm length (304 SS) Gainesville, FL	Yes	1.5	7
Breast tissue expanders and implants			
Becker Expander/Mammary Prosthesis (316L SS) Mentor H/S Santa Barbara, CA	No	1.5	10
Infall, breast implant (inflatable) (magnetic port) 3101198 Model Heyerschultzz	Yes	1.5	N/A
Radovan Tissue Expander (316L SS) Mentor H/S Santa Barbara, CA	No	1.5	10
Siltex Spectrum Post-Operatively Adjustable Saline-Filled Mammary Prosthesis (316L SS) Mentor H/S Santa Barbara, CA	No	1.5	10
Tissue expander with magnetic port McGhan Medical Corporation Santa Barbara, CA	Yes	1.5	N/A
Carotid artery vascular clamps			
Crutchfield (SS) Codman Randolf, MA	Yes*	1.5	11

APPENDIX I. *Continued.*

Implant, material, device, or object	Attraction/ deflection	Highest Field strength (T)	Reference
Kindt (SS) V. Mueller	Yes*	1.5	11
Poppen-Blaylock (SS) Codman Randolf, MA	Yes	1.5	11
Salibi (SS) Codman Randolf, MA	Yes*	1.5	11
Selverstone (SS) Codman Randolf, MA	Yes*	1.5	11
Dental devices and materials			
Brace band (SS) American Dental Missoula, MT	Yes*	1.5	3
Brace wire (chrome alloy) Ormco Corp. San Marcos, CA	Yes*	1.5	3
Castable alloy Golden Dental Products, Inc. Golden, CO	Yes*	1.5	12
Cement-in keeper Solid State Innovations, Inc. Mt. Airy, NC	Yes*	1.5	12
Dental amalgam	No	1.39	1
Gutta Percha Points	No	1.5	N/A
GDP Direct Keeper, Pre-formed post Golden Dental Products, Inc. Golden, CO	Yes*	1.5	12
Indian Head Real Silver Points Union Broach Co., Inc. New York, NY	No	1.5	N/A
Keeper, pre-formed post Parkell Products, Inc. Farmingdale, NY	Yes*	1.5	1
Magna-Dent, large indirect keeper Dental Ventures of America, Yorba Linda, CA	Yes*	1.5	1
Palladium clad magnet Parkell Products, Inc. Farmingdale, NY	Yes	1.5	13
Palladium/palladium keeper Parkell Products, Inc. Farmingdale, NY	Yes*	1.5	13
Palladium/platinum casting alloy Parkell Products, Inc. Farmingdale, NY	Yes*	1.5	13
Permanent crown (amalgam) Ormco Corp.	No	1.5	3
Stainless steel clad magnet Parkell Products, Inc. Farmingdale, NY	Yes	1.5	13

APPENDIX I. *Continued.*

Implant, material, device, or object	Attraction/ deflection	Highest field strength (T)	Reference
Stainless steel keeper Parkell Products, Inc. Farmingdale, NY	Yes*	1.5	13
Silver point Union Broach Co., Inc. New York, NY	No	1.5	3
Titanium clad magnet Parkell Products, Inc. Farmingdale, NY	Yes	1.5	13
Halo vests and cervical fixation devices			
Ambulatory Halo System AOA Co. Greenwood, SC	Yes[a]	1.5	14
Bremer standard halo crown and vest Bremmer Medical Co. Jacksonville, FL	No	1.0	15
Bremmer halo system MR compatible Bremmer Medical Co. Jacksonville, FL	No	1.0	15
Closed-back halo (titanium) Ace Medical Co. Los Angeles, CA	No	1.5	16
EXO adjustable coller Florida Manufacturing Co. Daytona, FL	Yes[a]	1.0	15
Guilford cervical orthosis Guilford & Son, Ltd. Cleveland, OH	Yes[a]	1.0	15
Guilford cervical orthosis, modified Guilford & Son, Ltd. Cleveland, OH	No	1.0	15
Mark III halo vest (aluminum superstructure, stainless steel rivets, titanium bolts) Ace Medical Co. Los Angeles, CA	No	1.5	16
Mark IV halo vest (aluminum superstructure and titanium bolts) Ace Medical Co. Los Angeles, CA	No	1.5	16
MR-compatible halo vest and cervical orthosis Lerman & Son Co. Beverly Hills, CA	No	1.5	N/A
Open-back halo (aluminum) Ace Medical Co. Los Angeles, CA	No	1.5	16

APPENDIX I. *Continued.*

Implant, material, device, or object	Attraction/ deflection	Highest field strength (T)	Reference
Open-back halo with Delrin inserts for skull pins (aluminum and Delrin) Ace Medical Co. Los Angeles, CA	No	1.5	16
Philadelphia coller Philadelphia Coller Co. Westville, NJ	No	1.0	15
PMT halo cervical orthosis PMT Corp. Chanhassen, MN	No	1.0	15
PMT halo cervical orthosis with graphite rods and halo ring PMT Corp. Chanhassen, MN	No	1.0	15
S.O.M.I. cervical orthosis U.S. Manufacturing Co. Pasadena, CA	Yes[a]	1.0	15
Trippi-Wells tong (titanium) Ace Medical Co. Los Angeles, CA	No	1.5	16
Heart valve prostheses			
Beall Coratomic Inc. Indiana, PA	Yes*	2.35	17
Bjork-Shiley (convexo/concave) Shiley Inc. Irvine, CA	No	1.5	3
Bjork-Shiley (universal/spherical) Shiley Inc. Irvine, CA	Yes*	1.5	3
Bjork-Shiley, Model MBC Shiley Inc. Irvine, CA	Yes*	2.35	18
Bjork-Shiley Model 22 MBRC 11030 Shiley Inc. Irvine, CA	Yes*	2.35	18
CarboMedics Heart Valve Prosthesis Aortic Reduced, Model R500 Size 19 CarboMedics Austin, TX	No	1.5	19
CarboMedics Heart Valve Prosthesis Aortic Reduced, Model R500 Size 21 CarboMedics Austin, TX	No	1.5	19
CarboMedics Heart Valve Prosthesis Aortic Reduced, Model R500 Size 23 CarboMedics Austin, TX	No	1.5	19

APPENDIX I. *Continued.*

Implant, material, device, or object	Attraction/ deflection	Highest field strength (T)	Reference
CarboMedics Heart Valve Prosthesis Aortic Reduced, Model R500 Size 25 CarboMedics Austin, TX	No	1.5	19
CarboMedics Heart Valve Prosthesis Aortic Reduced, Model R500 Size 27 CarboMedics Austin, TX	No	1.5	19
CarboMedics Heart Valve Prosthesis Aortic Reduced, Model R500 Size 29 CarboMedics Austin, TX	No	1.5	19
CarboMedics Heart Valve Prosthesis Aortic Standard, Model 500 Size 31 CarboMedics Austin, TX	No	1.5	19
CarboMedics Heart Valve Prosthesis Mitral Standard, Model 700 Size 23 CarboMedics Austin, TX	No	1.5	19
CarboMedics Heart Valve Prosthesis Mitral Standard, Model 700 Size 25 CarboMedics Austin, TX	No	1.5	19
CarboMedics Heart Valve Prosthesis Mitral Standard, Model 700 Size 27 CarboMedics Austin, TX	No	1.5	19
CarboMedics Heart Valve Prosthesis Mitral Standard, Model 700 Size 29 CarboMedics Austin, TX	No	1.5	19
CarboMedics Heart Valve Prosthesis Mitral Standard, Model 700 Size 31 CarboMedics Austin, TX	No	1.5	19
CarboMedics Heart Valve Prosthesis Mitral Standard, Model 700 Size 33 CarboMedics Austin, TX	No	1.5	19
Carpentier-Edwards Annuloplasty Ring, Model 4400 Baxter Healthcare Corporation Santa Ana, CA	No	1.5	N/A

APPENDIX I. *Continued.*

Implant, material, device, or object	Attraction/ deflection	Highest field strength (T)	Reference
Carpentier-Edwards Annuloplasty Ring, Model 4500 Baxter Healthcare Corporation Santa Ana, CA	No	1.5	N/A
Carpentier-Edwards Annuloplasty Ring, Model 4600 Baxter Healthcare Corporation Santa Ana, CA	No	1.5	N/A
Carpentier-Edwards Bioprosthesis Model 2625 Baxter Healthcare Corporation Santa Ana, CA	No	1.5	N/A
Carpentier-Edwards Bioprosthesis Model 6625 Baxter Healthcare Corporation Santa Ana, CA	No	1.5	N/A
Carpentier-Edwards, Model 2650 American Edwards Laboratories Santa Ana, CA	Yes*	2.35	18
Carpentier-Edwards (porcine) American Edwards Laboratories Baxter Healthcare Corporation Santa Ana, CA	Yes*	2.35	18
Carpenter-Edwards Pericardial Bioprothesis, Model 2700 Baxter Healthcare Corporation Santa Ana, CA	No	1.5	N/A
Carpentier-Edwards Physio Annuloplasty Ring, Model 4450 Baxter Healthcare Corporation Santa Ana, CA	No	1.5	N/A
Cosgrove-Edwards Annuloplasty Ring, Model 4600 Baxter Healthcare Corporation Santa Ana, CA	No	1.5	N/A
Duraflex Low Pressure Bioprosthesis, Model 6625E6R-LP Baxter Healthcare Corporation Santa Ana, CA	No	1.5	N/A
Duraflex Low Pressure Bioprosthesis, Model 6625LP Baxter Healthcare Corporation Santa Ana, CA	No	1.5	N/A
Edwards-Duromedics Bileaflet Valve, Model 3160 Baxter Healthcare Corporation Santa Ana, CA	No	1.5	N/A
Edwards-Duromedics Bileaflet Valve, Model 9120 Baxter Healthcare Corporation Santa Ana, CA	No	1.5	N/A

APPENDIX I. *Continued.*

Implant, material, device, or object	Attraction/ deflection	Highest field strength (T)	Reference
Edwards TEKNA Bileaflet Valve, Model 3200 Baxter Healthcare Corporation Santa Ana, CA	No	1.5	N/A
Edwards TEKNA Bileaflet Valve, Model 9200 Baxter Healthcare Corporation Santa Ana, CA	No	1.5	N/A
Hall-Kaster, Model A7700 Medtronic Minneapolis, MN	Yes*	1.5	3
Hancock I (porcine) Johnson & Johnson Anaheim, CA	Yes*	1.5	3
Hancock II (porcine) Johnson & Johnson Anaheim, CA	Yes*	1.5	3
Hancock extracorporeal Model 242R Johnson & Johnson Anaheim, CA	Yes*	2.35	19
Hancock extracorporeal Model M 4365-33 Johnson & Johnson Anaheim, CA	Yes*	2.35	19
Hancock Vascor, Model 505 Johnson & Johnson Anaheim, CA	No	2.35	19
Inonescu-Shiley, Universal ISM	Yes*	2.35	19
Lillehi-Kaster, Model 300S Medical Inc. Inver Grove Heights, MN	Yes*	2.35	17
Lillehi-Kaster, Model 5009 Medical Inc. Inver Grove Heights, MN	Yes*	2.35	19
Medtronic Hall Medtronic Inc. Minneapolis, MN	Yes*	2.35	18
Medtronic Hall Model A7700-D-16 Medtronic Inc. Minneapolis, MN	Yes*	2.35	18
Omnicarbon, Model 35231029 Medical Inc. Inver Grove Heights, MN	Yes*	2.35	18
Omniscience, Model 6522 Medical Inc. Inver Grove Heights, MN	Yes*	2.35	18
Smeloff-Cutter Cutter Laboratories Berkeley, CA	Yes*	2.35	18
Sorin, No. 23	Yes*	1.5	20
Starr-Edwards, Model 1000 Baxter Healthcare Corporation Santa Ana, CA	Yes*	1.5	N/A

APPENDIX I. *Continued.*

Implant, material, device, or object	Attraction/ deflection	Highest field strength (T)	Reference
Starr-Edwards, Model 1200 Baxter Healthcare Corporation Santa Ana, CA	Yes*	1.5	N/A
Starr-Edwards, Model 1260 American Edwards Laboratories Baxter Healthcare Corporation Santa Ana, CA	Yes*	2.35	17
Starr-Edwards, Model 2300 Baxter Healthcare Corporation Santa Ana, CA	Yes*	1.5	N/A
Starr-Edwards, Model 2310 Baxter Healthcare Corporation Santa Ana, CA	Yes*	1.5	N/A
Starr-Edwards, Model 2320 American Edwards Laboratories Baxter Healthcare Corporation Santa Ana, CA	Yes*	2.35	17
Starr-Edwards, Model 2400 American Edwards Laboratories Baxter Healthcare Corporation Santa Ana, CA	No	1.5	3
Starr-Edwards, Model Pre 6000 American Edwards Laboratories Baxter Healthcare Corporation Santa Ana, CA	Yes*	2.35	17
Starr-Edwards, Model 6000 Baxter Healthcare Corporation Santa Ana, CA	Yes*	1.5	N/A
Starr-Edwards, Model 6120 Baxter Healthcare Corporation Santa Ana, CA	Yes*	1.5	N/A
Starr-Edwards, Model 6300 Baxter Healthcare Corporation Santa Ana, CA	Yes*	1.5	N/A
Starr-Edwards, Model 6310 Baxter Healthcare Corporation Santa Ana, CA	Yes*	1.5	N/A
Starr-Edwards, Model 6320 Baxter Healthcare Corporation Santa Ana, CA	Yes*	1.5	N/A
Starr-Edwards, Model 6400 Baxter Healthcare Corporation Santa Ana, CA	Yes*	1.5	N/A
Starr-Edwards, Model 6520 Baxter Healthcare Corporation Santa Ana, CA	Yes*	2.35	19
St. Jude St. Jude Medical Inc. St. Paul, MN	No	1.5	3
St. Jude, Model A 101 St. Jude Medical Inc. St. Paul, MN	Yes*	2.35	19

APPENDIX I. *Continued.*

Implant, material, device, or object	Attraction/ deflection	Highest field strength (T)	Reference
St. Jude, Model M 101 St. Jude Medical Inc. St. Paul, MN	Yes*	2.35	19
Intravascular coils, filters, and stents			
Amplatz IVC filter Cook, Inc. Bloomington, IN	No	4.7	21
Cook occluding spring embolization coil, MWCE-338-5-10	Yes*†	1.5	N/A
Cook-Z Stent Gianturco-Rosch Biliary Design 10 mm × 3 cm Cook, Inc. Bloomington, IN	Yes*†	1.5	N/A
Cook-Z Stent Gianturco-Rosch Tracheobronchial Design 20 mm × 5 cm Cook, Inc. Bloomington, IN	Yes*†	1.5	N/A
Cragg Nitinol spiral filter	No	4.7	21
Flower embolization microcoil (platinum) Target Therapeutics San Jose, CA	No	1.5	22
Gianturco embolization coil Cook, Inc. Bloomington, IN	Yes*†	1.5	21
Gianturco bird nest IVC filter Cook, Inc. Bloomington, IN	Yes*†	1.5	21, 23
Gianturco zig-zag stent Cook, Inc. Bloomington, IN	Yes*†	1.5	21
Greenfield vena cava filter, Stainless steel MD Tech Watertown, MA	Yes*†	1.5	21, 24
Greenfield vena cava filter, Titanium alloy Ormco Glendora, CA	No	1.5	21
Gunther IVC filter William Cook, Europe	Yes*†	1.5	21
Hilal embolization microcoil Cook, Inc. Bloomington, IN	No	1.5	22
IVC venous clip (Teflon) Pilling Co.	No	1.5	N/A
Maas helical IVC filter Medinvent Lausanne, Switzerland	No	4.7	21

APPENDIX I. *Continued.*

Implant, material, device, or object	Attraction/ deflection	Highest field strength (T)	Reference
helical endovascular stent ...vent Lausanne, Switzerland	No	4.7	21
Mobin-Uddin IVC/umbrella filter American Edwards Santa Ana, CA	No	4.7	21
New retrievable IVC filter Thomas Jefferson University Philadelphia, PA	Yes*†	1.5	21
Palmaz endovascular stent Johnson & Johnson Interventional Warren, NJ	No	1.5	N/A
Palmaz endovascular stent Ethicon	Yes*†	1.5	21
Palmaz-Shatz balloon-expandable stent Johnson & Johnson Interventional Warren, NJ	Yes*†	1.5	N/A
Passager Stent (tantalum) 4 mm × 30 mm Meadox Surgimed Oakland, NJ	No	1.5	N/A
Passager Stent (tantalum) 10 mm × 30 mm Meadox Surgimed Oakland, NJ	No	1.5	N/A
Strecker stent (tantalum) MD Tech Watertown, MA	No	1.5	25
Wiktor coronary artery stent Medtronic Inverventional Vascular, Inc.	No	1.5	N/A
Ureteral stent	No	1.5	N/A
Ocular implants and devices			
Clip 50, double tantalum clip Mira Inc.	No	1.5	26
Clip 51, single tantalum clip Mira Inc.	No	1.5	26
Clip 52, single tantalum clip Mira Inc.	No	1.5	26
Clip 250, double tantalum clip Mira Inc.	No	1.5	26
Double tantalum clip Storz Instrument Co.	No	1.5	26
Double tantalum clip style 250 Storz Instrument Co.	No	1.5	26
Fatio eyelid spring/wire	Yes	1.5	27
Gold eyelid spring	No	1.5	N/A

APPENDIX I. *Continued.*

Implant, material, device, or object	Attraction/ deflection	Highest field strength (T)	Reference
Intraocular lens implant Binkhorst, iridocapsular lense, platinum-iridium loop	No	1.5	28
Intraocular lens implant Binkhorst, iridocapsular lense, platinum-iridium loop	No	1.0	28
Intraocular lens implant Binkhorst, iridocapsular lense, titanium loop	No	1.0	28
Intraocular lens implant Worst, platinum clip lense	No	1.0	28
Retinal tack (303 SS) Bascom Palmer Eye Institute	No	1.5	29
Retinal tack (titanium alloy) Coopervision Irvine, CA	No	1.5	29
Retinal tack (303 SS) Duke	No	1.5	29
Retinal tack (cobalt/nickel) Grieshaber Fallsington, PA	No	1.5	29
Retinal tack, Norton staple (platinum/ rhodium) Norton	No	1.5	29
Retinal tack (aluminum textraoxide) Ruby	No	1.5	29
Retinal tack (SS-martensitic) Western European	Yes	1.5	29
Single tantalum clip	No	1.5	26
Troutman magnetic ocular implant	Yes	1.5	N/A
Unitech round wire eye spring	Yes	1.5	N/A
Orthopedic implants, materials, and devices			
AML femoral component bipolar hip prothesis Zimmer Warsaw, IN	No	1.5	3
Cervical wire, 18 gauge (316L SS)	No	0.3	30
Charnley-Muller hip prosthesis Protasyl-10 alloy	No	0.3	N/A
Cortical bone screw, large (titanium, Ti-6A-4V alloy) Zimmer Warsaw, IN	No	1.5	31
Cortical bone screw, small (titanium, Ti-6A-4V alloy) Zimmer Warsaw, IN	No	1.5	31
Cotrel rods with hooks (316L SS)	No	0.3	30
Cotrel rod (SS-ASTM, grade 2)	No	1.5	N/A
DTT, device for transverse traction (316L SS)	No	0.3	30
Drummond wire (316L SS)	No	0.3	30

APPENDIX I. *Continued.*

Implant, material, device, or object	Attraction/ deflection	Highest field strength (T)	Reference
Endoscopic noncannulated interference screw (titanium) Acufex Microsurgical Norwood, MA	No	1.5	31
Fixation staple (cobalt chromium alloy, ASTM F 75) Richards Medical Co. Memphis, TN	No	1.5	31
Halifax clamps American Medical Electronics Richardson, TX	No	1.5	N/A
Harrington compression rod with hooks and nuts (316L SS)	No	0.3	30
Harrington distraction rod with hooks (316L SS)	No	0.3	30
Harris hip prosthesis Zimmer Warsaw, IN	No	1.5	3
Jewettt nail Zimmer Warsaw, IN	No	1.5	3
Kirschner intermedullary rod Kirschner Medical Timonium, MD	No	1.5	3
"L" Rod (cobalt-nickel) Richards Medical Co. Memphis, TN	No	1.5	N/A
Luque Wire	No	0.3	30
Moe spinal instrumentation Zimmer Warsaw, IN	No	1.5	N/A
Perfix interence screw (17-4 stainless steel, A 630-Cr17) Instrument Makar Okemos, MI	Yes	1.5	31
Rusch Rod	No	1.5	N/A
Spinal L-Rod DePuy Warsaw, IN	No	1.5	N/A
Stainless steel plate Zimmer Warsaw, IN	No	1.5	3
Stainless steel screw Zimmer Warsaw, IN	No	1.5	3
Staple plate, large (Zimaloy) Zimmer Warsaw, IN	No	1.5	3
Stainless steel mesh Zimmer Warsaw, IN	No	1.5	3
Stainless steel wire Zimmer Warsaw, IN	No	1.5	3

APPENDIX I. *Continued.*

Implant, material, device, or object	Attraction/ deflection	Highest field strength (T)	Reference
Synthes AO DCP 2, 3, 4, 5 hole plate	No	1.5	N/A
Zielke rod with screw, washer and nut (316L SS)	No	0.3	30
Otologic implants			
Austin tytan piston (titanium) Treace Medical Nashville, TN	No	1.5	32
Berger "V" bobbin ventilation tube (titanium) Richards Medical Co. Memphis, TN	No	1.5	32
Causse Flex H/A, notched, offset, partial ossicular prosthesis (titanium) Microtek Medical, Inc. Memphis, TN	No	1.5	33
Causse Flex H/A, notched, offset, total ossicular prosthesis (titanium) Microtek Medical Inc. Memphis, TN	No	1.5	33
Cochlear implant 3M/House	Yes	0.6	34
Cochlear implant 3M/Vienna	Yes	0.6	34
Cochlear implant Nucleus Mini 20-channel Cochlear Corporation Engelwood, CO	Yes	1.5	35
Cody tack	No	0.6	34
Ehmke hook stapes prosthesis (platinum) Richards Medical Co. Memphis, TN	No	1.5	32
Flex H/A notched offset total ossicular prosthesis (316LVM SS) Microtek Medical, Inc. Memphis, TN	No	1.5	33
Flex H/A offset partial ossicular prosthesis (316LVM SS) Microtek Medical, Inc. Memphis, TN	No	1.5	33
Fisch piston (Teflon, stainless steel) Richards Medical Co. Memphis, TN	No	1.5	35
House single loop (ASTM-318-76, Grade 2 stainless steel) Storz St. Louis, MO	No	1.5	28
House single loop (tantalum) Storz St. Louis, MO	No	1.5	32

APPENDIX I. *Continued.*

Implant, material, device, or object	Attraction/ deflection	Highest field strength (T)	Reference
House double loop (tantalum) Storz St. Louis, MO	No	1.5	32
House double loop (ASTM-318-76 Grade 2 stainless steel) Storz St. Louis, MO	No	1.5	32
House-type incus prosthesis	No	0.6	N/A
House-type wire loop stapes prosthesis (316L SS) Richards Medical Co. Memphis, TN	No	1.5	32, 35
House-type stainless steel piston and wire (ASTM-318-76 Grade 2 stainless steel) Xomed-Treace Inc. A Bristol-Myers Squibb Co.	No	1.5	32
House wire (tantalum) Otomed	No	0.5	36
House wire (stainless steel) Otomed	No	0.5	36
McGee piston stapes prosthesis (316L SS) Richards Medical Co. Memphis, TN	No	1.5	32, 35
McGee piston stapes prosthesis (platinum/316L SS) Richards Medical Co. Memphis, TN	No	1.5	32, 35
McGee piston stapes prosthesis (platinum/Cr17-Ni4, SS) Richards Medical Co. Memphis, TN	Yes	1.5	35
McGee Sheperd's Crook stapes prosthesis (316L SS) Richards Medical Co. Memphis, TN	No	1.5	32
Plasti-pore piston (316L SS/plasti-pore material) Richards Medical Co. Memphis, TN	No	1.5	32, 35
Platinum ribbon loop stapes prosthesis (platinum) Richards Medical Co. Memphis, TN	No	1.5	32
Reuter bobbin ventilation tube (316L SS) Richards Medical Co. Memphis, TN	No	1.5	32
Richards bucket handle stapes prosthesis (316L SS) Richards Medical Co. Memphis, TN	No	1.5	32, 35
Reuter drain tube	No	1.5	32

APPENDIX I. *Continued.*

Implant, material, device, or object	Attraction/ deflection	Highest field strength (T)	Reference
Richards Plasti-pore with Armstrong-style platinum ribbon Richards Medical Co. Memphis, TN	No	1.5	32
Richards platinum Teflon piston, 0.6 mm (Teflon, platinum) Richards Medical Co. Memphis, TN	No	1.5	35
Richards platinum Teflon piston, 0.8 mm (Teflon, platinum) Richards Medical Co. Memphis, TN	No	1.5	35
Richards piston stapes prosthesis (platinum/fluoroplastic) Richards Medical Co. Memphis, TN	No	1.5	32
Richards Shepherd's crook (platinum) Richards Medical Co. Memphis, TN	No	0.5	36
Richards Teflon piston (Teflon) Richards Medical Co. Memphis, TN	No	1.5	35
Robinson-Moon-Lippy offset stapes prosthesis (ASTM-318-76 Grade 2 stainless steel) Storz St. Louis, MO	No	1.5	32
Robinson-Moon offset stapes prosthesis (ASTM-318-76 Grade 2 stainless steel) Storz St. Louis, MO	No	1.5	32
Robinson incus replacement prosthesis (ASTM-318-76 Grade 2 stainless steel) Storz St. Louis, MO	No	1.5	32
Robinson stapes prosthesis (ASTM-318-76 Grade 2 stainless steel) Storz St. Louis, MO	No	1.5	32
Ronis piston stapes prosthesis (316L SS/fluoroplastic) Richards Medical Co. Memphis, TN	No	1.5	32
Schea cup piston stapes prosthesis (platinum/fluoroplastic) Richards Medical Co. Memphis, TN	No	1.5	32, 35
Schea malleus attachment piston (Teflon) Richards Medical Co. Memphis, TN	No	1.5	35

APPENDIX I. *Continued.*

Implant, material, device, or object	Attraction/ deflection	Highest field strength (T)	Reference
Schea stainless steel and Teflon wire prosthesis (Teflon, 316 L SS) Richards Medical Co. Memphis, TN	No	1.5	35
Scheer piston stapes prosthesis (316L SS/fluoroplastic) Richards Medical Co. Memphis, TN	No	1.5	32
Scheer piston (Teflon, 316L SS) Richards Medical Co. Memphis, TN	No	1.5	30
Schuknecht gelfoam and wire prosthesis, Armstrong style (316L SS) Richards Medical Co. Memphis, TN	No	1.5	37
Schuknecht piston stapes prosthesis (316L SS/fluoroplastic) Richards Medical Co. Memphis, TN	No	1.5	32
Schuknecht Tef-wire incus attachment (ASTM-318-76 Grade 2 stainless steel) Storz St. Louis, MO	No	1.5	32, 35
Schuknecht tef-wire malleus attachment (ASTM-318-76 Grade 2 stainless steel) Storz St. Louis, MO	No	1.5	32, 35
Schuknecht Teflon wire piston 0.6 mm (Teflon, 316L SS) Richards Medical Co. Memphis, TN	No	1.5	35
Schuknecht Teflon wire piston 0.8 mm (Teflon, 316L SS) Richards Medical Co. Memphis, TN	No	1.5	35
Sheehy incus replacement (ASTM-318-76 Grade 2 stainless steel) Storz St. Louis, MO	No	1.5	32
Sheehy incus strut (316L SS) Richards Medical Co. Memphis, TN	No	1.5	35
Sheehy-type incus replacement strut (Teflon, 316L SS) Richards Medical Co. Memphis, TN	No	1.5	32
Silverstein malleus clip, ventilation tube (Teflon, 316L SS) Richards Medical Co. Memphis, TN	No	1.5	35

APPENDIX I. *Continued.*

Implant, material, device, or object	Attraction/ deflection	Highest field strength (T)	Reference
Spoon bobbin ventilation tube (316L SS) Richards Medical Co. Memphis, TN	No	1.5	32
Stapes, fluoroplastic/platinum, piston Microtek Medical, Inc. Memphis, TN	No	1.5	33
Stapes, fluoroplastic/stainless steel piston (316LVM SS) Microtek Medical, Inc. Memphis, TN	No	1.5	33
Tantalum wire loop stages prosthesis (tantalum) Richards Medical Co. Memphis, TN	No	1.5	32, 35
Tef-platinum piston (platinum) Xomed-Treace Inc. A Bristol-Myers Squibb Co.	No	1.5	32
Total ossibular replacement prosthesis (TORP) (316L SS) Richards Medical Co. Memphis, TN	No	1.5	35
Trapeze ribbon loop stapes prosthesis (platinum) Richards Medical Co. Memphis, TN	No	1.5	32
Williams microclip (316L SS) Richards Medical Co. Memphis, TN	No	1.5	32
Xomed stapes (ASTM-318-76 Grade 2 SS) Xomed-Treace Inc. A Bristol-Myers Squibb Co.	No	1.5	32
Xomed ceravital partial ossicular prosthesis	No	1.5	N/A
Xomed Baily stapes implant	No	1.5	32
Xomed stapes prosthesis Robinson-style Richard's Co. Nashville, TN	No	1.5	32
Patent ductus arteriosus (PDA), atrial septal defect (ASD), and ventricular septal defect (VSD) occluders			
Rashkind PDA Occlusion Implant 12 mm, lot n. 07IC1391, (304V SS) C.R. Bard, Inc. Billerica, MA	Yes†	1.5	38
Rashkind PDA Occlusion Implant 17 mm, lot no. 514486, (304 V SS) C.R. Bard, Inc. Billerica, MA	Yes†	1.5	38

APPENDIX I. *Continued.*

Implant, material, device, or object	Attraction/ deflection	Highest field strength (T)	Reference
Lock Clamshell Septal Occlusion Implant 17 mm, lot no. 07BCO321, (304 V SS) C.R. Bard, Inc. Billerica, MA	Yes†	1.5	38
Lock Clamshell Septal Occlusion Implant 23 mm, lot no. 07CC1903, (304 V SS) C.R. Bard, Inc. Billerica, MA	Yes†	1.5	38
Lock Clamshell Septal Occlusion Implant 28 mm, lot no. 07BC1557, (304 V SS) C.R. Bard, Inc. Billerica, MA	Yes†	1.5	38
Lock Clamshell Septal Occlusion Implant 33 mm, lot no. 07AC1785, (304 V SS) C.R. Bard, Inc. Billerica, MA	Yes†	1.5	38
Lock Clamshell Septal Occlusion Implant 40 mm, lot no. 07AC1785, (304 V SS) C.R. Bard, Inc. Billerica, MA	Yes†	1.5	38
Bard Clamshell Septal Umbrella 17 mm, lot no. 09ED1230, (MP35n) C.R. Bard, Inc. Billerica, MA	No	1.5	38
Bard Clamshell Septal Umbrella 23 mm, lot no. 09ED1232, (MP35n) C.R. Bard, Inc. Billerica, MA	No	1.5	38
Bard Clamshell Septal Umbrella 28 mm, lot no. 09ED1233, (MP35n) C.R. Bard, Inc. Billerica, MA	No	1.5	38
Bard Clamshell Septal Umbrella 33 mm, lot no. 09ED1234, (MP35n) C.R. Bard, Inc. Billerica, MA	No	1.5	38
Bard Clamshell Septal Umbrella 40 mm, lot no. 09ED1231, (MP35n) C.R. Bard, Inc. Bellerica, MA	No	1.5	38

APPENDIX I. *Continued.*

Implant, material, device, or object	Attraction/ deflection	Highest field strength (T)	Reference
Pellets and bullets			
BB's (Daisy)	Yes	1.5	N/A
BB's (Crosman)	Yes	1.5	N/A
Bullet, .380 inch (copper, plastic, lead) Glaser	No	1.5	39
Bullet, .44 inch (Teflon, bronze) North American Ordinance	No	1.5	39
Bullet, 7.62 × 39 mm (copper, steel) Norinco	Yes	1.5	39
Bullet, .357 inch (copper, lead) Cascade	No	1.5	39
Bullet, .357 inch (lead) Remington	No	1.5	39
Bullet, .357 inch (aluminum, lead) Winchester	No	1.5	39
Bullet, 9 mm (copper, lead) Remington	No	1.5	39
Bullet, .380 inch (copper, nickel, lead) Winchester	Yes	1.5	39
Bullet, .357 inch (nylon, lead) Smith & Wesson	No	1.5	39
Bullet, .357 inch (nickel, copper, lead) Winchester	No	1.5	39
Bullet, .45 inch (steel, lead) Evansville Ordinance	Yes	1.5	39
Bullet, .357 inch (steel, lead) Fiocchi	No	1.5	39
Bullet, .357 inch (copper, lead) Hornady	No	1.5	39
Bullet, 9 mm (copper, lead) Norma	Yes	1.5	39
Bullet, .357 inch (bronze, plastic) Patton-Morgan	No	1.5	39
Bullet, .357 inch (copper, lead) Patton-Morgan	No	1.5	39
Bullet, .45 inch (copper, lead) Samson	No	1.5	39
Shot, 12 gauge, size: 00 (copper, lead) Federal	No	1.5	39
Shot, 7 1/2 (lead)	No	1.5	39
Shot, 4 (lead)	No	1.5	39
Shot, 00 buckshot (lead)	No	1.5	39
Penile implants			
Penile implant, AMS 700 CX Inflatable American Medical Systems Minnetonka, MN	No	1.5	40
Penile implant AMS Hydroflex self-contained	No	1.5	N/A

APPENDIX I. *Continued.*

Implant, material, device, or object	Attraction/ deflection	Highest field strength (T)	Reference
Penile implant AMS Malleable 600 American Medical Systems Minnetonka, MN	No	1.5	40
Penile implant, Duraphase	Yes	1.5	N/A
Penile implant, Flexi-Flate Surgitek Medical Engineering Corp. Racine, WI	No	1.5	40
Penile implant, Flexi-Rod (Standard) Surgitek Medical Engineering Corp. Racine, WI	No	1.5	40
Penile implant, Osmond, external	No	1.5	N/A
Penile implant, Flex-Rod II (Firm) Surgitek Medical Engineering Corp. Racine, WI	No	1.5	40
Penile implant, Jonas Dacomed Corp. Minneapolis, MN	No	1.5	40
Penile implant, Mentor Flexible Mentor Corp. Minneapolis, MN	No	1.5	40
Penile implant, Mentor Inflatable Mentor Corp. Minneapolis, MN	No	1.5	40
Penile implant, OmniPhase Dacomed Corp. Minneapolis, MN	Yes	1.5	40
Penile implant, Uniflex 1000	No	1.5	N/A
Vascular access ports and catheters			
A Port Implantable Access System (titanium) Therex Corporation Walpole, MA	No	1.5	41
Access Implantable (titanium/plastic) Celsa Cedex, France	No	1.5	41
Broviac Catheter single lumen (silicone, barium sulfate) Bard Access Systems Salt Lake City, UT	No	1.5	42
Button (polysulfone polymer, silicone) Infusaid Inc. Norwood, MA	No	1.5	41
CathLink LP (titanium) Bard Access Systems Salt Lake City, UT	No	1.5	42
CathLink SP (titanium) Bard Access Systems Salt Lake City, UT	No	1.5	42
Celsite Port and Catheter (titanium) B. Braun Medical Bethlehem, PA	No	1.5	41

APPENDIX I. *Continued.*

Implant, material, device, or object	Attraction/ deflection	Highest field strength (T)	Reference
Dome Port (titanium) Davol Inc., Subsidiary of C.R. Bard, Inc. Cranston, RI	No	1.5	41
Dual MicroPort (polysulfone polymer, silicone) Infusaid Inc. Norwood, MA	No	1.5	41
Dual MacroPort (polysulfone polymer, silicone) Infusaid Inc. Norwood, MA	No	1.5	41
Groshung Catheter	Yes*	1.5	N/A
Groshong Catheter, dual lumen, 9.5 Fr. (silicone, barium sulfact, tungsten) Bard Access Systems Salt Lake City, UT	No	1.5	42
Groshong Catheter, single lumen, 8 Fr. (silicone, barium sulfate, tungsten) Bard Access Systems Salt Lake City, UT	No	1.5	42
Hickman Catheter, single lumen, 3.0 Fr. Bard Access Systems Salt Lake City, UT	No	1.5	42
Hickman Catheter, dual lumen, 10.0 Fr. (silicone, barium sulfate) Bard Access Systems Salt Lake City, UT	No	1.5	42
Hickman Port (316L SS) Davol Inc., Subsidiary of C.R. Bard, Inc. Cranston, RI	Yes*	1.5	41
Hickman Port, Pediatric (titanium) Davol, Inc., Subsidiary of C.R. Bard, Inc. Salt Lake City, UT	No	1.5	41
Hickman subcutaneous port attachable venous catheter (titanium) Davol, Inc. Subsidiary of C.R. Bard, Inc. Salt Lake City, UT	No	1.5	42
Hickman subcutaneous port venous catheter preconnected (titanium) Davol Inc., Subsidiary of C.R. Bard, Inc. Salt Lake City, UT	No	1.5	41
Hickman subcutaneous port (SS, titanium, plastic components) Davol, Inc. Subsidiary of C.R. Bard, Inc. Salt Lake City, UT	No	1.5	42

APPENDIX I. *Continued.*

Implant, material, device, or object	Attraction/ deflection	Highest field strength (T)	Reference
HMP-Port (plastic) Horizon Medical Products Atlanta, GA	No	1.5	41
Implantofix II (polysulfone) Burron Medical Inc. Bethlehem, PA	No	1.5	41
Infusaid, Model 350 (titanium) Infusaid Inc. Norwood, MA	No	1.5	41
Infusaid, Model 600 (titanium) Infusaid Inc. Norwood, MA	No	1.5	41
Infuse-A-Kit (plastic) Infusaid Norwood, MA	No	1.5	41
LifePort, Model 6013 (Delrin) Strato Medical Corporation Beverly, MA	No	1.5	41
Lifeport, Model 1013 (titanium) Strato Medical Corp. Beverly, MA	No	1.5	41
LifePort Vascular Access System attachable catheter (plastic) Strato Medical Group Beverly, MA	No	1.5	41
LifePort Vascular Access System attachable catheter and bayonet lock ring (plastic) Strato Medical Group Beverly, MA	No	1.5	41
Low Profile MRI Port (Delrin) Davol, Inc., Subsidiary of C.R. Bard, Inc. Salt Lake City, UT	No	1.5	42
Low Profile MRI Port (titanium) Davol, Inc., Subsidiary of C.R. Bard, Inc. Salt Lake City, UT	No	1.5	42
Macroport (polysulfone, titanium) Infusaid Inc. Norwood, MA	No	1.5	N/A
Mediport Cormed	No	1.5	N/A
MicroPort (polysulfone, polymersilicone) Infusaid Inc. Norwood, MA	No	1.5	41
MRI Dual Port (Delrin, titanium) Davol, Inc., Subsidiary of C.R. Bard, Inc. Salt Lake City, UT	No	1.5	42

APPENDIX I. *Continued.*

Implant, material, device, or object	Attraction/ deflection	Highest field strength (T)	Reference
MRI Hard Base Implanted Port (plastic) Davol, Inc., Subsidiary of C.R. Bard, Inc. Salt Lake City, UT	No	1.5	41
MRI Port (Delrin, silicone) Davol, Inc., Subsidiary of C.R. Bard, Inc. Salt Lake City, UT	No	1.5	41
Norport-AC (titanium) Norfolk Medical Skokie, IL	No	1.5	41
Norport-DL (316L SS) Norfolk Medical Skokie, IL	No	1.5	41
Norport-LS (titanium) Norfolk Medical Skokie, IL	No	1.5	41
Norport-LS (316L SS) Norfolk Medical Skokie, IL	No	1.5	41
Norport-LS (polysulfone) Norfolk Medical Skokie, IL	No	1.5	41
Norport-PT (titanium) Norfolk Medical Skokie, IL	No	1.5	41
Norport-SP (polysulfone, silicone rubber, Dacron) Norfolk Medical Skokie, IL	No	1.5	41
OmegaPort Access System (titanium and 316L SS) Norfolk Medical Skokie, IL	No	1.5	41
OmegaPort-SR Access System (titanium and 316L SS) Norfolk Medical Skokie, IL	No	1.5	41
Open-ended Catheter, single lumen, 6 Fr. (ChronoFlex) Davol, Inc., Subsidiary of C.R. Bard, Inc. Salt Lake City, UT	No	1.5	42
Open-ended Catheter, single lumen, 8 Fr. (ChronoFlex) Davol, Inc., Subsidiary of C.R. Bard, Inc. Salt Lake City, UT	No	1.5	42
OptiPort Catheter, single lumen (silicone) Simms-Deltec St. Paul, MN	No	1.5	42

APPENDIX I. *Continued.*

Implant, material, device, or object	Attraction/ deflection	Highest field strength (T)	Reference
PeriPort (polysulfone, titanium) Infusaid Inc. Norwood, MA	No	1.5	41
Phantom Norfolk Medical Skokie, IL	No	1.5	41
Plastic Port (polysulfone, titanium) Cardial Saint-Etienne, France	No	1.5	42
Port-A-Cath, P.A.S. Port Portal (titanium) Pharmacia Deltec St. Paul, MN	No	1.5	41
Port-A-Cath Titanium Dual Lumen Portal (titanium) Pharmacia Deltec St. Paul, MN	No	1.5	41
Port-A-Cath Titanium Peritoneal Portal (titanium) Pharmacia Deltec St. Paul, MN	No	1.5	41
Port-A-Cath Titanium Venous Low Profile Portal (titanium) Pharmacia Deltec St. Paul, MN	No	1.5	41
Port-A-Cath Titanium Venous Portal (titanium) Pharmacia Deltec St. Paul, MN	No	1.5	41
Porto-cath Pharmacin, NUTECH Pharmacia Deltec St. Paul, MN	No	1.5	41
Q-Port (316L SS) Quinton Instrument Co. Seattle, WA	Yes*	1.5	41
S.E.A. (titanium) Harbor Medical Devices, Inc. Boston, MA	No	1.5	41
Snap-Lock (titanium, polysulfone polymer, silicone) Infusaid Inc. Norwood, MA	No	1.5	41
Synchromed, Model 8500-1 (titanium, thermoplastic, silicone) Medtronic, Inc. Minneapolis, MN	No	1.5	41
Triple Lumen Arrow International, Inc. Reading, PA	No	1.5	N/A
Vasport (titanium/fluoropolymer) Gish Biomedical, Inc. Santa Ana, CA	No	1.5	41

APPENDIX I. *Continued.*

Implant, material, device, or object	Attraction/ deflection	Highest field strength (T)	Reference
Vascular Access Catheter With Repair Kit PMT Corporation Chanhassen, MN	No	1.5	N/A
Vital-Port (polysulfone, titanium) Cook Pacemaker Corp. Leechburg, PA	No	1.5	42
Vital-Port, Dual (polysulfone, titanium) Cook Pacemaker Corp. Leechburg, PA	No	1.5	42
Miscellaneous			
Accusite pH Enteral Feeding System pH Site Locator 10 Fr Zinetics Medical Salt Lake City, UT	No††††	1.5	N/A
Artificial urinary sphincter AMS 800 American Medical Systems	No	1.5	3
Biosearch endo-feeding tude	No	1.5	N/A
Cerebral ventricular shunt tube connector, Accu-Flow, straight Codman Randolf, MA	No	1.5	3
Cerebral ventricular shunt tube connector, Accu-flow right angle Codman Randolf, MA	No	1.5	3
Cerebral ventricular shunt tube connector, Accu-flow, T-connector Codman Randolf, MA	No	1.5	3
Cerebral ventricular shunt tube connector (type unknown)	Yes	0.147	1
Contraceptive diaphragm All Flex Ortho Pharmaceutical Raritan, NJ	Yes*	1.5	3
Contraceptive diaphragm Flat Spring Ortho Pharmaceutical Raritan, NJ	Yes*	1.5	3
Contraceptive diaphragm Koroflex Young Drug Products Piscataway, NJ	Yes*	1.5	3
Cranial Ceramic Drill bit (ceramic) MicroSurgical Techniques Inc. Fort Collins, CO	No	1.5	43

APPENDIX I. *Continued.*

Implant, material, device, or object	Attraction/ deflection	Highest field strength (T)	Reference
Deponit (nitroglycerin transdermal delivery system) aluminized plastic Schwarz Pharma Milwaukee, WI	No†††	1.5	N/A
EEG electrodes, Pediatric E-5-GH (gold plated silver) Grass Co. Quincy, MA	No	0.3	44
EEG electrodes, Adult E-6-GH (gold plated silver) Grass Co. Quincy, MA	No	0.3	44
Endotracheal tube with metal ring marker Trachmate	No	1.5	N/A
Flex-tip Plus Epidural catheter (304V SS) Arrow International Inc. Reading, PA	Yes††††	1.5	N/A
Forceps (titanium)	No	1.39	1
Forceps (ceramic) MicroSurgical Techniques Inc. Fort Collins, CO	No	1.5	43
Hakim valve and pump	No	1.39	1
Intraflex Feeding Tube tungstun weight, plastic	No	1.5	N/A
Intrauterine contraceptive device (IUD), Copper T Searle Pharmaceuticals Chicago, IL	No	1.5	45
Intrauterine contraceptive device (IUD) Lippey loop, plastic	No	1.5	N/A
Intrauterine contraceptive device (IUD) Perigard Gyne Pharmaceuticals	No	1.5	N/A
Mercury Duotube-feeding	No	1.5	N/A
Mitek anchor	No	1.5	N/A
Scalpel, Microsharp Ceramic Scalpels (#10, #11, #11c, #15, #15c) MicroSurgical Techniques Inc. Fort Collins, CO	No	1.5	43
Scalpel (SS)	Yes	1.5	N/A
Shunt valve, Holtertype The Holter Co. Bridgeport, PA	Yes*	1.5	46
Shunt valve, Holter-Hausner type Holter-Hausner, Inc. Bridgeport, PA	No	1.5	46

APPENDIX I. *Continued.*

Implant, material, device, or object	Attraction/ deflection	Highest field strength (T)	Reference
Sophy adjustable pressure valve	Yes	1.5T	47
SychroMed, implantable drug infusion device Medtronic	No†††	1.5T	N/A
Super ArrowFlex PSI 9 Fr × 11 cm (304V SS) Arrow International Inc. Reading, PA	Yes††††	1.5	N/A
Super ArrowFlex PSI 10 Fr × 65 cm (304V SS) Arrow International Inc. Reading, PA	Yes††††	1.5	N/A
Swan-Ganz thermodilution catheter American Edwards Laboratories Irvine, CA	No††	1.5	48
Swan-Ganz triple-lumen thermodilution catheter American Edwards Laboratories Irvine, CA	No††	1.5	N/A
Tantalum powder	No	1.39	1
TheraCath (304 V SS) Arrow International Inc. Reading, PA	Yes††††	1.5	N/A
Tweezers (ceramic) MicroSurgical Techniques Inc. Fort Collins, CO	No	1.5	43
Vascular marker, O-ring washer (302 SS) PIC Design, Middlebury, CT	Yes*	1.5	N/A
Vitallium implant	No	1.5	N/A
Winged infusion set MRI compatible E-Z-EM Inc. Westbury, NY	No	1.5	49

TABLE FOOTNOTES

"Highest field strength" refers to the highest intensity of the static magnetic field that was used for the evaluation of deflection force, or magnetic field attraction of the various metallic implant materials, devices, or objects tested.

*Denotes the metallic implants, materials, devices, or objects that were considered to be safe for patients undergoing MR procedures despite being attracted by static magnetic fields. For example, certain prosthetic heart valves were attracted to the magnetic fields but the attractive forces were considered to be less than the forces exerted on the prosthetic heart valves by the beating heart.

†Ferromagnetic coils, filters, stents, and cardiac occluders typically become firmly incorporated into the vessel wall several weeks following placement. Therefore, it is unlikely that they will be moved or dislodged by attraction to magnetic fields. Patients with coils, filters, and stents marked "*†" in the attraction/deflection column should wait a minimum 6 weeks prior to an MR procedure to assure firm implantation of the implant into the vessel wall.

††Although the triple-lumen thermodilution Swan-Ganz catheter has no attraction to a static magnetic field there was a report of a catheter "melting" in a patient during an MR procedure. Therefore, this catheter would be considered a relative contraindication for patients undergoing MR procedures. This is also a potential problem with devices that have a similar design.

†††The Deponit, nitroglycerin transdermal delivery system, although not attracted to the static magnetic field of an MR system, has been found to heat excessively during MR imaging. This excessive heating may burn a patient wearing this patch. Therefore, it is recommended that the patch be removed prior to the MR procedure and a new patch should be applied immediately after the examination.

††††These devices are attracted to the static magnetic field of the MR system, however, because of the relative amount of attractive force and their in vivo use, these devices are unlikely to pose a hazard associated with dislodgement. The potential risk to performing MR procedures in patients with these devices is related to induced current and excessive heating. Therefore, it is inadvisable to perform MR procedures patients with these devices.

[a] These halo vests are known to have ferromagnetic components. However, the relative amount of attraction to the magnetic field was not determined.

N/A, Not applicable. These implants, materials, devices, or objects were tested for ferromagnetism using standardized techniques. However, the data has not been published.

Manufacturer information was provided if known.

SS, Stainless steel.

REFERENCES

1. New PFJ, Rosen BR, Brady TJ, et al. Potential hazards and artifacts of ferromagnetic and nonferromagnetic surgical and dental materials and devices in nuclear magnetic resonance imaging. *Radiology* 1983;147:139–148.
2. Becker RL, Norfray JF, Teitelbaum GP, et al. MR imaging in patients with intracranial aneurysm clips. *AJR Am J Roentgenol* 1988;9:885–889.
3. Shellock FG, Crues JV. High-field strength MR imaging and metallic biomedical implants: an ex vivo evaluation of deflection forces. *AJR Am J Roentgenol* 1988;151:389–392.
4. Brown MA, Carden JA, Coleman RE, et al. Magnetic field effects on surgical ligation clips. *Magn Reson Imag* 1987;5:443–453.
5. Dujovny M, Kossovsky N, Kossowsky R, et al. Aneurysm clip motion during magnetic resonance imaging: in vivo experimental study with metallurgical factor analysis. *Neurosurgery* 1985;17:543–548.
6. Barrafato D, Henkelman RM. Magnetic resonance imaging and surgical clips. *Can J Surg* 1984;27:509–512.
7. Moscatel M, Shellock FG, Morisoli S. Biopsy needles and devices: assessment of ferromagnetism and artifacts during exposure to a 1.5 Tesla MR system. *J Magn Res Imag* 1995;5:369–372.
8. Shellock FG, Shellock VJ. Additional information pertaining to the MR-compatibility of biopsy needles and devices. *J Magn Res Imag* 1996;6:441.

9. Hathout G, Lufkin RB, Jabour B, et al. MR-guided aspiration cytology in the head and neck at high field strength. *J Magn Res Imag* 1992;2:93–94.
10. Fagan LL, Shellock FG, Brenner RJ, Rothman B. Ex vivo evaluation of ferromagnetism, heating, and artifacts of breast tissue expanders exposed to a 1.5 T MR system. *J Magn Res Imag* 1995;5:614–616.
11. Teitelbaum GP, Lin MCW, Watanabe AT, et al. Ferromagnetism and MR imaging: safety of cartoid vascular clamps. *AJNR Am J Neuroradiol* 1990;11:267–272.
12. Gegauff A, Laurell KA, Thavendrarajah A, et al. A potential MRI hazard: forces on dental magnet keepers. *J Oral Rehabil* 1990;17:403–410.
13. Shellock FG. Ex vivo assessment of deflection forces and artifacts associated with high-field strength MRI of "mini-magnet" dental prostheses. *Magn Reson Imag* 1989;7(suppl 1):P38.
14. Shellock FG, Slimp G. Halo vest for cervical spine fixation during MR imaging. *AJR Am J Roentgenol* 1990;154:631–632.
15. Clayman DA, Murakami ME, Vines FS. Compatibility of cervical spine braces with MR imaging. A study of nine nonferrous devices. *AJNR Am J Neuroradiol* 1990;11:385–390.
16. Shellock FG. MR imaging and cervical fixation devices: assessment of ferromagnetism, heating, and artifacts. *Magn Reson Imag* 1996 (in press).
17. Soulen RL, Budinger TF, Higgins CB. Magnetic resonance imaging of prosthetic heart valves. *Radiology* 1985;154:705–707.
18. Shellock FG, Morisoli SM. Ex vivo evaluation of ferromagnetism, heating, and artifacts for heart valve prostheses exposed to a 1.5 Tesla MR system. *J Magn Res Imag* 1994;4:756–758.
19. Hassler M, Le Bas JF, Wolf JE, et al. Effects of magnetic fields used in MRI on 15 prosthetic heart valves. *J Radiol* 1986;67:661–666.
20. Frank H, Buxbaum P, Huber L, Globits S, Glogar D, Wolner E, Mayr H, Imhof H. In vitro behavior of mechanical heart valves in 1.5 T superconducting magnet. *Eur J Radiol* 1992;2: 555–558.
21. Teitelbaum GP, Bradley WG, Klein BD. MR imaging artifacts, ferromagnetism, and magnetic torque of intravascular filters, stents, and coils. *Radiology* 1988;166:657–664.
22. Marshall MW, Teitelbaum GP, Kim HS, et al. Ferromagnetism and magnetic resonance artifacts of platinum embolization microcoils. *Cardiovasc Intervent Radiol* 1991;14:163–166.
23. Watanabe AT, Teitelbaum GP, Gomes AS, et al. MR imaging of the bird's nest filter. *Radiology* 1990;177:578–579.
24. Leibman CE, Messersmith RN, Levin DN, et al. MR imaging of inferior vena caval filter: safety and artifacts. *AJR Am J Roentgenol* 1988;150:1174–1176.
25. Teitelbaum GP, Raney M, Carvlin MJ, et al. Evaluation of ferromagnetism and magnetic resonance imaging artifacts of the Strecker tantalum vascular stent. *Cardiovasc Intervent Radiol* 1989;12:125–127.
26. Shellock FG, Myers SM, Schatz CJ. Ex vivo evaluation of ferromagnetism determined for metallic scleral "buckles" exposed to a 1.5 T MR scanner. *Radiology* 1992;185(P):288–289.
27. de Keizer RJ, Te Strake L. Intraocular lens implants (pseudo-phakoi) and steelwire sutures: a contraindication for MRI? *Doc Ophthalmol* 1984;61:281–284.
28. Albert DW, Olson KR, Parel JM, et al. Magnetic resonance imaging and retinal tacks. *Arch Ophthalmol* 1990;108:320–321.
29. Joondeph BC, Peyman GA, Mafee MF, et al. Magnetic resonance imaging and retinal tacks (letter). *Arch Ophthalmol* 1987;105:1479–1480.
30. Lyons CJ, Betz RR, Mesgarzadeh M, et al. The effect of magnetic resonance imaging on metal spine implants. *Spine* 1989;14:670–672.
31. Shellock FG, Mink JH, Curtin S, et al. MRI and orthopedic implants used for anterior cruciate ligament reconstruction: assessment of ferromagnetism and artifacts. *J Magn Res Imag* 1992;2: 225–228.
32. Shellock FG, Schatz CJ. High-field strength MR imaging and metallic otologic implants. *AJNR Am J Neuroradiol* 1991;12:279–281.
33. Nogueira M, Shellock FG. Otologic bioimplants: ex vivo assessment of ferromagnetism and artifacts at 1.5 Tesla. *AJR Am J Roentgenol* 1995;163:1472–1473.
34. Mattucci KF, Setzen M, Hyman R, et al. The effect of nuclear magnetic resonance imaging on metallic middle ear protheses. *Otolaryngol Head Neck Surg* 1986;94:441–443.
35. Applebaum EL, Valvassori GE. Further studies on the effects of magnetic resonance fields on middle ear implants. *Ann Otol Rhinol Laryngol* 1990;99:801–804.
36. White DW. Interation between magnetic fields and metallic ossicular prostheses. *Am J Otol* 1987;8:290–292.

37. Leon JA, Gabriele OF. Middle ear prothesis: significance in magnetic resonance imaging. *Magn Reson Imag* 1987;5:405–406.
38. Shellock FG, Morisoli SM. Ex vivo evaluation of ferromagnetism and artifacts for cardiac occluders exposed to a 1.5 Tesla MR system. *J Magn Reson Imag* 1994;4:213–215.
39. Teitelbaum GP, Yee CA, Van Horn DD, et al. Metallic ballistic fragments: MR imaging safety and artifacts. *Radiology* 1990;175:855–859.
40. Shellock FG, Crues JV, Sacks SA. High-field magnetic resonance imaging of penile prostheses: in vitro evaluation of deflection forces and imaging artifacts (abstr.) In: *Book of Abstracts, Society of Magnetic Resonance in Medicine.* Berkeley, CA: Society of Magnetic Resonance in Medicine; 1987;3:915.
41. Shellock FG, Nogueira M, Morisoli S. MR imaging and vascular access ports: Ex vivo evaluation of ferromagnetism, heating, and artifacts at 1.5 T. *J Magn Reson Imag* 1995;4:481–484.
42. Shellock FG, Shellock VJ. Vascular access ports and catheters tested for ferromagnetism, heating, and artifacts associated with MR imaging. *Magn Reson Imag* 1996 (in press).
43. Shellock FG, Shellock VJ. Evaluation of MR compatibility of 38 bioimplants and devices. *Radiology* 1995;197(P):174.
44. Lufkin R, Jordan S, Lylcyk M. MR imaging with topographic EEG electrodes in place. *AJNR Am J Neuroradiol* 1988;9:953–954.
45. Mark AS, Hricak H. Intrauterine contraceptive devices: MR imaging. *Radiology* 1987;162: 311–314.
46. Go KG, Kamman RL, Mooyaart EL. Interaction of metallic neurosurgical implants with magnetic resonance imaging at 1.5 Tesla as a cause of image distortion and of hazardous movement of the implant. *Clin Neurosurg* 1989;91:109–115.
47. Fransen P, Dooms G, Thauvoy. Safety of the adjustable pressure ventricular valve in magnetic resonance imaging: problems and solutions. *Neuroradiology* 1992;34:508–509.
48. ECRI, Health devices alert. A new MRI complication? May 27, 1988.
49. To SYC, Lufkin RB, Chiu L. MR-compatible winged infusion set. *Comput Med Imag Graphics* 1989;13:469–472.

Appendix II

Safety Recommendations for MR Procedures

FOOD AND DRUG ADMINISTRATION*

AGENCY: Food and Drug Administration.

ACTION: Notice

SUMMARY: The Food and Drug Administration (FDA) is issuing for public comment the recommendation of the Radiologic Devices Panel (the Panel) that FDA reclassify the magnetic resonance diagnostic device from class III (premarket approval) into class II (performance standards). The Panel made this recommendation after review of reclassification petitions filed by 13 manufacturers. The FDA is also issuing for public comment its tenative findings on the recommendation. After reviewing any public comment on the recommendation and FDA's tenative findings, FDA will approve or deny the reclassification petitions by order in the form of a letter to each petitioner. FDA's decision on these reclassification petitions will be announced in the **Federal Register.**

DATE: Comments by May 9, 1988

ADDRESS: Written comments to the Dockets Management Branch (HFA-305), Food and Drug Administration, Rm. 4-62, 5600 Fishers Lane, Rockville, MD 20857.

FOR FURTHER INFORMATION CONTACT: Joseph M. Sheehan, Center for Devices and Radiological Health (HFZ-84), Food and Drug Administration, 5600 Fishers Lane, Rockville, MD 20857, 301-443-4874.

SUPPLEMENTARY INFORMATION: On June 18, 1987, FDA filed reclassification petitions submitted by the 13 manufacturers below. Twelve manufacturers

*Docket Nos. 87P-0214/CP through 87P-0214/CP0013. Magnetic Resonance Diagnostic Device; Panel Recommendation and Report on Petitions for MR Reclassification. [FR Doc. 88-5116 Filed 2-8-88; 8:45 am].

requested reclassification of the magnetic resonance diagnostic device from class III into class II and one requested reclassification into class I. The petitions were submitted under section 513(f) of the Federal Food, Drug and Cosmetic Act (the act) (21 U.S.C. 360c(f) and 21 CFR 860.120).

Petitioner	Model
Advanced NMR Systems, Inc.	Instascan
Bruker Medical Instruments	Tomikon BMT-1100
Diasonics MRI Division	Diasonics MT/S
Fonar Corp.	Beta-3000, Beta-3000M
General Electric Co.	Signa
Instrumentarium	ULF MR Imaging System
NMR Imaging, Inc.	PermaScan
Philips Medical Systems	Gyroscan R, Gyroscan S5
	Gyroscan S15, Gyroscan S20
Picker International, Inc.	Vista MR 1100, Vista MR 2055
	Vista MR 2055HP
Resonex, Inc.	Rx-4000
Siemens Medical Systems, Inc.	Magnetom M, Magnetom H
Stuart Medical, Inc.	MD800-1A
Thomson-GGR Medical Corp.	Magnascan 5000

The versions of the generic type of device (magnetic resonance diagnostic device) listed above are automatically classified into class III under section 513(f)(1) of the act because they are not preamendments devices (i.e., devices which were in commercial distribution before May 28, 1976), and they are neither substantially equivalent to a preamendments device, nor substantially equivalent to any postamendments device (i.e., a device that has been placed in commercial distribution since May 28, 1976) which subsequently has been reclassified to class II or class I.

Section 513(f)(2) of the act provides that the manufacturer or importer of a device classified into class III under section 513(f)(1) of the act may file a petition for reclassification of the device into class I or class II. FDA's regulations in 21 CFR 860.134 set forth the procedures for filing and review of a petition for reclassification of such class III devices. For the purpose of reclassification of the magnetic resonance diagnostic device, it is necessary to show that the proposed new class has sufficient controls to provide reasonable assurance of the safety and effectiveness of the device.

Consistent with the act and the regulations, the agency referred the reclassification petitions to the Panel and on July 27, 1987, during an open public meeting, the Panel recommended that FDA reclassify the magnetic resonance diagnostic device from class III into class II, and that it be assigned a low priority for the establishment of a performance standard for the device. The Panel's recommendation appears as part II below.

I. DEVICE HISTORY AND DESCRIPTION

Laboratory magnetic resonance instruments have been routinely used since the early 1950s by chemists and physicists to study the molecular structure and dynamics of small homogeneous specimens (Ref. 1). The basic scientific principles of nuclear magnetic resonance were scientifically established well before devices using these same principles were developed for use on humans to obtain medical diagnostic information.

The fundamental scientific technology of magnetic resonance diagnostic devices is the phenomenon of magnetic resonance whereby certain nuclei when placed in a magnetic field experience a resonance condition and can absorb and emit energy at well-defined frequencies. In 1946, Felix Block and Edward Purcell first demonstrated the nuclear magnetic resonance principle, and they jointly received the Nobel Prize for physics in 1952 for their discoveries. In 1971 Raymond Damadian of the State University of New York, Brooklyn, proposed use of measured magnetic relaxation times to discriminate between malignant tumors and normal tissue. In 1973, Paul Lauterbur of the State University of New York, Stony Brook, proposed using the basic principles of tomography to form a two- or three-dimensional magnetic resonance image. Since that time, a variety of other imaging and spectroscopic techniques have been used with the device.

As described by the Panel (part II, below), the magnetic resonance diagnostic device present images or nuclear magnetic resonance parameters of the human body such as density or flow of resonant nuclei, relaxation times T1 and T2, and chemical shift. Electromagnetic signals are acquired from the body using nuclear magnetic resonance phenomena with a static magnetic field, gradient magnetic fields, and radiofrequency magnetic fields. Computers process this information and present an image, a spectrum, or localized nuclear magnetic resonance parameter data. Various imaging techniques and spectroscopy acquisition protocols are used.

The device consists of a main magnet system, magnetic gradient coil assemblies, radio frequency coil assemblies, associated power supplies, filters, amplifiers, signal analysis, display, recording, storage, and communication equipment, patient support and positioning equipment, as well as physiological motion gating and compensating devices and accessories. The main (static) magnetic field is generated by either a permanent magnet, a resistive magnet, or superconducting magnet. The systems subject to the petitions may include radiofrequency coils for use on the whole body, head, and various surfaces.

II. RECOMMENDATION OF THE PANEL

At its meeting on July 27, 1987, the Panel considered petitions submitted by the following 13 manufacturers of magnetic resonance diagnostic devices: Advanced NMR Systems, Inc., Bruker Medical Instruments, Diasonics MRI Division, Fonar Corp., General Electric Co., Instrumentarium, NMR Imaging, Inc., Philips Medical Systems, Picker International, Inc., Resonex, Inc., Siemens Medical Systems, Inc., Stuart Medical, Inc., and Thomson-CGR Medical Corp.

Twelve of the petitioners requested reclassification of the magnetic resonance diagnostic device from class III into class II, and one requested reclassification into class I. The Panel was asked to: (1) Identify risks to health posed by the devices, (2) determine which class could reduce these risks, (3) decide whether or not to recommend reclassification, and (4) if reclassification to class II is recommended, recommend the priority for development of a performance standard. After considering the petitions and answering the questions posed to it, the Panel recommends that the magnetic resonance diagnostic device be reclassified from class III to class II and that FDA assign a low priority to development of a performance standard for the device.

III. SCOPE OF THE PANEL'S RECOMMENDATION

The reclassification covers the 20 petitioned models of the device and all devices substantially equivalent to them.

The magnetic resonance diagnostic device presents images which reflect the spatial distribution, and magnetic resonance spectra which reflect the frequency distribution, of nuclei exhibiting nuclear magnetic resonance. Other physical parameters derived from the images and spectra may also be produced. The functions of the device for which reclassification is requested include hydrogen-1 (proton) imaging, sodium-23 imaging, hydrogen-1 spectroscopy, phosphorus-31 spectroscopy, and chemical shift imaging (preserving simultaneous frequency and spatial information).

The magnetic resonance diagnostic devices for which reclassification is recommended meet the following exposure characteristics: (1) The head or trunk of a patient is exposed to static magnetic fields insufficient to produce significant adverse effect; (2) the patient is exposed to time-varying magnetic fields insufficient to produce peripheral nerve stimulation or other adverse effects; (3) the patient is exposed to radiofrequency magnetic fields insufficient to produce a core temperature increase in excess of 1°C and localized heating to greater than 38°C in the head, 39°C in the trunk, and 40°C in the extremities, or other adverse effect. A device which meets these characteristics and is accompanied by adequate labeling (Ref. 2) is expected to be safe and effective.

IV. SUMMARY OF THE PANEL'S REASONS FOR THE RECOMMENDATION

The panel recommends reclassification from class III into class II of the magnetic resonance diagnostic device for the following reasons:

1. General controls by themselves are insufficient to provide reasonable assurance of the safety and effectiveness of the device.

2. There is sufficient publicly available information to demonstrate that the risks to health have been determined for the magnetic resonance diagnostic devices for which reclassification has been requested. The relationships between the device's safety and performance parameters and risks have been established by valid scientific evidence, and there is sufficient publicly available information to establish a performance standard to control the device's safety and effectiveness.

The Panel recommended that FDA assign a low priority to the establishment of a performance standard for the generic type of device under section 514 of the act (21 U.S.C. 360(d)). The Panel believes the quality of the data in the petitions was sufficiently strong in describing the safety and effectiveness of the devices subject to the petitions, so that assigning a low priority for standards development is appropriate. All currently marketed magnetic resonance diagnostic devices have undergone premarket approval, and as a result there is a reasonable assurance of the device's safety and effectiveness. Additionally, devices subject to the petitions but not currently marketed are supported by substantial amounts of valid scientific evidence describing device safety and effectiveness.

The Panel based its recommendation for reclassification of the generic type of device on data in the petitions (Refs. 3 to 15) and additional valid scientific data presented to the Panel during its open meeting held on July 27, 1987 (Refs. 16 and 17). In sum, the Panel believes that premarket approval of the generic type of device is unnecessary to provide reasonable assurance of the device's safety and effectiveness, and that lesser controls can be expected to assure safety and effectiveness of the device.

V. THE PANEL'S VIEW OF DEVICE RELATED RISKS AND BENEFITS

A. Risks to Health

Risks to health identified in the petitions include: (1) Adverse effects of whole or partial body exposure to the static magnetic field, (2) adverse effects of exposure to time-varying magnetic fields, (3) adverse effects of absorption of energy from radiofrequency magnetic fields, (4) hazards from high acoustic noise levels, (5) hazards from laser beams, (6) electrical and mechanical hazards, (7) insufficient image or spectral quality resulting in reduced clinical utility, and (8) other potential hazards addressed by labeling.

Sufficient publicly available information exists to write a performance standard for the magnetic resonance diagnostic device to obviate these concerns.

B. Benefits

In the past few years, magnetic resonance imaging of hydrogen protons has become a well-established diagnostic technique. Its clinical uses are particularly numerous for the diagnostic evaluation of disorders of the head, spine, and central nervous system (Ref. 18). Because of the abundance of hydrogen protons in water throughout the body, the technique is useful for imaging all major organ systems and tissues (Ref. 19). Since sodium is one of the more abundant elements in the body, it is used to image many different anatomical sites. Sodium imaging is of clinical relevance due to the correlation of relative sodium concentrations in extra- and intracellular space as a function of disease or trauma (Ref. 20). Hydrogen proton spectroscopy is used in detection of ischemia, investigating metabolic pathways and kinetics, and cancer detection (Ref. 21). Phosphorus-31 spectroscopy is used to study normal energy metabolism in tissue, to describe diseased tissue energy metabolism, and to better understand and diagnose diseases (Ref. 22). In sum, use of the magnetic resonance diagnostic device allows, with minimal risk, access to diagnostic information not available by any imaging techniques.

VI. SUMMARY OF DATA UPON WHICH THE PANEL RECOMMENDATION IS BASED

The Panel considered a number of potential concerns regarding the safe and effective operation of a magnetic resonance diagnostic device. The following identifies the Panel's concerns and its determination, based on data, that a standard and general controls can provide a reasonable assurance of safety and effectiveness:

1. The static magnetic field produced by the main magnet determines the resonant radiofrequency of the nuclei of interest. Available literature indicates a consensus that no adverse effects are expected from whole body exposure or exposure of the head to magnetic fields with strength of 2 tesla or less for a period of 1 hour or less (Ref. 16). Many thousands of patients have been exposed to 2 tesla or less

static magnetic fields with no adverse effects. A standard could be written to limit the static field to a level less than that which would produce significant biological hazard.

2. Time-varying magnetic fields (dB/dt) occur during switching of the magnetic gradients used for spatial localization of the acquired NMR signal. Circulating currents in biological systems may be induced, causing peripheral nerve stimulation. This risk can be reduced by limiting patient exposure to time-varying magnetic fields with strengths significantly less than those required to produce peripheral nerve stimulation (Refs. 3-18). Many thousands of patients have been exposed to such limited strength time-varying magnetic fields without exhibiting deleterious effects attributable to these fields. A standard could be written to limit the time-varying magnetic fields to levels less than those that would produce significant biological hazard.

3. Radiofrequency magnetic fields occur at the resonant frequency of the nuclei of interest. Radiofrequency energy absorption in the patient may cause systemic thermal overload and local thermal injury. Limiting that thermal increase to a rise in a patient's core body temperature of less than 1°C controls this risk (Ref. 16). Standards could be written to adequately address this risk. In addition, radiofrequency power deposition may cause heating around metallic implants, tattoos, or permanent eyeliner. These risks can be controlled by placing appropriate warnings in the labeling.

4. High acoustic noise levels may be generated upon pulsing of the electrical current energizing the gradient coils. Acoustic noise may be annoying, cause discomfort, or beyond certain levels be hazardous (Ref. 23). These risks can be reduced by following a standard which limits acoustic noise to levels below the occupational limits recommended by the American Conference of Governmental Industrial Hygienists for exposures of up to 1 hour per day (Ref. 24), or below the permissible time-averaged and peak noise exposure given by the Occupational Safety and Health Association (Ref. 23).

5. A laser system may be used in patient positioning. A laser has the potential for causing permanent eye injury, although no such injury has been reported. The lasers, which are considered electronic products capable of producing a beam of low power visible light radiation, meet power output limits of the Federal performance standard for class II laser products under the Radiation Control for Health and Safety Act of 1968.

6. Potential electrical and mechanical hazards can be controlled by a standard that requires that devices have adequate design specifications and adherence to good design practices.

7. Reduced clinical utility may result from insufficient image or spectral quality. Sufficient information, included in the petitions (refs. 3-15), exists to write a performance standard for image quality and spectroscopy performance measures. Indeed, the petitions referenced draft standards developed by the National Electrical Manufacturers Association that specifically address image quality measures, including signal-to-noise ratio, geometric distortion, uniformity, and slice

thickness and spacing (Ref. 25), and spectroscopy performance measures, including spectral resolution, spectral calibration and labeling, and localization (Ref. 26), which could be used in writing a performance standard.

8. Concerns addressed by labeling (Ref. 2):

a. The field near the magnet, that is, the fringe field, may be strong enough to attract ferromagnetic objects such as tools with great force, causing a collision. This potentially hazardous situation can be controlled by placing warning statements in the labeling, such as warnings to restrict access to only authorized personnel and requiring in-place procedures for emergency services of patients in areas where the fringe field is weaker. The field in or near the magnet may fatally interfere with the operation of devices such as cardiac pacemakers. This risk can be controlled by placing contraindications in the labeling prohibiting use of the magnetic resonance diagnostic device on patients with these devices. The static magnetic field may move or dislodge ferromagnetic materials within the patient's body, such as intracranial aneurysm clips, shrapnel fragments, and prostheses constructed of ferromagnetic material, which could cause life-threatening situations. The risk can be controlled by placing contraindications in the labeling against scanning patients with intracranial aneurysm clips or warning of the risk of scanning patients with other implanted ferromagnetic material.

b. Special concerns arise when scanning fetuses or infants who are particularly susceptible to thermal overload and require careful monitoring for signs of cardiocirculatory and respiratory distress. The risk can be controlled by placing appropriate warnings in the labeling.

c. Liquid helium and nitrogen cryogens are used to cool the superconducting wire in a superconducting magnet. Some boiloff of the gases occurs during normal operation. If the magnet quenches, the boiloff rate of the cryogens will increase, and gas could suddenly be released into the room causing asphyxiation of site personnel or patients. Labeling can describe proper venting of the system to ensure safety should this problem occur.

d. Due to the configuration of the system and the length of the exam, some patients become claustrophobic. Labeling to include a precautions section addressing the scanning of patients who are likely to develop claustrophobic reactions controls this risk.

e. Operator quality assurance tests and routine preventive maintenance procedures are required in the device labeling. These routine checks and maintenance procedures assist in optimizing image or spectral quality.

REFERENCES

The petitions, the transcript of the Panel meeting, and the following material are on public file in the Dockets Management Branch (address above), where they may be seen by interested persons between 9 a.m. and 4 p.m., Monday through Friday.

1. Andrew, E. R., *Nuclear Magnetic Resonance*, Cambridge University Press, Cambridge, 1955.
2. Draft of magnetic resonance diagnostic device labeling, September 1987.
3. Reclassification petition from General Electronic Company, 87P-0214/CP.
4. Reclassification petition from Bruker Medical Instruments, 87P-0214/CP0002.
5. Reclassification petition from Stuart Medical, Inc., 87P-0214/CP0003.
6. Reclassification petition from Siemens Medical Systems, Inc., 87P-0214/CP0004.
7. Reclassification petition from Diasonics MRI Division, 87P-0214/CP0005.
8. Reclassification petition from Fonar Corp., 87P-0214/CP0006.
9. Reclassification petition from Philips Medical Systems, 87P-0214/CP0007.
10. Reclassification petition from NMR Imaging, Inc., 87P-0214/CP0008.
11. Reclassification petition from Thomson-CGR Medical Corp., 87P-0214/CP0009.
12. Reclassification petition from Instrumentarium, 87P-0214/CP00010.
13. Reclassification petition from Resonex, Inc., 87P-0214/CP0011.
14. Reclassification petition from Picker International, 87P-0214/CP0012.
15. Reclassification petition from Advanced NMR Systems, Inc., 87P-0214/CP0013.
16. Czerski, P., and T.W. Athey, "Safety of Magnetic Resonance In Vivo Diagnostic Examinations: Theoretical and Clinical Considerations," presented July 27, 1987.
17. Reilly, J. Patrick, "Peripheral Stimulation by Pulsatile Currents: Applications to Time-Varying Magnetic Field Exposure," Report MT 87-100; June 1987.
18. Kressel, Herbert Y., editor, *Magnetic Resonance Annual 1987*, Raven Press, New York, 1987.
19. ACR Commission on MRI, "Clinical Applications of Magnetic Resonance, " November 1985.
20. Perman, William H.; Patrick A. Turski; Lanning W. Houston; Gary H. Glover; and Cecil E. Hayes, "Methodology of in Vivo Human Sodium MR Imaging at 1.5 T," Radiology, 160: 811-820, 1986.
21. Luyten, P.R. and J.A. den Hollander, "H-1 MR Observation of Metabolites in Human Tissues In Situ," presented at the Society of Magnetic Resonance in Medicine, fifth annual meeting, Montreal, August 18 to 22, 1986.
22. Radda, George K., "The Use of NMR Spectroscopy for the Understanding of Disease," *Science*, 233: 640-645, 1986.
23. Occupational Safety and Health (OSHA) 1910.95, "Occupational Noise Exposure."
24. American Conference of Governmental Industrial Hygienists, "TLVs, Threshold Limit Values for Chemical Substances in the Work Environment, Adopted by ACGIH for 1983-84, Noise and Impulsive or Impact Noise, " pp. 80-82.
25. National Electrical Manufacturers Association (NEMA) draft of performance standards, "Determination of Signal-to-Noise Ratio in Diagnostic Magnetic Resonance Imaging," "Determination of Two-Dimensional Geometric Distortion in Diagnostic Magnetic Resonance Imaging," "Determination of Slice Thickness in Diagnostic Magnetic Resonance Imaging," and "Determination of Uniformity in Diagnostic Magnetic Resonance Imaging," 1987.
26. National Electrical Manufacturers Association, draft document of "Measurement Methods for MR Spectroscopy," 1987.

FDA'S TENTATIVE FINDINGS

FDA tentatively agrees with the Panel's recommendation that the magnetic resonance diagnostic device described in the petitions be reclassified from class III into class II and that it be assigned a low priority for the establishment of a performance standard for the device.

Economic Considerations

After considering the economic consequences of approving this reclassification, FDA certifies that this notice requires neither a regulatory impact analysis, as specified in Executive Order 12291, nor a regulatory flexibility analysis, as defined in the Regulatory Flexibility Act (Pub. L. 96-354). Approval of this petition would not have a significant economic impact on a substantial number of small entities. However, it may permit small potential competitors to enter the marketplace by lowering the barriers to entry. The petitioners and all future manufacturers of the reclassified magnetic resonance diagnostic devices would be relieved of the costs of complying with the premarket approval requirements in section 515 of the act (21 U.S.C. 360(e)). There are no offsetting costs that the petitioners would incur from reclassification into class II other than those associated with meeting a standard once established. The actual cost of complying with a standard cannot be determined until the standard is developed. The magnitude of the economic savings from approval of this petition depends on the extent of the studies that the petitioners would have conducted in support of new premarket approval applications or supplements to existing premarket approval applications, and the number of future competitors satisfying the requirements of premarket approval. None of these parameters can be reliably calculated to permit quantification of the economic savings. Because of statutory deadlines (section 513(f)(2) of the act) and requirements in the regulations (21 CFR 860.134(b)(5), FDA is required to publish this notice in the **Federal Register** as soon as practicable. As authorized by section 8(a)(2) of Executive Order 12291, FDA is publishing in the **Federal Register** this notice without clearance of the Director, Office of Management and Budget. FDA will notify that office of the publication of this notice.

Interested persons may, on or before May 9, 1988, submit to the Dockets Management Branch (address above) written comments on this recommendation. Two copies of any comments are to be submitted, except that individuals may submit one copy. Comments are to be identified with the name of the device and the docket number found in brackets in the heading of this document. Received comments may be seen in the office above between 9 a.m. and 4 p.m., Monday through Friday.

Dated February 27, 1988.

Frank E. Young,
Commissioner of Food and Drugs.

FOOD AND DRUG ADMINISTRATION MRI GUIDANCE UPDATE FOR dB/dt

Background

On April 21, 1995, the Center for Devices and Radiological Health (CDRH) released a document for public comment containing draft revisions to the "Guidance for the Content and Review of a Magnetic Resonance Diagnostic Device 510 (k) Application" dated August 2, 1988. The revisions relate to operation at dB/dt levels beyond the levels of concern listed in that original guidance.

Comments were solicited from MRI manufacturers, user groups, and technical experts regarding the provisions contained in the April 21, 1995 draft. Also, a public meeting of the Radiological Devices Panel was held on September 11, 1995 to discuss the proposed guidance. This document incorporates the revisions in the draft guidance of April 21, 1995 that have been made in response to the comments received.

The original 1988 guidance required manufacturers to provide valid scientific evidence to establish the safety of operating with changing magnetic field gradients in excess of levels of concern identified in Attachment I of that document. The MRI Guidance Update for dB/dt contains an outline of the types of evidence needed to establish the safety of operating at these levels. This evidence includes the results of laboratory measurements, human studies, special labeling, and device features to ensure safety.

The Guidance Update incorporates some of the requirements contained in IEC-601-2-33. However, changes have been made to reflect additional scientific data that have become available since the drafting of that standard.

Thank you to all whose comments and criticisms have helped in the development of this document. If you have any questions please contact:

Robert A. Phillips, Ph.D.
Chief, Computed Imaging Devices Branch
ODE/CDRH
9200 Corporate Blvd.
Rockville, MD 20850
Phone: (301) 594-1212
Fax: (301) 480-4224

Comments on 4-21-95 Draft

Laboratory Data

There was general agreement among manufacturers and technical experts that the rate of change of the imaging component of the gradient, dB_z/dt, is not the best measure of the probability of peripheral nerve stimulation. The NEMA MR Technical Committee has offered to develop a measurement method to replace the existing NEMA standard, and to forward the new method as an amendment to IEC-601-2-33. In the interim, the method proposed in the 4-21-95 draft, which is based on |B| and sequence timing information, will be retained as the recommended method of characterizing the gradient fields and determining dB/dt values.

Clinical Studies

In the draft guidance limited volunteer studies were proposed to determine if a system has the potential for producing peripheral nerve stimulation. These studies were to be conducted under conditions that produce the maximum dB/dt based on laboratory data. Comments were made regarding the inherent limitations of such pilot studies. However, no objections were raised and this provision will be retained.

A recommendation has been added that manufacturers also report the level of stimulation experienced by the volunteers in these limited studies under maximum dB/dt conditions. There was a general consensus at the Panel meeting that painful stimulation should be avoided. Consequently, it is assumed that systems will be limited so that painful stimulation is not induced. The limited volunteer studies will also provide a check that this is the case.

Questions were raised regarding the need for more extensive volunteer studies that were to provide the relationship between operating parameters and the percentage of patients who experience stimulation. Concern was expressed by manufacturers that there are too many combinations of amplitude, frequency, pulse width, and spacing in MRI pulse sequences to perform a study of this type for each 510 (k). Also, it was pointed out that the operator can be informed of the potential for stimulation without performing such studies.

Because mild stimulation is not hazardous and the more extensive studies would be time consuming, the provision regarding more extensive volunteer studies has been deleted from the revised guidance. However, it is recommended that if a system is observed to produce stimulation in the limited volunteer studies, manufacturers conduct additional studies to verify that the warning to the operator is provided below a value at which peripheral nerve stimulation is produced.

As noted below, the recommendation that operators complete a report of any incidents of stimulation during clinical use has been removed from the guidance. However, in lieu of this it is recommended that manufacturers include in their premarket notification the results of their clinical experience with a gradient system to the extent such information is available (e.g., from beta testing).

Manufacturers are also encouraged to provide any available information regarding their clinical experience in scanning the special patient groups identified by the panel (e.g., children, pregnant women, epileptics, patients with metallic implants, cardiac arrhythmia, peripheral neuropathy, comatose patients, or patients unable to communicate).

Labeling

The Radiology Devices Panel recommended that special patient groups should be examined in controlled clinical settings under IRB supervision when fast gradient procedures are used. This recommendation has been included in the suggested labeling.

Manufacturers, technical experts, and panel members agreed that mild peripheral nerve stimulation is a subjective perception, and that it is not possible to obtain reliable information regarding the threshold of stimulation from patients in a general clinical setting. Consequently, the recommendation that operators complete a report of any incidents of stimulation has been deleted. Also, the associated recommendation that companies track the total number of patients who are scanned with procedures that have the potential for producing stimulation has been eliminated. The purpose of tracking the total number of patients scanned was to validate if the operator warning was set such that less than 1% of patients were stimulated below the warning level. Comments received on this issue indicate that such a validation is not feasible.

There was agreement that a scan need not be terminated if a patient experiences mild peripheral nerve stimulation. There was also a general consensus that a scan should be terminated if a patient complains of severe discomfort or pain. The guidance has been revised accordingly.

As noted in the discussion of the comments regarding clinical data above, the recommended reporting of incidents of peripheral nerve stimulation has been eliminated. However, reporting of incidents of severe discomfort or pain is recommended.

Device Characteristics

There was general agreement with the recommendation that the operator and patient be warned when the possibility of stimulation exists. The draft guidance had recommended that this warning be given at a level at which fewer than 1% of patients experience stimulation. This warning was to be set based on premarket testing and validated from the reports of patient stimulation received after the product was placed in general clinical service.

Since the recommendation that clinical incidents of stimulation be reported to the company has been removed from the guidance, the 1% criterion would no longer apply. Consequently, it is suggested that manufacturers choose the level at which the operator warning is initiated based on volunteer testing and available premarket clinical experience. This warning level is not considered to be critical because there are no known harmful effects associated with mild peripheral nerve stimulation. However, it should be chosen conservatively to ensure that ample warning is given.

Informal comments were received suggesting that CDRH choose a curve of dB/dt level versus frequency for the operator warning based on current available information. The agency has reviewed the information in published studies and the data provided in premarket notifications submitted to date and has concluded that there is insufficient information at present to establish such a curve.

The recommendation that a record of the dB/dt value be included with the image data is consistent with IEC-601-2-33. It was inadvertently omitted from the draft guidance. A record of dB/dt will be useful in the analysis of cases of reported painful stimulation.

As noted above, panel members, industry representatives, and technical experts have agreed that painful stimulation is to be avoided in routine clinical MRI procedures. Consequently, it is recommended that equipment output be limited so that painful stimulation is not induced.

Guidance

Laboratory Data

The purpose of the laboratory data for evaluating dB/dt is to characterize the magnetic field produced by each gradient coil, including the components not related to imaging. The volume to be examined for maxima of the gradient fields is limited to the region that could be occupied by the largest patient.

Manufacturers should provide an estimate of the maximum $|B|$ produced by each gradient coil (x, y, and z) that could be experienced by a patient, where $|B|$ denotes the magnitude of the vector sum of the gradient field components (B_x, B_y, and B_z). The location of the maximum value of $|B|$ for each gradient coil and the values of the individual field components at that location also should be reported. Samples of field plots used in these determinations should be included in the submission.

Manufacturers should provide worst case sequence timing information and use this to estimate the shape and amplitude of the worst case $d|B|/dt$ pulse for each gradient coil. Measurements should be made and submitted to verify these estimates.

Human Studies

Applicability

The provisions of this section are applicable to manufacturers of magnetic resonance diagnostic devices that are capable of producing levels of dB/dt in excess of the following values:

for tau > 120 μs	dB/dt > 20 T/s
for 120 μs > tau > 12 μs	dB/dt > 2400/tau T/s
for 12 μs > tau	dB/dt > 200 T/s

where tau is the pulse width in microseconds of a rectangular dB/dt pulse or the half period of a sinusoidal dB/dt pulse.

This is the level of concern for axial gradients identified in the previous guidance. Based on current knowledge, a separate level of concern for transverse gradients is not warranted.

Volunteer Studies

Manufacturers of devices capable of producing dB/dt levels in excess of the above values should submit limited human volunteer studies of peripheral nerve stimulation using equipment as similar as possible to the system submitted for marketing clearance. Studies should consist of at least 20 volunteers, and should include conditions (patient position and scan parameters) that produce the maximum dB/dt based on laboratory data. The number of patients who experience stimulation and the level of stimulation (mild, moderate, or painful) should be reported.

For those systems found to produce stimulation in these limited volunteer studies, additional studies are recommended to verify that the operator notification regarding the possibility of stimulation (see below) is provided at an appropriate level.

Clinical Experience

Manufacturers of gradient systems capable of producing dB/dt values in excess of the levels specified above should provide a summary of the preliminary clinical experience with these systems (i.e., beta testing). This summary should include the number of patients scanned, the dB/dt values used, and a description of the patient reactions (mild, moderate, and painful stimulation). The summary should also provide a description of the types of disease conditions included in the patient population.

Labeling

Warnings

Manufacturers of systems capable of producing peripheral nerve stimulation should include warnings to the operator regarding the risk of scanning special patient groups with fast scanning techniques. These groups include children, pregnant women, epileptics, patients with metallic implants, cardiac arrhythmia, peripheral neuropathy, comatose patients, or patients unable to communicate. Such patients should be examined in controlled clinical settings under IRB supervision.

Instructions to Operators

Manufacturers of systems capable of producing peripheral nerve stimulation should include instructions to the operator that describe the types of imaging techniques available on the system (e.g., echo planar) that may produce peripheral nerve stimulation. A description of the types of sensations of peripheral nerve stimulation should be included in these instructions. Instructions describing the operation of any related special equipment features (e.g., monitors or displays) also should be provided.

Instructions to Patients

Operators should be instructed that when techniques that may produce peripheral nerve stimulation are used, they should:

1. inform the patient that peripheral nerve stimulation may occur
2. describe the nature of the sensation to the patient
3. instruct patients not to claps their hands, because this may create a conductive loop that will increase the possibility of stimulation
4. maintain constant contact with the patient
5. instruct patients to inform the operator if they experience severe discomfort or pain
6. terminate the scan if the patient complains of severe discomfort or pain
7. complete a report of any incidents involving severe discomfort or pain, including a description of the associated circumstances (imaging parameters, dB/dt value, level of pain, etc.), and submit this report immediately to the company.

Device Characteristics

Manufacturers of equipment capable of producing peripheral nerve stimulation should provide means to notify the operator when this is possible. This notification should be provided below the lowest dB/dt level at which stimulation has been observed in volunteer and clinical studies. Deliberate action by the operator should then be necessary to proceed with the scan. A record of the dB/dt value should be included with the image data.

Equipment intended for routine clinical MRI use should be limited so that painful stimulation is not induced.

STATEMENT BY THE NATIONAL RADIOLOGICAL PROTECTION BOARD*

Principles for the Protection of Patients and Volunteers During Clinical Magnetic Resonance Diagnostic Procedures

SCOPE

1. The Board has the responsibility for advising the Department of Health on acceptable limits of exposure of patients and volunteers to magnetic fields encountered during clinical diagnosis by magnetic resonance (MR) systems for imaging (MRI) or spectroscopy (MRS). Such examinations may last up to about 1 h and result in exposure to static, extremely low frequency (ELF) gradient and radiofrequency (RF) magnetic fields. Previous advise was issued in 1984. The following revised recommendations are based on a reassessment of the possible effects on human health derived from new information from studies of the experimental exposure of humans and animals to electromagnetic fields and from extensive operational experience. These recommendations consider both whole-body and partial-body exposure and the implications of heterogeneous patterns of energy depositon. Restrictions on staff exposure to time-varying magnetic fields (including ELF and RF fields) are covered by separate guidance; this advice is presently under revision and will include restrictions on exposure to static magnetic fields.

PRINCIPLES

2. The data available at present are insufficient to allow thresholds for adverse effects of acute exposure of humans to electromagnetic fields to be accurately defined. As an interim measure, a two-tier system of restriction is recommended: a lower level identifies exposures considered to be safe and which may be exceeded under certain controlled circumstances; an upper level identifies exposures which present evidence suggests it would be inadvisable to exceed. The adoption of a two-tier standard is to provide some flexibility and to allow the cautious development of MR diagnostic techniques in which humans may be exposed to magnetic fields greater than those commonly used at present. Any effects of exposure between the lower and upper levels are expected to be small, although such exposure should be under carefully controlled conditions. The assessment of patient responses at exposures between these two levels of restriction and the publication of these data will provide valuable information for future revision of this advice.

---

*Documents of the NRPB. Includes: Board Statement on Clinical Magnetic Resonance Diagnostic Procedures, vol. 2 NO. 1, 1991. National Radiological Protection Board, Chilton, Didcot, Oxon OX11 ORQ.

3. Restrictions on exposure to static magnetic fields are intended to prevent the possibility of adverse health effects resulting from reduced aortic blood flow, increased blood pressure, cardiac arrhythmia and impaired mental function. These effects have been observed experimentally or predicted at high levels of exposure but are not well established. A degree of caution in patient and volunteer exposure is therefore needed until further operational experience becomes available.

4. Restrictions on gradient (ELF) magnetic field exposure are intended to prevent the stimulation of peripheral nerves and muscles, particularly cardiac muscle, by magnetically induced electric currents. Threshold current densities for peripheral nerve or cardiac muscle stimulation are estimated to be similar at low frequencies. Both can be avoided by setting a basic restriction on induced current densities to below threshold values for these responses. Relaxation of this restriction can be envisaged for short periods of magnetic field change due to the progressively shorter time available for the accumulation of the electric charge necessary for stimulation of the nerve cell membrane. The threshold for cardiac muscle stimulation rises at longer wavelengths (or lower frequencies) of magnetic field change than do thresholds for peripheral nerve stimulation. Thus, in this region, stimulation of peripheral nerves should give adequate warning of cardiac stimulation. Restrictions intended to avoid the stimulation of cardiac muscle but not peripheral nerves should be exceeded only under controlled conditions. Secondary restrictions on the rate of change of magnetic flux density can be derived from these basic restrictions but may be exceeded where it can be shown that the basic restrictions will not be exceeded.

5. Heating is a major consequence of exposure to the RF frequencies used in MR. Restrictions on RF magnetic field exposure are intended to prevent adverse responses to increased heat load and elevated body temperature. These responses include increased cardiac output, associated with elevated skin blood flow, and sweating, and may be contraindicated in patients with decreased thermoregulatory ability or cardiovascular problems. Increased body temperature is also associated with decreased mental function and with other physiological changes. These adverse effects of whole-body heat load can be adequately avoided by setting basic restrictions on the rise in body temperature. Secondary restrictions on the specific energy absorption rate (SAR)* averaged over the whole body can be derived from these basic restrictions and may be exceeded provided that the appropriate restriction on rise in body temperature is not exceeded. Despite the effects of cooling, body temperature increases with an increase in the total amount of RF energy absorbed, at least for the first 30 min of exposure, so that for a given rise in body temperature, progressively higher rates of energy absorption (SARs) can be applied for decreasing periods of exposure.

---

*The specific energy absorption rate (SAR) represents the rate of absorption of electromagnetic energy, for example by tissue, normalised to the mass under consideration and is expressed in watts per kilogram (W kg^{-1}). In terms of thermal loading, the SAR can be equated with the rate of metabolic heat production.

6. In practice, exposure to RF magnetic fields during MRI and particularly during MRS is predominantly to a region of the body such as the head or abdomen. In addition, the distribution of RF absorption and the rise in tissue temperature within the exposed region will be non-uniform due to tissue inhomogeneities and variation in blood flow. Restrictions on this localised absorption of RF energy are intended to prevent adverse effects on tissues and organs resulting from elevated temperatures. Basic restrictions are needed for the maximum temperature in different regions of the body. The head and, in pregnant women, the embryo or fetus are regarded as particularly vulnerable to elevated temperature; tissues in the trunk and limbs are regarded as less sensitive. Secondary restrictions on localised SAR are intended to prevent tissue temperatures exceeding basic restrictions.

7. Patients with certain medical disorders or under medication may be at some risk from exposure above the lower advised levels of static, ELF or RF magnetic fields. In particular, patients with compromised thermoregulatory abilities may be particularly susceptible to RF heating; such patients may well include those with cardiac problems or with a fever and those taking certain drugs. In addition, infants, pregnant women and old people may be considered compromised in this respect. In these circumstances, the doctor in charge must make this judgment and weigh the benefit of diagnosis against any possible risk. Since the potentially sensitive categories of patient are not well defined, it is advised that all patients exposed above the lower level of restriction have simple physiological parameters, such as body temperature, blood pressure and heart rate, routinely monitored.

8. Patients should be exposed only with the approval of a registered medical practitioner who should be satisfied either that the exposure is likely to result in a net benefit to the patient or that it is part of a research project which has been approved by a local research ethical committee.

9. The exposure of volunteers participating in experimental trials of MR imaging or spectroscopic techniques should be approved by a local ethical committee. Volunteers should be medically assessed for general fitness. They should be freely consenting and fully informed. Additional guidance is given in the WHO Technical Report 611.

10. Although there is no good evidence that mammalian embryos are sensitive to the magnetic fields encountered in magnetic resonance systems, it is prudent, until further information becomes available, to exclude pregnant women during the first three months of pregnancy. However, MR diagnostic procedures should be considered where the only reasonable alternative to MR diagnosis requires the use of X-ray procedures. There is no need to exclude women for whom a termination of pregnancy has been indicated. It is advised that pregnant women should not be exposed above the advised lower levels of restriction.

11. Metallic implants may present a hazard because of RF induced heating. In addition, implants made of ferromagnetic material will experience a force exerted on them by the static magnetic field which may result in movement of the implant and local tissue damage. In general, exposure is contraindicated unless a careful evaluation has been carried out. The exposure of persons with large metallic

implants such as hip prostheses should be stopped immediately if any discomfort is experienced.

12. Pacemakers and other electrically, mechanically or magnetically activated implants may be subject to electromagnetic interference, heating and a mechanical force if made of magnetic material; persons fitted with such implants should not be exposed unless the particular implant has been demonstrated to be unperturbed by MR fields.

REFERENCES

1. NRPB. Advice on acceptable limits of exposure to nuclear magnetic resonance clinical imaging. Chilton, NRPB, ASP5 (1984) (London, HMSO).
2. NRPB. Guidance as to restrictions on exposure to time-varying electromagnetic fields and the 1988 recommendations of the International Non-Ionizing Radiation Committee. Chilton, NRPB-GS11 (1989) (London, HMSO).
3. WHO. Use of ionizing radiation and radionuclides on human beings for medical research, training, and nonmedical purposes. Reports of a WHO Expert Committee. Geneva, World Health Organization, Technical Report Series 611 (1977).

ENVIRONMENTAL PROTECTION AGENCY: FEDERAL RADIATION PROTECTION GUIDANCE; PROPOSED ALTERNATIVES FOR CONTROLLING PUBLIC EXPOSURE TO RADIOFREQUENCY RADIATION*

AGENCY: U.S. Environmental Protection Agency (EPA).

ACTION: Notice of proposed recommendations, request for written comments on alternatives.

SUMMARY: The Environmental Protection Agency (EPA) is proposing four alternative approaches to limit the public's exposure to radiofrequency (RF) radiation. Three options are regulatory. For frequencies above 3 Megahertz (MHz), Options 1, 2, and 3 would limit whole-body average specific absorption rates (SARs) to 0.04, to 0.08, and to 0.4 watts per kilogram (W/kg), respectively. Electric field intensity (volts per meter, V/m) and magnetic field intensity (amperes per meter, A/m) would be limited for frequencies below 3 MHz. The limits are 87 V/m and 0.23 A/m, 275 V/m and 0.73 A/m, and 614 V/m and 1.63 A/m for Options 1, 2, and 3, respectively. The fourth option is nonregulatory; information and technical assistance programs would be conducted in lieu of adopting Federal Guidance. Depending on the Agency's final decision, any of the first three options could be recommended to the President as Federal Radiation Protection Guidance for Federal agencies, and whole-body SAR would be directly related to frequency dependent exposure power density values for implementation.

The EPA is considering this action for several reasons. The number and type of RF radiation sources have increased, and the population is continuously exposed to varying degrees; environmental levels of RF radiation and the number of persons exposed to higher levels has grown. Concerns over potential health effects from RF radiation have also heightened. Effects occur in test animals exposed at RF radiation intensities found in the environment. The need for Federal Guidance for RF radiation has been expressed to the Agency by Federal and other governmental bodies, by industry, and by the public.

DATES: The Agency is seeking written comments on this Notice, and all written comments will be carefully considered in preparing final recommendations to the President. Written comments must be received on or before October 28, 1986.

ADDRESSES: Written comments should be submitted to the Central Docket Section (LE-131), U.S. Environmental Protection Agency, Attn.: Docket Number A-81-43, Washington, DC 20460.

Docket No. A-81-43, containing material relevant to this proposal, is located in the West Tower Lobby, Gallery 1, Central Docket Section, U.S. Environmental Protection Agency, 401 M Street, SW., Washington, DC. The Docket may be inspected between 8 A.M. and 4 P.M. on weekdays, except holidays. A reasonable fee may be charged for copying.

---

*Environmental Protection Agency: Federal Radiation Protection Guidance; Proposed Alternatives for Controlling Public Exposure to Radiofrequency Radiation; Notice of Proposed Recommendations:July 30, 1986.

Single copies of background reports on environmental levels of RF radiation, biological effects, and the potential costs of Federal Guidance for RF radiation may be requested in writing from the Program Management Office (ANR-458), U.S. Environmental Protection Agency, Washington, DC 20460, or by calling (202) 475-8388.

A copy of each of the reports is also available for inspection at EPA's Central Docket Section (address above) and at the library in each of the 10 EPA Regional Offices. See SUPPLEMENTARY INFORMATION for the locations of the 10 regional libraries.

FOR FURTHER INFORMATION CONTACT: David E. Janes, Director, Analysis and Support Division (ANR-461), Office of Radiation Programs, U.S. Environmental Protection Agency, 401 M Street, SW., Washington, DC 20460, (202) 475-9626.

SUPPLEMENTARY INFORMATION

I. Statutory Authority

Federal radiation protection guides are developed by the Environmental Protection Agency (EPA) under the Federal Radiation Council Authority (Pub. L. 86-373), transferred to EPA by Reorganization Plan No. 3 of 1970, as codified at 42 U.S.C. 2021(h). The Administrator of the Environmental Protection Agency is charged to advise the President with respect to radiation matters, directly or indirectly affecting health, including Guidance for all Federal agencies in the formulation of radiation standards and in the establishment and execution of programs of cooperation with States. Upon Presidential approval of EPA recommendations, the pertinent Federal agencies are responsible for implementing Guidance. The Agency's authorities for Federal Radiation Guidance also require the Administrator to consult with the National Council on Radiation Protection and Measurements (NCRP) and other expert bodies.

II. Basic Terms Used in This Notice

Various technical terms are used throughout this Notice and are defined below. The reader is also referred to other reference documents (1,2) for description of technical terms.

(a) *Consumer Electronic Product* For the purpose of this Notice, any consumer product that emits, or has the potential to emit, radiofrequency radiation, e.g., a microwave oven.

(b) *Continuous Exposure* Exposure equal to or greater than 6 continuous minutes. Exposure less than 6 minutes is called short-term.

(c) *Electric Field Strength* (E) The force exerted on a stationary unit of positive charge at a point in an electric field. Electric field strength may be expressed in volts per meter (V/m).

(d) *Energy Density* The instantaneous power density integrated over its duration. Energy density may be expressed in units of power density-time, e.g., microwatt-minute per square centimeter or Watt-second per square meter.

(e) *Equivalent Plane-Wave Power Density* (S) The power density derived from electric (E) or magnetic (H) field strengths with the assumption that the relationship between power density and field strength is the same as that for plane waves in free space. In free space, E/H=377 ohms. [See also the definition for power density.]

(f) *Exposure* Exposure occurs whenever and wherever a member of the public is subjected to external electric, magnetic, or electromagnetic fields, and/or is subjected to low frequency electric shock when making contact with an electrically grounded object. [See also the definitions for power density and specific absorption rate.]

(g) *Far Field Region* A region in the field of an antenna, located far enough from the antenna so that the electric and magnetic fields have essentially a plane-wave character, i.e., locally very uniform distributions of electric field strength and magnetic field strength in planes transverse to the direction of propagation. For large antennas especially, the far field region is also called the Fraunhofer region.

(h) *Hertz (Hz)* A unit for expressing frequency (f) in units of cycles per second, i.e., one Hz is defined as one cycle per second. For RF radiation in air, the frequency of electromagnetic waves is related to wavelength by the relationship f=c/wavelength where c, the velocity of radiowaves, is 3×10^8 meters/second, and wavelength is in units of meters. This relationship is illustrated below where the frequency may be expressed in multiplicative units of Hz as shown. See Table 1.

(i) *Magnetic Field Strength* (H) The force on a hypothetical stationary unit magnetic north pole at a point in a magnetic field. Magnetic field strength may be expressed in amperes per meter (A/m) or milliamperes per meter (mA/m).

TABLE 1.

Frequency	Wavelength (meters)
10 kilohertz (kHz) = 10,000 Hz	30,000.0
100 kz	3,000.0
1 megahertz (MHz) = 1000 kHz	300.0
10 MHz	30.0
100 MHz	3.0
1 gigahertz (GHz) = 1000 MHz	0.3
10 GHz	0.03
100GHz	0.003

(j) *Mixed Frequency Fields* Exposure fields which consist of more than one RF radiation frequency.

(k) *Near-Field Region* A region in the field of an antenna, located near the antenna, in which the electric and magnetic fields do not have essentially a plane-wave character but vary considerably from point to point. The near-field region has a different size and geometry (shape) for large and small antennas. The near-field region is further subdivided into the reactive near-field region, which is closest to the antenna and contains most or nearly all of the stored energy associated with the field of the antenna, and the radiating near-field region.

(l) *Plane Wave* An electromagnetic wave with parallel or nearly parallel planar surfaces of constant phase.

(m) *Power Density* (S) The magnitude of the electromagnetic energy flux density at a point in space, expressed in power per unit area such as watts per square meter, milliwatts per square centimeter, or microwatts per square centimeter. For plane waves, E, H, and direction of propagation are mutually orthogonal (perpendicular). E^2 and H^2 are simply related to power density, i.e., $S=E^2/3770$ or $S=37.7\ H^2$ in units of milliwatts per square centimeter where E=electric field strength (V/m) and H=magnetic field strength (A/m). E^2 and H^2 are the actual quantities measured by many survey meters even though the instrument is calibrated to indicate power density units. The general relationship between power density and SAR is discussed in Section IV.B.

(n) *Product Performance Standard* Refers to a standard which limits RF radiation emitted from a specific product under specified operating conditions; these standards establish tests to be performed by a manufacturer during or immediately after product assembly. The specific maximum allowable emission values are set so as to provide appropriate protection of the public during normal operation of the product. Such values are not the same as exposure limits, as considered by this Notice. Product performance standards are promulgated under the Radiation Control for Health and Safety Act of 1968 (Pub. L. 90-602) and are administered by the Food and Drug Administration (FDA).

(o) *Public* The term public in this Notice means all persons except: (a) workers, to the extent they are occupationally exposed to RF fields produced by activities of their employer at the place of employment whether or not their duties directly involve RF radiation, (b) patients, to the extent they are exposed due to prescribed medical treatment or procedures using RF fields, and (c) persons, to the extent they are exposed as a result of the use of consumer electronic products (see definition (m), Product Performance Standard). The intent is to consider these people as members of the public except when they are exposed from occupational activities, medical procedures, and/or consumer electronic products, respectively.

(p) *Pulse Modulated Field* An electromagnetic field which is caused by the modulation of a carrier by a series of pulses.

(q) *Radiofrequency (RF) Radiation* Defined as electromagnetic fields within the frequency range of 10 kHz to 100 GHz in these recommendations.

(r) *Root-Mean-Square (RMS)* Certain electrical effects are proportional to the square root of the mean value of the square of a periodic function (over one period). This value is known as the effective value or the root-mean-square (RMS) value since it is derived by first squaring the function, determining the mean value of this squared value, and extracting the square root of the mean value to determine the end result.

(s) *Short-Term Exposure* Exposure for less than 6 continuous minutes.

(t) *Specific Absorption Rate (SAR)* The time derivative of the incremental energy (dW) absorbed by (dissipated in) an incremental mass (dm) contained in a volume element (dV) of a given density (D).

$$SAR = \frac{d}{dt}\left(\frac{dW}{dm}\right) = \frac{1}{D}\frac{d}{dt}\left(\frac{dW}{dV}\right)$$

The specific absorption rate is expressed in units of watts per kilogram (W/kg). Conventionally, the SAR in tissue in expressed as:

$$SAR = \frac{C_t E_t^2}{D}$$

where

Ct=tissue conductivity at the irradiation frequency (mhos per meter),

Et=RMS electric field strength in the tissue (volts per meter), and

D=tissue density (kilograms per cubic meter).

Note that Et is not the same as the external electric field (E) which is specified by the proposed limits discussed in this Notice.

The general relationship between exposure, measured as power density, and SAR is discussed in Section IV.B.

III. Background

The Concern

Manmade RF radiation is part of modern society. Applications are found in communications, transportation, defense, industry, consumer products, security, and medicine. Essentially everyone in the United States is continuously exposed to low levels of RF radiation, and some people who live or work near powerful sources are exposed to higher levels. RF radiation sources have steadily increased in number, and their uses have diversified so that a general increase in exposure levels in the environment has occurred. Various effects occur in experimental animals exposed to intensities which are found in the general environment. The increase in source coupled with a better understanding of biological effects has heightened concerns about potential adverse effects on public health from exposure to RF radiation.

Existing Standards

There are no Federal standards or guidelines for controlling exposure of the public to RF radiation in the environment. As a result, in 1982 the Federal Communications Commission (FCC) proposed the adoption of interim standards for public exposure to RF radiation until Federal guides were adopted, or standards were promulgated by EPA (3). The FCC recently decided to use the 1982 voluntary American National Standards Institute (ANSI) standard (discussed below) in processing license applications and facility modifications under its National Environmental Policy Act (NEPA) responsibilities (4). The Food and Drug Administration (FDA) has established a product performance standard for microwave ovens to limit leakage of radiation (21 CFR 1010.10); this is a performance standard rather than an exposure standard.

The lack of a Federal public exposure standard has led to diverse regulatory activity by State and local governments. The city of Portland (5) and Multnomah County (6) in Oregon have enacted amendments to zoning ordinances to control construction of new facilities. The town of Onondaga, New York (7) has issued a moratorium on construction of new RF radiation transmitting systems until Federal public exposure guidance is available. The City of New York has had a proposal to control population exposures under consideration for a number of years (8). Massachusetts (9), Texas (10) and New Jersey (11) have enacted statutes to limit exposure. In Connecticut, Public Act No. 84-383 (effective June 8, 1984) directs the Connecticut Commissioner of Environmental Protection to adopt the 1982 American National Standards Institute voluntary standard.

The American National Standards Institute (ANSI) developed a voluntary standard for occupational exposure in 1966 (12) which was reaffirmed with minor changes in 1974 (13). The ANSI is a private, non-profit organization that, among other things, coordinates the development of voluntary national standards, primarily for technical, industrial, and manufacturing practices. ANSI standards are intended as guides to aid manufacturers, consumers, and the public. The Occupational Health and Safety Administration (OSHA) adopted the 1966 ANSI standard for occupational exposure in 1971 (14), permitting an exposure of up to 10 milliwatts per square centimeter for frequencies between 10 MHz and 100 GHz. The OSHA standard was determined to be merely advisory in 1976 (15) and was implemented by OSHA under the General Duty Clause of the Occupational Safety and Health Act (16) until March 1982 at which time OSHA proposed to revoke its standard (47 FR 23477). In February 1984, OSHA determined to retain its standard because it provided useful advice for employers (49 FR 5318).

The ANSI revised its voluntary standard in 1982. This standard is now frequency dependent with more stringent levels of exposure in certain frequency ranges. For example, a maximum exposure level of 1 milliwatt per square centimeter is specified for frequencies between 30 and 300 MHz (17).

Occupational exposure standards in most Western countries range from 1 to 10 milliwatts per square centimeter. These levels limit the amount of heat that is generated when RF radiation is absorbed in human tissue. Eastern European countries, e.g., USSR, Poland, and Czechoslovakia, have lower exposure standards for most occupational situations. In the USSR, for example, the occupational standard is 0.025 milliwatts per square centimeter (25 microwatts per square centimeter) for frequencies above 300 MHz (18). These Eastern European standards are largely based on behavioral and clinical studies that, for the most part, have not been repeated or replicated in other countries because reports on these studies generally lack sufficient description of needed technical details.

The National Council on Radiation Protection and Measurements (NCRP) recently recommended RF exposure criteria for the public (19). A draft proposal was first reported at the 1984 Annual Meeting of the NCRP on April 5, 1984 in Washington, DC. The NCRP is a nonprofit corporation chartered by Congress that collects, analyzes, develops, and disseminates information and recommendations about radiation protection and radiation measurements, quantities, and units. The International Radiation Protection Association (IRPA) published interim guidelines for exposure to radiofrequency radiation in April 1984 (20). The IRPA is an international scientific union of various national health physics and radiation protection associations. Although the limits recommended by NCRP and IRPA are generally similar to the 1982 ANSI standard in derivation and form, they are five times more stringent for exposure of the public. In addition, the Applied Physics Laboratory of Johns Hopkins University, based on results of research there, established an exposure limit of 100 microwatts per square centimeter for frequencies between 30 MHz and 100 GHz for all employees regardless of whether their jobs directly involved exposure to RF radiation (21).

The exposure levels recommended by the ANSI, IRPA, NCRP, Massachusetts, Multnomah County, Portland, New Jersey, and Connecticut are all based on the concept that whole-body average specific absorption rates (SARs) should be the same for all frequencies above 3 MHz. This approach requires different exposure levels at different frequencies. Also, the guidelines developed to date are based largely on the same assessment criterion used by ANSI, i.e., whole-body average SARs greater than 4 W/kg cause behavioral effects in irradiated animals. Behavioral disruption was selected by ANSI as the most reliable indicator of a potentially harmful health effect although other harmful effects including lethality occur around 4 W/kg and various other biological effects have also been experimentally determined or theoretically predicted to occur at lower SAR values. The ANSI then applied a safety factor of 10 to specify a permissible whole-body average SAR of 0.4 W/kg which provided the basis for limiting power densities for human exposures (17). The other standards are lower than the ANSI standard primarily because a larger margin of safety was determined to be necessary for the general population; the safety factors applied to derive exposure limits range from 50 to 100.

One important reason for the different determinations of appropriate margins of safety is the judgment on whether a distinction should be made between occupational and public exposures. Previous ANSI guides have been widely interpreted as occupational standards, but ANSI intended its 1982 guide to apply to both occupational and nonoccupational exposures and stated its guides were offered as upper limits of exposure, particularly for the population at large (17). The use of a single standard for both occupational and public exposures is a departure from traditional practices in public health protective regulations which usually differentiate between occupational and general populations. Environmental health criteria for RF radiation published by the World Health Organization (WHO), used as the scientific basis for the IRPA guidelines, state that exposure of the general population should be kept as low as readily achievable and exposure limits should generally be lower than those for occupational exposure (22). It is also a practice of the NCRP to differentiate between occupational and general populations (23). Among the reasons cited by groups such as IRPA or NCRP for more stringent general population exposure standards are that the general public comprises individuals of all ages, different health status, and varying susceptibilities and there is the possibility of continuous and lifelong exposure.

Related Activities by EPA

An Advance Notice of Proposed Recommendations (ANPR) published in the Federal Register on December 23, 1982 (47 FR 57338), announced the Agency's intent to develop guidance for Federal agencies to sue to limit exposure of the public to RF radiation (24). The ANPR provided background information relevant to the development of Federal guidance. Comments were received from the public in response to the ANPR. These comments supported the development of Federal Exposure Guidance for RF Radiation and, in some cases, recommended specific exposure limits. These comments are available for public examination in Docket Number A-81-43 in the Central Docket Section of the EPA (see ADDRESSES).

An Interagency Work Group was established to provide information to EPA on issues of concern to Federal agencies and to comment on drafts of this Notice. Though the draft reviewed by the Work Group consisted of only Option 1, most of the comments received are pertinent to all options. This group is comprised of sixteen Federal agencies and three governmental advisory bodies. The Interagency Work Group includes the Federal Communications Commission, Central Intelligence Agency, Federal Aviation Administration (FAA) in the Department of Transportation, Occupational Safety and Health Administration (Department of Labor), National Bureau of Standards (Department of Commerce), National Science Foundation, National Aeronautics and Space Administration, Department of Energy, Food and Drug Administration (Department of Health and Human

Services), Department of State, Department of Agriculture, Voice of America (United States Information Agency), Department of Defense (DOD), Coast Guard (Department of Transportation), Veterans Administration, National Telecommunications and Information Administration (Department of Commerce), National Academy of Sciences, National Council on Radiation Protection and Measurements, and the Conference of Radiation Control Program Directors.

The Environmental Protection Agency operates an environmental monitoring and assessment program on RF radiation and has supported a biological effects research program in this area. These activities have enabled the Agency to develop the information necessary for this Notice. Three background reports have been prepared and are largely based on results from the Agency's research and environmental assessment programs. *Biological Effects of Radiofrequency Radiation* provides an in-depth critical review of the biological effects literature (25). *The Radiofrequency Radiation Environment: Environmental Exposure Levels and RF Radiation Emitting Sources* evaluates sources and levels of RF radiation in the environment (26). *An Engineering Assessment of the Potential Impact of Federal Radiation Guidance on the AM, FM and TV Broadcast Services* analyzes the potential impact of various proposed control levels on affected RF sources and users of the electromagnetic spectrum (27). Another report, *An Estimate of the Potential Costs of Guidelines Limiting Public Exposures to Radiation from Broadcast Sources,* details economic impact analyses (28). Information on how to obtain these reports is given in Section IX of this Notice.

Under the aegis of the Agency's Science Advisory Board (SAB), a Subcommittee on the Biological Effects of RF Radiation was established to evaluate the scientific adequacy and technical merit of drafts of the report *Biological Effects of Radiofrequency Radiation.* The final report was revised in accordance with the comments of this Subcommittee. Subcommittee reports and meeting transcripts are also available for public review in EPA Docket No. A-81-43 (see ADDRESSES).

Issues Addressed

EPA has received numerous comments on the ANPR and a published draft of *Biological Effects of Radiofrequency Radiation* (29). Comments have also come from the Interagency Work Group. Overall, the comments expressed a need for the development by EPA of Radiation Protection Guidance for limiting exposure of the public to RF radiation. Analysis of the comments identified at least seven major issues of concern.

1. Future efforts to develop and carry out implementation programs will require resources to acquire and develop personnel and capabilities which most Federal agencies do not now have. Several agencies, including the FCC and FAA, have indicated they may request assistance from EPA. If Guidance is established, the Administrator of EPA will establish a capability to develop and evaluate the measurement techniques and systems needed to allow EPA to exercise oversight

responsibilities to assist Federal agencies in developing implementation and compliance programs.

2. Many Federal agencies expressed concern that it may be difficult to distinguish between public exposure and occupational exposure when implementing Guidance in Federal facilities. Is an individual to be classified as a "member of the public" or as a "worker": (a) If duties when working at a facility do not directly involve RF radiation, but exposure to levels exceeding the Guidance limits occurs, or (b) when visiting a facility where exposure levels generally exceed environmental exposure limits? To clarify this situation in part, we propose to exclude all persons who are occupationally exposed to RF fields produced by activities of their employer at the place of employment whether or not their duties directly involve RF radiation. But, EPA is soliciting comment on this matter and is especially interested in how to treat exposures to members of the general public who may visit Federal facilities.

3. The Food and Drug Administration (FDA) did not want any EPA Guidance to conflict with their responsibilities for developing product performance standards. EPA proposes, therefore, to exclude from consideration those exposures of the public resulting from electronic consumer products. Certain electronic consumer products may cause exposures that exceed the various limits discussed in this Notice, but any such exposures might be more readily controlled by product performance standards.

4. Several Federal agencies were concerned that EPA Guidance for general population exposure will mistakenly be viewed by their employees as an occupational exposure standard. Notwithstanding these concerns, EPA believes the target population is explicitly and sufficiently delineated in this proposal.

5. Some Federal agencies are concerned the compliance with general population exposure guidance will affect some Federal operations involving RF sources. Even for the most stringent control levels under consideration, EPA analyses indicate relatively minor impact on Federal operations; unofficial estimates by certain agencies are in disagreement. However, one major DOD organization suggested its analyses were consistent with EPA's assessment of little impact. But, the extent of impact is apparently related to issue 2, above, i.e, whether employees not directly working with RF sources should be classified as occupationally exposed. The EPA asked the Federal agencies to identify sites they consider might present potential compliance problems. The EPA hopes to measure exposure levels at some of these sites to help provide information which may be useful in resolving the questions raised.

6. The Report on Biological Effects and the composition of the SAB subcommittee that reviewed the report were criticized (30). Effects due to modulated RF fields and at frequencies below 10 kHz were of particular concern. This proposal makes no special provision for modulated RF fields because the scientific data on how such fields interact with biological systems is not considered to be sufficiently developed to permit an assessment of the potential human health consequences of exposure to such fields. Modulation is an important issue in need of more research, and if more adequate information becomes available modulation may be addressed

in the future. Additionally, EPA intends to treat exposures to fields at frequencies less than 10 kHz as a separate subject for possible future Guidance.

7. A need for Federal Guidance to control exposure of the public to RF radiation was expressed to EPA by local and State governments, other Federal regulatory agencies, industrial groups, and private citizens. For example, the National Telecommunications and Information Administration (NTIA) has urged EPA to devote all resources necessary to support its research and efforts to promulgate these guidelines as soon as possible (31). Two major concerns have been identified: (1) a concern for the potential public health consequences of increasing and continuous exposure to RF radiation in the environment, and (2) a desire that local and State standards should be based on Federal Guidance rather than many diverse standards developed individually.

The need for Federal exposure guidance to protect public health has emerged as an important issue as RF radiation sources, uses, and, thus, exposures have increased and as our understanding of the biological effects from RF radiation exposure has improved. Essentially everyone in the United States is continuously exposed to very low levels of RF radiation. People who live or work near powerful sources are exposed to higher levels. It is now known that various effects occur in experimental animals exposed to certain intensities that are found in the general environment and to which people are exposed. In addition, levels of RF radiation in the environment are expected to continue to increase with continued growth in telecommunications and other sources. From a public health perspective, therefore, any establishment of Federal exposure guidance could be viewed as both a corrective and preventive action to (1) correct existing exposure problems by reducing potentially harmful levels and eliminating easily avoidable exposures to levels believed to be safe and (2) assure that environmental levels of RF radiation in the future do not increase above acceptable levels.

Federal Guidance has become important also because its absence has led to varying State and local government actions affecting the construction and use of new transmitting facilities, particularly in the telecommunications industry, as well as to enactment of several different public exposure standards. Segments of the telecommunications industry have urged establishment and adoption of a uniform Federal exposure standard to forestall what is viewed as the disruptive and costly impact of diverse local regulatory activity on the development of telecommunications facilities (32–36).

IV. Basis for This Proposal

A. RF Radiation in the Environment

EPA has conducted monitoring and measurement programs and extensively analyzed sources and levels of RF radiation in the environment. The results of these studies, summarized below, are discussed in detail in the technical report, *The*

Radiofrequency Radiation Environment: Environmental Exposure Levels and Radiofrequency Radiation Emitting Sources, which has been placed in the docket. Typical sources of RF radiation include AM and FM radio and television broadcast stations, radars, satellite communication and microwave relay systems, land mobile radio, and amateur radio. The number, types, and uses of RF radiation sources have rapidly expanded.

Extensive environmental RF measurements made by EPA have shown that the sources most likely to produce the highest population exposure levels are domestic broadcast stations with frequencies between 535 kHz and 806 MHz. Some of the most intense public exposures result from emissions within the FM radio broadcast band as frequencies between 88 and 108 MHz. It is significant that this frequency band falls within the range for resonant absorption (a concept discussed in the next section on dosimetry) for humans resulting in maximal rates of energy absorption by the body.

Levels of exposure are determined by how close people are to a RF source, i.e., exposure intensity generally decreases as the distance from a radiating source increases. Exposure may result from one source or many sources. Most people, particularly in urban areas, receive their exposure from the superposition of RF fields emitted from many sources that operate at different frequencies.

Data in Tables 1 and 2 are presented in terms of power density (microwatts per square centimeter). Power density can be related to the rate at which energy is absorbed. For example, for FM and VHF frequencies, 1,000 microwatts per square centimeter corresponds to about 0.4 W/kg. Dosimetric relationships are described in detail in the next section and in Chapter 3 of reference 25.

TABLE 2. *Estimated Population Exposure for 15 U.S. Cities in Microwatts Per Square Centimeter*

City	Median Exposure	Percent exposed to less than 1 microwatt/cm^2
Boston	0.018	98.50
Atlanta	0.016	99.20
Miami	0.0070	98.20
Philadelphia	0.0070	99.87
New York	0.0022	99.60
Chicago	0.0020	99.60
Washington	0.009	97.20
Las Vegas	0.012	99.10
San Diego	0.010	99.85
Portland	0.020	99.70
Houston	0.011	99.99
Los Angeles	0.0048	99.90
Denver	0.0074	99.85
Seattle	0.0071	99.81
San Francisco	0.002	97.66
All Cities	0.0048	99.44

Based upon analyses of extensive measurements in 15 metropolitan areas (see Table 1), EPA estimates that the typical median exposure in urban areas is 5 nanowatts per square centimeter and that typical exposures for most of the population, over 99 percent, is less than 1 microwatt per square centimeter. It is important to note that these "typical" population exposure estimates represent exposures for individuals living or working close to the RF sources. Also, these exposures do not take into account population mobility, exposures at heights of greater than six meters above ground, building attenuation, and periods when the sources are not transmitting.

In contrast to these typical exposures, higher values than those shown in Table 2 can occur at locations near to the antennas of broadcast stations and other sources. Some representative exposures obtained from EPA studies near antennas are summarized in Table 3. From present information it is not possible to estimate the number of people continuously or intermittently exposed to these higher levels. However, the number of sources capable of producing various levels were estimated in analyzing the costs of different control levels, and the results are summarized in Section VII.B.

In summary, if an individual's exposure is predominantly due to a nearby source(s), it can be significantly higher than exposures associated with the multisource environments as described. The EPA has determined that approximately one percent of the U.S. population is exposed to RF fields from VHF broadcasting with intensities greater than one microwatt per square centimeter (37). Exposures due to nearby sources in publicly accessible areas may reach maximum values in the 1–10 milliwatts per square centimeter range or higher, but the number of people exposed to these levels is not yet well characterized.

TABLE 3. *Range of Measurements Located Near Broadcast Antennas*[1]

	Power Density Microwatts per square Centimeter	
Tall Buildings:		
F.M. TV	0.2–375	
AM	2,650–10,600	Electric Fields.
	(100–200 V/m)	
	570–2,170	Magnetic Fields.
	(0.123–0.240 A/m	
Ground Levels:		
FM, TV	10–7,000	
AM	106–23,900	Electric Fields.
	(20–300 V/m)	
	1,510–3.05×10^4	Magnetic Fields.
	(0.2–9A/m)	

[1] Abstracted from various EPA measurement survey reports. Measurements were made very near antennas, usually within 200 feet or less. For AM frequencies, the electric and magetic field strength equivalents of the power density are given for ease in comparison to the field strengths given in the various options.

B. Electromagnetic Field Interactions and Dosimetry

RF radiation can be absorbed, reflected, or transmitted by the body. The amount of radiation that is absorbed is what is important when determining whether given levels of RF radiation exposure are harmful. It is, thus, necessary to be able to relate the intensity (power density) of exposure to the actual rate at which energy can be absorbed by an individual. The rate of energy absorption is called "specific absorption rate" or SAR and is given in units of watts per kilogram of body mass (W/kg). Except under controlled experimental conditions, SAR cannot be directly determined by measurements on humans, but it is proportional to the intensity of incident electromagnetic fields, or power density, which can be measured.

The SAR is the rate of energy absorption at any point within an absorbing body and will vary from point to point within the body. The maximum value of the SAR is called the peak SAR. The conventional use of SAR is in reference to the energy absorption rate of the body as a whole; called "whole-body average SAR" indicating that the SAR has been averaged over the entire body mass. It is this whole-body average SAR that is most commonly specified in studies of the biological effects of RF radiation. The value of the whole-body average SAR for man or laboratory animals depends on the interaction of several factors such as the size, shape, electrical properties, and position of the body in relation to the polarization and frequency of the RF radiation field (for example, AM versus FM radio waves). These various factors determine the frequency at which the whole-body average SAR of an absorbing object reaches its maximum value, the so called resonant frequency. The resonant frequency for humans lies in the range of 30–300 MHz. For example, in this range, which includes the frequencies for FM radio and VHF-TV broadcasts, exposure at an incident power density of 1,000 microwatts per square centimeter can result in a whole-body average SAR of approximately 0.4 W/kg. Dosimetric relationships are described in detail in Chapter 3 of reference 25.

The SAR given in biological effects research is commonly averaged over time as well as averaged over the body mass of test animals. In the following discussion of biological effects the terminology "whole-body average SAR" means that the SAR is averaged over time unless noted otherwise.

To summarize, in contrast to power density, SARs better describe how energy is absorbed in the body, are more reliable predictors of biological effects, and permit comparison of one health effects study to another. Specific absorption rates instead of power densities are, thus, used below to discuss health effects.

C. Health Effects of Radiofrequency Radiation

1. The Relationship Between Effects and Specific Absorption Rates (SARs)

The scientific literature on the biological effects of RF radiation has been critically reviewed by the Agency in *Biological Effects of Radiofrequency Radiation,* and the major findings from the report are excerpted and given below (25). It should be noted that epidemiological data are currently very limited and, thus, are not useful for deriving environmental exposure limits. Great reliance, therefore, must be placed on experiments with animals to derive environmental exposure limits. The results discussed below are obtained from animal experiments unless specifically noted to be drawn from human data. The reader is referred to *Biological Effects of Radiofrequency Radiation* for citations (25).

(a) High level RF radiation is a source of thermal energy (as seen with, for example, microwave ovens) that carries all of the known implications of heating for biological systems. At a given incident field strength, maximal heating occurs at the resonant frequency (D Andrea et al. 1977). In general, the data are consistent with the hypothesis that the SAR required to raise the body temperature of laboratory animals decreases as body mass increases; that is, a lower SAR is needed to produce a given significant increase in the temperature of a large laboratory animal than is required to achieve the same temperature rise in a small animal.

(b) Relatively short duration whole-body exposure of laboratory animals at whole-body average SAR values greater than 30 W/kg can be lethal; lethal SAR levels vary with species and exposure conditions. [Additional information on lethality is given further in this Section.]

(c) Brief exposures (less than 5 minutes) of the whole body to high intensity RF radiation may result in significant biological damage, e.g., birth defects, increased embryonic and fetal resorptions, lowered birth weights, and reduced survival of infant animals irradiated both before and after birth. Localized exposure to very high intensity RF radiation can result in burns; for example, facial burns on monkeys have been reported at 115 W/kg.

(d) A single short exposure of the eye to high-intensity RF radiation, if applied for sufficient time, is cataractogenic in some experimental animals. In the rabbit, the animal most often used in ocular studies, the cataractogenic threshold for a 100-minute exposure is 150 milliwatts per square centimeter (138 W/kg peak SAR in the lens). The cataractogenic potential of microwave radiation varies with frequency; the most effective frequencies for producing cataracts in the rabbit eye appear to be in the 1 to 10 GHz range. Cataracts have not been produced in primates acutely exposed to RF radiation under conditions that caused cataracts in lower mammals. This is attributed to the different facial structure in primates that causes a different pattern of absorbed energy in the eye. No cataracts have been reported in rabbits after whole-body, far-field RF radiation exposures, at SARs of 42 W/kg for 15 minutes. No data at present support a conclusion that low-level, chronic exposure to microwave radiation induces cataracts in human beings, although some studies have associated ocular-lens defects with microwave radiation exposure.

(e) In most of the animal studies that report a biological effect of RF radiation, exposures occurred at ambient temperatures of 20–25 degrees Celsius and relative humidities of 50–70 percent. At more thermally stressful conditions, e.g., higher ambient temperature and the same or higher relative humidity, the experimental results show that lower SARs cause a similar biological effect. For example, Rugh et al. (1974) found that the lethal dose of 2450-MHz radiation for mice was inversely related to a temperature-humidity index. Gage (1979b) showed that a 2450-MHz exposure at 22 degrees Celsius resulted in a reduced behavioral response rate in rats at 3 W/kg, but that similar exposures at 28 degrees Celsius caused reduced response rates at 1, 2, and 3 W/kg.

(f) No consistent biological effect has yet been found with molecular and subcellular systems exposed in vitro to RF radiation other than effects occurring at SARs that cause general temperature increases. Conclusions regarding effects of in vitro exposure of higher-order biological systems, such as single cells and brain tissue, are given below.

(g) The electrophysiological properties of single cells, especially the firing rates of neurons in isolated preparations, may be affected by RF radiation at SARs as low as 1 W/kg in a manner different from generalized heating.

(h) In general, no changes in chromosomes, DNA, or reproductive potential of RF-exposed animals have been reported and corroborated in the absence of significant rises of temperature. Similarly, RF radiation does not appear to cause mutations or genetic changes in bacterial test systems unless temperatures well above the normal physiological range are produced.

(i) Effects on the hematologic and immunologic systems have been reported at SARs equal to and greater than 0.5 W/kg; however, there is a lack of convincing evidence for RF radiation effects on these systems without some form of thermal involvement. Some of the reported effects of RF radiation on the hematologic and immune systems are similar to those resulting from a stress response involving the hypothalamic-hypophyseal-adrenal axis or following administration of glucocorticoids. In those few cases where the reversibility of RF radiation effects on the hematologic and immunologic systems has been examined, the effects have proved to be transient.

(j) RF radiation is teratogenic at high SARs (greater than 15 W/kg) that approach lethal levels for the pregnant animal. High maternal body temperatures are known to be associated with birth defects. There appears to be a threshold for the induction of experimental birth defects when a maternal rectal temperature of 41–42 degrees Celsius is reached. Any agent capable of producing elevated internal temperatures in this range, including RF radiation, is a potential teratogen. [Additional information on teratology is given further in this Section.]

(k) Reduced fetal mass (low birth weight) seems to occur consistently in rodents exposed during gestation to teratogenic levels of RF radiation, or at SARs somewhat less than those which cause death or malformation.

(l) There is evidence that exposure of rodents during gestation to RF radiation may cause functional changes later in life. For example, Johnson et al. (1978) observed lower body weight at weaning and in young adult rats exposed at 2.5 W/kg for 20 h/day during 19 days of gestation, and Chernovetz et al. (1975) found increased postnatal survival of mice exposed at 38 W/kg for 10 minutes during gestation. These studies illustrate the different effects that have been observed for chronic low-level versus acute high-level exposures. Also, Rugh (1976a) has shown that RF irradiation on select days in vitro can alter later (sometimes much later) effects of reirradiation with microwaves.

(m) Permanent changes in reproductive efficiency have been directly associated with RF radiation exposures that caused temperatures in animal testes greater than 45 degrees Celsius. At temperatures of 37–42 degrees Celsius, mature sperm may be killed with a temporary loss of spermatogenic epithelium. Irradiation of rats at an SAR of 5.6 W/kg, which produced a core temperature of 41 degrees Celsius, resulted in temporary infertility.

(n) Neurons in the central nervous system (CNS) of experimental animals have been reported to be altered by acute high-level and by chronic low-level exposures (equal to or greater than 2 W/kg). Pulsed RF radiation may have a potentiating effect on drugs that affect nervous system function. Some of the early reports of RF radiation effects on the blood-brain barrier (BBB) at SARs equal to or less than 2 W/kg have not been substantiated by later investigations.

(o) An increased mobilization of calcium ions occurs in brain tissue exposed in vitro to RF radiation, amplitude modulated at frequencies recorded in the electroencephalogram (EEG) of awake animals. The response appears to be based on the intensity of the electric field within the tissue, which can be related to SAR; the lowest effective SAR in in vitro samples is estimated to be 0.0013 W/kg. Calcium-ion efflux is a nonlinear effect in terms of both AM frequency and field intensity; that is, the response occurs at specific frequencies and electric field strengths. The physiological significance of this effect has not been established.

(p) Some types of animal behavior are disrupted at SARs that are approximately 25–50 percent of the resting metabolic rates of many species. For example, changes in locomotor behavior in rats occur at an SAR of 1.2 W/kg, and alterations in thermoregulatory behavior in squirrel monkeys occur at an SAR of 1 W/kg. Decreases in other operant or learned behavioral responses during exposure have been found at an SAR of 2.5 W/kg in the rat and at 5.0 W/kg in the rhesus monkey. The reported behavioral alterations appear to be reversible with time.

(q) Changes reported in endocrine gland function and blood chemistry are similar to those observed during increased thermoregulatory activity and heat stress, and are generally associated with SARs greater than 1 W/kg. Exposures of sufficient intensity to produce whole-body heating produce an increase in heart rate similar to that caused by heating from other sources. Changes in whole-body metabolism have been reported following exposures at thermal levels (approximately 10 W/kg), and brain energy metabolism is altered at levels as low as 0.1 W/kg following irradiation of the exposed surface of the brain of anesthetized animals.

(r) Pulsed RF radiation in the range 216–6500 MHz can be heard by some human beings. The sound associated with the RF hearing varies with pulse width and pulse-repetition rate and is described as a click, buzz, or chirp. The threshold for human perception of this effect is approximately 40 microjoules per square centimeter (incident energy density per pulse), or 40 microwatt-seconds per square centimeter per pulse. The most generally accepted mechanism for the RF-auditory sensation is that the incident pulse induces a minuscule but rapid thermoelastic expansion within the skull, which results in a pressure wave that is conducted by the bone to the cochlear region of the ear.

(s) For the broad range of frequencies between 0.5 MHz and 100 GHz, cutaneous perception of heat and thermal pain may be an unreliable sensory mechanism for protection against potentially harmful RF radiation exposure levels. Many frequencies deposit most of their energy at depths below the cutaneous thermal receptors.

(t) There is no convincing evidence that exposure to RF radiation shortens the life span of human beings or experimental animals or that RF radiation is a primary carcinogen (cancer inducer); however, (1) few studies have used longevity or cancer incidence as end points, and (2) human studies have lacked statistical power to exclude life shortening or cancer. There is evidence from one group of investigators that chronic exposure to RF radiation (SAR=2 to 3 W/kg) resulted in cancer promotion or co-carcinogenesis in three different types of tumors in mice; the incidence of cancer was comparable to that observed in mice exposed to chronic stress.

(u) Human data are currently limited and incomplete but do not indicate any obvious relationship between prolonged low-level RF radiation exposure and increased morality or morbidity, including cancer incidence.

(v) The prospects for revision and refinement of the major conclusions and generalizations stated above are considerable because of limited knowledge of (1) effects of most frequencies in the range 0.5 MHz to 100 GHz; (2) effects of chronic low-level exposures on human beings and laboratory animals; (3) which segments of the population are most sensitive; (4) the influence of ambient environmental conditions and of potential synergistic interaction with other agents; (5) the implication of nonhomogeneous RF-energy deposition; (6) the existence and significance of frequency-specific effects and power-density windows; and (7) the physical mechanisms of interaction at low exposure levels, including field-specific phenomena.

(w) The central nervous system, the hematologic and immunologic systems, and behavior appear to be most sensitive to disturbance by RF radiation exposure. In particular, behavior is considered to be a sensitive function to evaluate adverse responses to hazardous agents since it indicates how well the whole organism, and especially the nervous system, is functioning. The ANSI, for instance, concluded both that the most sensitive measures of biological effects were based on behavior, whole-body average SARs between 4–8 W/kg were associated with thresholds of behavioral disruption, and reliable evidence of hazardous effects is associated with whole-body average SARs above 4 W/kg (17). The decrease in behavioral response rates cited by ANSI were based on studies done at ambient temperatures of 20 to 25 degrees Celsius. Additional research at EPA has shown that similar change in behavior occur at lower SARs when exposures are conducted at higher ambient temperature; that is, at 22 degrees Celsius (25). The effective SAR was 3 W/kg, whereas at 28 degrees Celsius SARs of 1 and 2 W/kg were effective (25).

(x) In summary, the data currently available on the relation of SAR to biological effects show evidence for biological effects at an SAR of about 1 W/kg. This value is lower by a factor of 4 than 4 W/kg, the value above which reliable evidence of hazardous effects was found by ANSI (1982) following a review of the literature in February 1979. The above conclusion is based on: (a) the findings that more thermally stressful conditions result in lower threshold SARs for behavioral changes similar to those changes determined by ANSI (1982) to be the most sensitive measures of biological effects, (b) the effects of endocrine gland function, blood chemistry, hematology, and immunology that appear to result from some form of thermal involvement due to absorbed RF energy, and (c) data from one laboratory showing that RF radiation can act as a cancer promoter or carcinogen and results from another laboratory describing changes in brain cellularity.

The SAB Subcommittee on the Biological Effects of Radiofrequency Radiation reviewed the document, *Biological Effects of Radiofrequency Radiation*, and concluded that "... it represents an adequate statement of the current scientific literature and can serve as a scientifically defensible basis for the Agency's development of radiation protection guidance...." Since then, some additional information is now available for consideration by the Agency and is discussed below.

The Agency received information and comment on biological effects from the National Institute of Occupational Safety and Health (NIOSH) that included the following (38):

(a) Certain data on teratogenicity were not available for inclusion in EPA's health effects review document. Based on research at NIOSH, malformations have been seen at SARs as low as 8–9 W/kg, and severe teratogenic effects center around SARs of 10 W/kg, rather than the 15 W/kg cited in the EPA report.

(b) The EPA report stated that acute whole-body exposure of laboratory animals at SAR values greater than 30 W/kg is lethal; however, the report did not specifically analyze lethal levels of exposure and lethality data. The NIOSH identified relevant reports in the scientific literature and noted that exposures can lead to death in animals at SARs as low as 4 W/kg. NIOSH also stated it is helpful to point out that SARs resulting in lethality are generally lower for larger animals than for smaller animals and are quite low for monkeys (and presumably man).

(c) Severe heat stress has been reported in multiple species at dose rates (SARs from 4–8 W/kg) that are lethal if exposure is of sufficient duration. Core temperature increases resulting from such exposures generally are 3 degrees Celsius or more.

(d) Whole-body average SARs from 2–30 W/kg cause death, embryonic and fetal resorption, cellular necrosis, severe heat stress, excessive increases in core temperature, reduced body and organ weight, extreme agitation, suppression of behavior, fatigue, inhibition of mitosis, and other clearly adverse effects in laboratory animals. A study at the University of Washington was recently completed and examined the long-term effects in rats exposed throughout their lifetime to pulsed microwave radiation at a maximum average SAR of 0.4 W/kg. The eighth report in a series of published reports on this study details these latest results (39). There were generally no differences between control and exposed animals except for some evidence of (1) altered immune function, (2) increased weight of adrenal glands in exposed animals, and (3) a statistically higher incidence of primary malignancies in exposed animals.

Because of the potential significance of these data for human health, EPA intends to review this study. The following issues are important to consider:

(a) Many clinical and biological measurements were made in the University of Washington study. It is, thus, possible that some differences would be noted that are due to chance alone.

(b) The reported tumor incidence in the exposed group of animals was not significantly different than unexposed groups of the same type of animals reported in the scientific literature; that is, the cancer incidence in the study's control animals was lower than expected from historical data on the same strain and species. The validity of comparisons to historical controls will be considered by EPA.

(c) The tumors occurred at multiple sites and were of multiple types, leaving biological interpretation open to question. On the other hand, many of the tumors were in organs susceptible to stress or to the action of cancer promoters.

(d) The study was designed to simulate chronic exposure of man to 450-MHz radiation at an incident power density of 1 milliwatt per square centimeter with an absorbed dose rate of 0.4 W/kg and, thus, to test the safety afforded by the 1982 ANSI guideline.

Other recent studies also need to be carefully evaluated by EPA. Some of these are: (a) a study on the potential carcinogenic activity of 2.45 GHz pulsed microwave radiation with an in vitro assay (40), (b) a reported increase in cancer, especially for blood-forming organs and lymphatic tissue, in a population of career servicemen in the Polish military (41), (c) a preliminary report on altered protein patterns in cerebrospinal fluid of radar workers in Sweden (42), and (d) corneal endothelial (eye) abnormalities in primates exposed to 2.45 GHz microwaves (43).

2. *Consequences of Elevated Body Temperature*

Heating has been the most generally understood and accepted explanation for most RF radiation effects. It is, thus, important to examine biological effects in relation to increases in body temperature (also referred to as core or rectal temperature) whether from RF radiation exposure or other sources of heat. The following information is also drawn from *Biological Effects of Radiofrequency Radiation* (25).

The average core temperature is approximately 37.0 degrees Celsius (98.6 degrees Fahrenheit) for humans and ranges from 36–38 degrees Celsius for most other mammals. In general, the lethal temperature is approximately 6 degrees Celsius above the average core temperature. Prolonged elevation of core temperature at 5 degrees Celsius above normal (42 degrees Celsius or 107.6 degrees

Fahrenheit) is associated with heat stroke and brain damage in people. A temperature of 41.2 degrees Celsius (106.2 degrees Fahrenheit) occurs in only 1 of 1,000 people during fever. Elevated body temperature in men is associated with reduced fertility, and high maternal body temperatures are associated with birth defects.

Since high body temperatures are related to reproductive and teratologic effects, it is important to consider these effects in relation to RF radiation-induced temperature increases. It is known that when mammalian testes, which have a normal temperature of 33–35 degrees Celsius, are heated to temperatures approaching abdominal temperatures (37–38 degrees Celsius), sterility can occur. At temperatures of 37–42 degrees Celsius, mature sperm may be killed with a temporary loss of spermatogenic tissue. Permanent changes in reproductive efficiency have been directly associated with RF radiation exposures that caused temperatures in animal testes greater than 45 degrees Celsius. In studies of healthy young men whose average body temperature was increased to 41 degrees Celsius by RF radiation exposure up to three hours, sperm numbers decreased by 60 percent at 40 to 60 days after the exposure. Also at this core temperature (41 degrees Celsius), temporary infertility in male rats exposed to RF radiation has also been reported; the whole-body average SAR was 5.6 W/kg. It can, thus, be concluded that adverse effects, albeit possibly reversible, on male fertility may occur if RF radiation exposure raises body temperature to 41 degrees Celsius. The whole-body average SAR in humans associated with this temperature is not known, but, based on mathematical models, it is expected to be greater than 4 W/kg under average environmental conditions.

RF radiation is teratogenic at whole-body average SARs of approximately 10 W/kg or greater, and there appears to be a threshold for the induction of experimental birth defects when a maternal rectal temperature of 41–42 degrees Celsius is reached. Any agent capable of producing elevated internal temperatures in this range, including RF radiation, is a potential teratogen. Reduced fetal mass (stunting or low birth weight) also seems to occur consistently in rodents exposed during gestation to SARs at 6 W/kg or greater for short-term exposures and at 4.8 W/kg for longer term exposures.

Other kinds of effects have also been reported in various animal species when exposure to RF radiation resulted in lower core temperature increases in the range of 1–3 degrees Celsius. These effects include, for example, hormonal and immunologic effects, changes in blood chemistry, and changes in behavior. But, as a general rule, exposures that produce an increase in core temperature less than 0.5 degrees Celsius have not been found to cause detectable effects.

In most of the animal studies that report a biological effect of RF radiation, the exposures occurred at ambient temperatures of 20–25 degrees Celsius and relative humidities of 50–70 percent. Experimental results show that lower SARs will cause similar biological effects under more thermally stressful conditions, e.g., higher ambient temperature and the same or higher relative humidity. In other words, it is reasonable to expect that the above described biological effects associated with core temperature increases greater than 0.5 degrees Celsius, will also occur at lower SARs if the combination of RF radiation exposure and ambient conditions is such that a similar core temperature increase results.

The results just discussed indicate that core temperature increases of 1 degree Celsius or more are associated with various health effects, and exposure to RF radiation is a source of heat which can increase core temperature. As a comparison, the Threshold Limit Value (TLV) for heat stress in the work environment established by the American Conference of Governmental Industrial Hygienists states that workers should not be permitted to continue their work when their core temperature exceeds 38 degrees Celsius, that is, 1 degree Celsius above the average normal temperature for adult human beings (44). One may conclude, therefore, that exposure to an environmental agent such as RF radiation that may cause a 1 degree Celsius rise in core temperature should be considered hazardous to relatively healthy individuals (25). It is important, then, to consider the SARs that may be required to produce a 1 degree Celsius rise in the core temperature of human beings exposed to RF radiation.

There are few data that exist on the RF radiation exposure conditions that cause core temperature changes of up to 1 degree Celsius in human beings. Estimates, however, have been obtained from mathematical modeling (24). The results of these modeling analyses indicate that whole-body average SARs of 1–4 W/kg for relatively short durations (1 hour) produce significant increases of about 1.0 degree Celsius in human body temperature at ambient temperatures of 25–30 degrees Celsius (77–86 degrees Fahrenheit). It is also reasonable to conclude that increases in body temperature are likely to occur at lower SARs if exposure occurs under more thermally stressful conditions, e.g., higher ambient temperature and/or higher relative humidity. Data from experimental studies with primates are in close agreement with the results of the modeling experiments.

The evidence indicates that exposure of human beings at frequencies in the resonant region at an SAR of approximately 1 W/kg produces significant changes in body temperature under some environmental conditions. Three additional factors should also be considered. First, a measurable increase in body temperature can be interpreted as an indication that the body is under stress. Exposure to RF radiation at SARs below those that cause an increase in core temperature may be activating the heat-dissipating thermoregulatory mechanisms of the body to try to maintain core temperature within the normal range. Second, under many conditions of RF exposure, it is probable that some regions of the body will experience an increase in temperature due to localized RF energy absorption while the core temperature remains near normal. For example, an EPA mathematical model has shown that a whole-body average SAR of 1.4 W/kg produced a 3.6 degrees Celsius rise in temperature of the thigh although the core temperature rose only 0.5 degrees Celsius (25). Localized energy absorption is, however, not yet well characterized. Third, the general population has groups of individuals particularly susceptible to heat. [See Section 4 below.]

In summary, based chiefly on experiments with animals, RF radiation exposures which elevate core temperature by 1 degree Celsius can produce adverse effects.

Results from animal experiments, especially with primates, and from thermal models of humans, indicate the SARs associated with such core temperature increases may vary from 1 to 4 W/kg, depending on species differences and environmental variables.

3. Low-Level and Nonthermal Effects

The public health significance of biological effects at whole-body average SARs lower than 1 W/kg is, at present, not well understood partly because the underlying mechanism(s) responsible for these low-level effects is not known. In some cases, results are from single studies and, thus, are not yet confirmed by replication. Most notable are neurological effects and effects from exposure to modulated fields, e.g., metabolic and histologic changes in the brain tissues of animals and of cells in vitro. Some of these effects are discussed below.

Many reports of effects of RF fields that are amplitude modulated at very low frequencies have not been independently corroborated (25). The major exception is calcium-ion efflux from chick brain tissue in vitro at intensity levels far below those that cause heating. This, combined with the results of studies of brain biochemistry and electroencephalograms (EEGs) in animals and with synaptosomes and human neuroblastoma cells in culture, provides evidence that central nervous system (CNS) tissue from several species, including human beings, is affected by low-intensity RF fields sinusoidally amplitude modulated at specific low frequencies or by those low frequencies directly. The physiological significance of these field-induced effects is not established. In addition to the CNS-related changes, amplitude-modulated RF fields have been reported to alter an immune response and a pancreatic tissue function.

These reports with diverse biological systems are without apparent connection to each other except for the physical agent causing the change. The critical parameter common to all these experiments is the specificity of the low frequency electromagnetic signal. However, in most cases, dose response curves, namely, magnitude of the response as a function of frequency, have not been obtained.

No report has yet described a mechanism of action in sufficient detail to identify the conditions necessary and sufficient to explain unequivocally calcium ion efflux in the brain or the other biological changes caused by low frequency signals or by modulated RF fields. The response to specific frequencies and intensities is unusual and at present unexplained. This response to amplitude modulated RF radiation may be a true field effect at a very low SAR and at biologically relevant frequencies, i.e., in the range of frequencies normally present in the EEG. The evidence is against heat as the underlying cause. These unusual, multiple-intensity-range responses challenge standard dose-response analyses and, by their very nature, may prohibit the invocation of threshold levels.

Pulsed RF radiation can be perceived ("heard") by some people. The perception of sound associated with "RF hearing" varies with pulse width and pulse-repetition rate and is described as a click, buzz, or chirp. Because this effect is a function of instantaneous peak energy deposition and pulse width, average whole-body SARs are not useful exposure parameters. Although the effects of RF hearing on health are not now known, the experience may be annoying and stressful.

4. Potential Human Health Effects

A. Introduction. Exposure to RF radiation produces various biological effects. Most studies use experimental animals exposed for relatively short periods of time, rather than long-term continuous exposures, and few health studies of people have been done. At relatively high rates of energy absorption, health effects are due to heating of cells and tissues and increases in temperature depend on duration of exposure. Absorption of sufficient RF radiation energy, as with other sources of external heat such as sunlight, can be harmful.

Effects have also been found in experimental animals at levels that do not produce detectable temperature increases in tissue. It is not known whether these effects occur in humans or if they are harmful. Most people are exposed to even lower levels that have not been shown to result in adverse effects in experiments with animals. Despite various uncertainties in the understanding of how RF radiation exposure effects human health, it is still possible to evaluate the potential for adverse health effects in exposed people and to identify groups in the population who may be particularly sensitive to RF radiation. The potential health effects of RF radiation can best be discussed from two perspectives: thermal effects and potential nonthermal effects.

B. Thermal Effects. Humans have a "thermostat" that maintains the body's temperature at 37 degrees Celsius. The ability of the body to reach and maintain a characteristic temperature is called thermoregulation. There are a variety of thermoregulatory processes by which body temperature is maintained despite widely varying environmental temperatures. Two major ways of dissipating excess heat from the body are: (1) the diversion of blood circulation to the surface of the body to radiate body heat and (2) sweating and other fluid-dependent processes. These are involuntary physiological processes, but people also react to the perception of heat or cold with a variety of voluntary actions including changing location, altering temperature settings in contained spaces, and changing clothing. We also respond to the thirst caused by sweating. An understanding of thermoregulatory processes helps to interpret the levels of RF radiation that are likely to produce adverse effects and to estimate what types of people would be particularly susceptible to such effects. Two levels of RF radiation are important to consider: (1) The level that significantly raises deep body temperature, called the core temperature, and (2) the level that is of sufficient intensity to produce a detectable change in involuntary human thermoregulatory responses.

For the first level of concern, increases in body core temperature of roughly 1 degree Celsius appear to occur at SARs of 1–4 W/kg. The actual increase in temperature is strongly dependent on exposure duration and ambient conditions. Raising the body core temperature could be adverse for a healthy individual. At the least, such an effect can be considered an abnormal stress on bodily processes that would be particularly serious to those individuals with preexisting significant acute or chronic disease. The health consequences would obviously be more severe at higher levels of RF energy absorption. But RF radiation levels that only begin to increase body temperature on an acute basis should not be automatically considered to pose an acute health threat because there is a normal daily variation in body temperature as well as changes in body temperature due to hormonal rhythms. Furthermore, people are subject to increased body temperature as a result of illness fever. The onset of increased body temperature should be considered to be a potential adverse health effect to be avoided, but, at its lowest levels, the effect will rarely be adverse.

The second RF radiation level of concern is the lower level of exposure that activates the body's thermoregulatory responses. The onset of this effect appears to occur roughly at or above 0.4 W/kg. Merely turning on or off usual thermoregulatory mechanisms should not in itself adversely affect health, but it is most certainly a measurable physiological change, and certain people might be more susceptible to such changes. Also, of obvious concern would be individuals who have lost one or more of the thermoregulatory responses that normally help dissipate heat. Such people would be anticipated to have an increase in body core temperature at a level of RF radiation exposure lower than the level required to increase body core temperature in individuals with uncompromised thermoregulatory mechanisms. The people most at risk would be those who are unable to move voluntarily; that is, lack of voluntary motion would preclude obtaining liquids in response to sweat-induced loss of fluid, changing locations, changing clothing, altering indoor temperature settings, or moving about to dissipate body heat. Infants would have to cry and would depend on an adult to provide relief. Presumably, people with vascular disease would be particularly affected because their circulatory problems could affect their thermoregulation. One could also speculate that an individual who was already thermally stressed, for example, with a fever, also may be at risk. Furthermore, it is also possible that pregnant women may be more susceptible to heat stress. The people most likely to be most severely affected by RF radiation below the SARs of 1–4 W/kg that raise body temperature would be elderly infirm individuals who are also immobile. Also, dehydration is a factor that can aggravate a number of adverse conditions in such individuals.

Groups of individuals particularly susceptible to heat stress were identified by Ellis (45) who examined the Vital Statistics Reports of the U.S. Public Health Service for the years 1952–67. Heat waves had occurred in five different years during that period. Excess deaths, especially for various forms of heart and circulatory disease, were found to be associated with the heat-wave periods. It was also concluded that infants less than one year of age are the most heat-susceptible group below age 50 and adults over 50 years of age are more heat-susceptible than infants and become progressively more susceptible with advancing age. Consideration should perhaps be given to the health impact of the thermal extremes that can exist in the U.S. during summer months.

C. Nonthermal Effects. There are a number of effects described in the scientific literature that occur at levels equal to or less than 0.4 W/kg, and these are generally not associated with increases in temperature. For example, it has been experimentally observed that the efflux of calcium ions from animal brain tissue is enhanced after exposure to low intensity RF energy under certain discrete conditions. Calcium ions are important to several physiological functions, particularly in the nervous system. There are many reasons why there could be changes in ion movement, and the extent to which this effect might indicate a hazard to humans is not presently known. Further research is needed to determine the relevance, if any, of this phenomenon to human health.

Other studies have endpoints that may be of more concern. One example is the recently reported study involving long-term exposure at 0.4 W/kg in which rats were found to have enlarged adrenal glands and an increase in overall tumor incidence, although there was no statistical increase in any particular type of tumor.

The overall implications for human health of low-level nonthermal effects is not clear, and in some cases there are conflicting data on whether a given effect occurs. Further research is required to determine the generality of these low-level effects and whether they constitute a hazard to human health.

D. Summary. One mechanism by which RF radiation produces effects is by heating the human body. The increase in body core temperatures due to RF radiation is reported to occur at SARs of 1–4 W/kg. This should be considered an adverse health effect. But short-term small increases in body temperature should be of relatively minimal health concern. It is possible that lower SARs could also increase core body temperature in hot and humid environments, especially in those people with impaired thermoregulatory processes and particularly in individuals who are immobile; the threshold would be expected to be that RF radiation level that causes the onset of thermoregulatory processes and apparently could occur at about 0.4 W/kg or above.

The scientific literature also contains evidence intimating nonthermal effects from RF radiation, but whether such effects would affect the health of people is not yet clear. Several recent studies, including one said to show a nonspecific increase in tumors in laboratory animals chronically exposed at 0.4 W/kg, need to be analyzed.

5. Conclusion

Based on the currently available biological effects data, EPA has concluded that adverse human health effects are associated with whole-body average SARs of 1 to 4 W/kg or greater. However, data are insufficient to assess the adversity and human health implications of effects that occur below this level, and this leaves potentially significant issues unresolved. Effects in question include, among others, those associated with low-frequency modulated RF fields, the potential for cancer promotion, and frequency specific effects such as changes in brain energy metabolism.

D. Approach to the Derivation of Exposure Limits

Because they are believed to have mechanisms of action that exhibit thresholds, agents producing noncarcinogenic health effects are generally evaluated differently than carcinogens. For noncarcinogens, public health regulatory agencies, including EPA, typically have applied preselected safety factors to non-observed-effect-levels (NOELs) or other parameters to determine the level below which human exposure should fall (46–50). A safety factor in health protection standard does not guarantee safety; it represents, instead, an attempt to compensate for unknowns and uncertainties. Safety factors or, more appropriately, uncertainty factors typically range from 10 to 1000, depending on the type of available data, e.g., human versus animal, acute versus chronic, and so forth. Although selection of the actual level of a factor is largely judgmental, uncertainty factors are used to account for several areas of uncertainty such as intra- and inter-species variations in response to an agent; sensitive human sub-populations, e.g., the ill; possible synergistic interactions; the greater probability or risk in the human population that is larger than the number of animals that can be tested; and other considerations. Uncertainty factors of 100 have most traditionally been used and essentially contain a 10-fold factor to account for interspecies differences and a 10-fold factor to account for uncertainties when extrapolating from high to low doses. Also, in establishing standard for many agents, a common practice has been to assign a 10-fold factor to occupational exposures and an additional 10-fold factor to exposures in the general population. The difference is related primarily to the lack of consent to and knowledge of the exposures and the greater diversity in the general population which contains a wider range of ages and more susceptible subgroups than does a presumably more healthy working population.

Developed from reviews of basically the same information, the various existing criteria or recommendations for RF radiation exposure essentially differ only in terms of the applied margin of safety. Using a starting point of an SAR of 4 W/kg, the ANSI applied an uncertainty factor of 10 to develop its recommendation of 0.4 W/kg for workers and the general population but stated that this level should be viewed as an upper limit of exposure especially for the general population (17). The Massachusetts standard, the IRPA interim guideline, and the NCRP recommendation each used an uncertainty factor of 50 to derive an exposure limit of 0.08 W/kg, a level five times more stringent than ANSI to afford greater protection for the general population. Portland, Oregon has used zoning guidance of 0.04 W/kg; this is 10 times more stringent than the ANSI voluntary standard and is equivalent to applying an uncertainty factor of 100 to a SAR level of 4 W/kg.

On the basis of the available data, the Agency believes RF radiation should, for now, be treated as a noncarcinogen, and an uncertainty factor should be used in deriving exposure limits, especially in view of the remaining uncertainties in our knowledge of the health effects of RF radiation exposure. But, because of the degree of judgment involved in selecting any uncertainty factor, comments are solicited on this matter and specifically on the following issues that relate to the magnitude of an uncertainty factor:

(1) Reasonably precise and reproducible information is typically obtained from experimental animals. Nevertheless, there are still likely to be sensitivities that may go undetected and results can vary even under the best of conditions (46). Any series of experiments can yield false-positive and false negative results (47). Use of a safety factor helps compensate for experimental and statistical uncertainties.

(2) The extent and validity of animal data is an important consideration in determining an appropriate margin of safety. For RF radiation, there are multiple studies in different animal species. This body of data has led to some degree of consensus within the scientific community on what constitutes adverse effects levels, and this would tend to lessen the need for a large margin of safety.

(3) Much of the biological effects data from animal experiments is, however, based on relatively short exposures. There are uncertainties associated with extrapolating data from short duration exposure to long-term exposure both in animals and people. Lack of data on long-term exposures could be highly significant since environmental exposure of the public generally occurs continuously over a long period of time.

(4) There are also uncertainties associated with extrapolating data from test animals to human beings. Because of interspecies differences, human responses may not correspond to animal responses to comparable exposures.

(5) Unlike experimental animals, humans are genetically very diverse, exhibit varying susceptibilities, and live in a heterogeneous environment. Use of a safety factor is indicated since it is not possible to estimate effects of all the genetic and environmental variation in the general population (46). Subpopulations at potentially greater risk from exposure to RF radiation have not yet been well characterized, although it is known that the body's ability to handle high temperatures and humidity depends on age and health condition.

(6) In experimental animals, the whole-body average SAR required to produce a given effect depends on the environmental conditions accompanying the RF radiation exposure. The SAR level at which adverse effects occur in humans might also be expected to depend on environmental conditions, but actual data are not presently available. A safety factor might, then, be needed to account for the predictable influence of adverse environmental conditions on both healthy and susceptible populations exposed to RF radiation.

(7) Certain biological effects that do not seem to be due to heating occur below the 1 to 4 W/kg range, but there is no evidence to indicate whether and under what conditions these effects are adverse or persistent. Prudence would seem to dictate use of a safety factor because of the possibility that the effects observed below 1 W/kg may prove to be biologically significant.

(8) In setting health protection standards, there has been a tradition of differential margins of safety between occupational and general population standards on the basis that different levels of knowledge, consent, and health, as well as exposure time, exist in the affected groups. As mentioned in the discussion of existing standards, the ANSI selected a safety factor of 10 to derive its recommended expo-

sure limit. Both the IRPA and NCRP concluded that a larger margin of safety should be applied to derive exposure limits for the public, and we seek comment on this issue.

(9) At some frequencies, RF radiation energy is generally deposited deep in the body below cutaneous thermal receptors; therefore, cutaneous perception of heat and thermal pain may be an unreliable sensory mechanism for protection against potentially harmful RF radiation exposure levels. This means the body may not "recognize" or react to RF radiation energy as quickly or in the same way as it does to other sources of thermal loading or heating. This bypass or delay in response of the body's adaptive protective mechanism would argue for a larger margin of safety.

(10) On the other hand, the human thermoregulatory system is more adaptive than most fur-bearing animals, primarily because of the ability to secrete sweat on the skin. Extrapolating thermoregulatory data from animals to humans is, therefore, difficult and a one-to-one relationship may be overly conservative. This would tend to argue for a smaller margin of safety.

(11) The biological effects data indicate that the larger the animal, the lower the effective SAR required to produce many types of effects. This might indicate that any uncertainty factor should account for the greater mass of humans compared to experimental animals. But, for thermoregulatory responses, this is a much debated issue, related to the concerns noted in #10 above.

(12) The whole-body average SAR is an estimate of absorbed energy averaged over the whole-body mass. It is currently the parameter most used to describe energy absorption in biological systems. Because of limits associated with measurement of the SAR in individuals, the whole-body SAR must be computed on a theoretical basis, and it does not directly address the existence of localized areas in the body of increased energy deposition ("hot spots"). For example, the SAR within a specific body tissue can exceed the whole-body average SAR by a factor of 100 or more, depending on frequency and orientation of the body (51). The uncertainties associated with localized versus whole-body energy absorption would tend to argue for a larger margin of safety.

(13) Analytical and experimental studies have shown that SAR is dependent on whether an individual is electrically grounded or ungrounded. For grounded conditions, SAR may be as much as twice the ungrounded value at identical exposure conditions, and the maximum value typically occurs at a new lower resonant frequency. Virtually all of the SARs derived from animal experiments described in the literature where direct assessment of SAR was not reported are based on the assumption of ungrounded conditions. Since people are generally grounded, consideration of the SARs for grounded conditions could be made in deriving permissible RF radiation exposure field strengths.

(14) The severity and health consequence of any given effect is an important consideration, e.g., cancer has more severe consequences for the individual than does transient respiratory illness. But one of the major problems in attempting to assess the health risks from RF radiation exosure is that the observed biological

effects are diverse and have not yet been linked, through research, to a given disease, condition, or set of distinct symptoms in people. (The scientific literature from the Soviet Union and Eastern Europe has, however, discussed the occurrence of "microwave sickness" or a "neurasthenic syndrome".) In fact, there is accumulating evidence that RF radiation acts as a generalized environmental stressor, via the mechanism of heating, and, as such, could precipitate or exacerbate a host of physiological conditions and clinical states with varying degrees of severity. This makes the choice of an appropriate margin of safety very difficult.

(15) Human exposure to low levels of RF radiation has occurred without obvious untoward effects, and this should also be considered in establishing a margin of safety. On the other hand, very few carefully controlled analytical epidemiological or clinical studies have been done. It is difficult in epidemiological studies to detect low probability risks in general and if RF radiation can produce varied effects as a generalized stressor (see #14 above), it would be difficult to identify and detect subtle or diverse changes even in a well-designed study with a large sample size.

(16) Nonreversible effects may require a larger margin of safety than do reversible effects. When evaluated, many of the biological effects from RF radiation exposure are reversible after exposure stops. Low birth weight may, however, persist for a significant period of time in young animals after exposure ceases (52). Reversibility would argue for a smaller margin of safety. The ANSI, however, took the position that, for behavioral effects, "reversible disruption during an acute exposure is tantamount to irreversible injury during chronic exposure." (17) [See also #3 above.]

(17) Integral to any uncertainty factor analysis is determination of the pertinent threshold to be used as a starting point, be it a non-observed-adverse-effect-level (NOAEL) or a no-observed-effect-level (NOEL). For thermal effects, RF radiation would appear to be a threshold pollutant. But much of the research to date has not fully defined dose-response relationships because exposure levels (and resultant SARs) have often been selected arbitrarily rather than selected to define thresholds. The biological effects data may, then, be more in line with the concept of lowest-observed-adverse-effect-levels (LOAEL). A variable uncertainty factor between 1 and 10 is often applied to bring a LOAEL into the range of a NOAEL, depending on the severity of the effect (48).

(18) A smaller margin of safety may be required if the mechanism of action for an agent is well understood (48). This is the case for the thermal effects of RF radiation exposure but the mechanism of action has not been established for the presumed nonthermal effects. Because the mechanisms of action and human health implications of the low-level or nonthermal effects are not known, EPA proposes to restrict the use of these results to margin of safety considerations.

(19) The EPA has considered biological effects *in toto* to determine where an overall cut off point or threshold for adverse effects appears to lie. This approach was also used by ANSI, IRPA, and NCRP. For chemical toxicants, it is more usual to select one health effect in the most sensitive species. The Agency is, therefore,

interested in comments on which approach is more suitable when evaluating the effects of RF radiation exposure.

V. Additional Consideration for Frequencies Below 3 MHz

Exposure to RF radiation below 3 MHz, and particularly below 200 kHz, requires special consideration and treatment. Practical experience has shown that prevention of electrical shock can be a significant safety consideration (53). The principal area of concern for public exposure arises from the induction of RF currents in conductive objects. These induced currents may flow through the body of an individual who contacts them. The amount of current that will flow through the body of a person depends upon how well the individual is electrically grounded and the impedance between the current source and the individual. Low-frequency fields can cause potentially hazardous electric currents to flow in capacitive objects such as vehicles, fencing, metal roofing, and other ungrounded conducting objects, including the human body, when these objects become adequately grounded. EPA advise that, as a minimum, low-frequency fields should be limited to intensities that prevent accident-causing startle reactions in ungrounded individuals who may momentarily contact grounded objects while exposed to high intensity RF fields, but is soliciting comments on this issue. This subject is discussed in greater detail in the following section.

VI. Discussion of Proposals

A. Approaches To Control Exposure to Radiofrequency Radiation

The increase in the number and type of RF radiation sources has created a RF radiation environment to which the population is continuously exposed to varying degrees, and the number of RF radiation sources is expected to continue to increase in the future. People live, work, or pass through areas near RF radiation emitting sources that can produce levels of exposure that are now known to be associated with various effects in laboratory animals. Although EPA cannot yet fully enumerate or characterize the populations exposed to differing levels of RF radiation, measurement and modeling analyses by the Agency have provided information on the number and characteristics of sources likely to produce high exposures. For example, it is predicted that over 1,100 existing broadcast sites exceed the current ANSI guideline.

EPAs overall objective is to prevent adverse health effects that may be associated with exposure to RF radiation in the environment. By this Notice, EPA solicits comment on four options, three regulatory and one nonregulatory, that it has developed as alternative approaches to control exposure to RF radiation. Depending on how they are implemented, all options should achieve the Agency's objective of reducing or preventing adverse health effects, although with varying degrees of confidence. It is assumed that a margin of safety is needed given current uncertainties in translating from experimental animal data to human exposures and effects and in predicting sensitive populations and effects under conditions of environmental extremes. It is also assumed that the greater the margin of safety, the greater the likelihood that adverse health effects can be reduced or prevented.

The proposed options encompass the range of limits recommended or adopted by various advisory groups such as the International Radiation Protection Association (IRPA), the National Council on Radiation Protection and Measurements (NCRP), and the American National Standards Institute (ANSI), and include:

(1) Controlling public exposure by limiting whole-body average specific absorption rates (SAR) to 0.04 watts per kilogram (W/kg) for frequencies above 3 megahertz (MHz) and by limiting electric field intensity to 87 volts per meter (V/m) and magnetic field intensity to 0.23 amperes per meter (A/m) at frequencies below 3 MHz.

(2) Controlling public exposure by limiting whole-body average SARs to 0.08 W/kg for frequencies above 3 MHz and by limiting electric field intensity to 275 V/m and magnetic field intensity to 0.73 A/m for frequencies below 3 MHz.

(3) Controlling public exposure by limiting whole-body average SARs to 0.4 W/kg for frequencies above 3 MHz and by limiting electric field intensity to 614 V/m and magnetic field intensity to 1.63 A/m for frequencies below 3 MHz.

(4) In lieu of adopting Federal Guidance for RF radiation, establishing public awareness programs to distribute information on health effects and environmental measurements as well as provide technical assistance to States and Federal agencies.

The nonregulatory option, Option 4, would not establish Federal Guidance but would provide and continue to develop technical information that others could use to establish controls. Option 3 would protect healthy people in normal environments against the adverse thermal effects of RF radiation exposure. Options 1 and 2 incorporate respectively larger safety factors and, thus, offer increasing degrees of assurance that adverse health effects would be prevented and the potential for other effects would also be reduced.

Because of the substantial uncertainties in the available health effects information and the complex character of RF radiation exposures, the Administrator wishes to solicit the fullest possible participation and comment by the public before deciding which Guidance levels, if any, should be recommended to the President. The EPA seeks comments on its overall objective, on the adequacy of each of the proposed approaches for protecting public health, and on the following specific issues and questions:

1. Each of the alternative approaches has advantages or disadvantages, discussed below, that will be considered by the Administrator:

(a) *Option 1: Guidance Based on an SAR of 0.04 W/kg.* This option represents a "no effects" level by protecting against thermally-related health effects in humans, including most sensitive subgroups of the population. No measurable changes in core temperature would occur at this level nor would any thermoregulatory responses be initiated. This level is consistent with the usual practice of providing substantially more protective standards (here, by a factor of 10, when compared to, for example, the 1982 ANSI voluntary standard of 0.4 W/kg) for the public than those recommended for occupational exposures. This level might be viewed as unnecessarily stringent in that the health protection provided may not be commensurate with its cost, particularly in view of the present uncertainties surrounding low-level and nonthermal effects.

(b) *Option 2: Guidance Based on an SAR of 0.08 W/kg.* This option also effectively represents a "no effects" level by protecting against thermally related health effects in humans, including most sensitive subgroups of the population. No changes in core temperature should occur at this level nor should any thermoregulatory responses be initiated. Also consistent with the usual practice of generally providing more protective standards for the public than those recommended or occupational exposures, this level differs from Option 1 in that it is lower than, for example, the 1982 ANSI guide by a factor of 5 rather than a factor of 10, as given in Option 1. This option is similar to the Massachusetts standard, to the IRPA guideline in the resonant frequency range, and to the exposure limits recently recommended by the NCRP. The Agency is particularly interested in comment on this option, because 42 U.S.C. 2021(h) states that the Administrator shall consult with the NCRP, among others, on radiation matters.

(c) *Option 3: Guidance Based on an SAR of 0.4 W/kg.* This option should protect against thermal effects except in possibly more susceptible or sensitive people or possibly at high ambient temperatures and humidities. This level corresponds to the lower end of the range postulated to be associated with the onset of thermoregulatory responses in humans. Effects that occur below this level do not, for the most part, seem to be caused by generalized heating. The 1982 ANSI standard, set at this level, does not differentiate between occupational and public exposure but noted, "... these guides are offered as upper limits of exposure, particularly for the population at large." (17) Various groups in the broadcasting industry have indicated to EPA their willingness to comply with a guideline at this level (letters placed in the Central Docket). The agency is particularly interested in comment on this option, because it is similar to the 1982 ANSI guide voluntarily adopted by much of the broadcast industry and is to be used by the FCC to determine the need for environmental impact analyses for new and renewal license applications.

(d) *Option 4: Conduct Other Activities in Lieu of Adopting Federal Radiation Protection Guidance for RF Radiation.* This is a nonregulatory option, and it would provide public health protection only as it is realized indirectly through the advice and technical assistance provided by EPA to Federal agencies, States, or industry. Taking no regulatory action at this time could permit any further regulatory action to be based on more refined biological, technical, and economic analyses. For example, allowing more time for additional research to identify and quantify adverse health effects in the population may result in more improved risk estimates. It is not clear whether this approach will meet the perceived need of Federal agencies, States, or industry that have requested uniform Federal exposure guidelines, and EPA seeks comments on this issue.

2. An analysis of the potential economic impacts associated with each of the regulatory approaches indicates that the range of costs differs by about a factor of three. The estimated costs and number of affected sites are discussed in Part VIII of this Notice. The Agency solicits comment on its analysis of the potential economic impacts of establishing Federal Guidance for radiofrequency radiation.

In addition, EPA is also interested in comments on costs relative to the degree of health protection afforded by each option. As the degree of stringency or health protection increases, the estimated costs of compliance also increase. Costs roughly double between each option while the presumed gain in health protection increases five-fold between Option 2 and 3 but only two-fold between Option 1 and 2. Also, changes in regulations over time can impose additional costs of compliance as for example, systems are adapted or retrofitted to comply with updated regulations, be they more restrictive or loosened. If any future research more clearly indicates adverse human health effects could result at low levels of exposure, it is least likely that any RF radiation Guidance initially set at the level of Option 1 would have to be lowered. Option 1, then, should minimize the possibility of industry incurring additional incremental costs of compliance in the future but its current projected costs are higher than the other options. Similarly, if Guidance were ever revised downward from the level proposed under Option 3, there could be some disruption to industry, involving additional incremental costs for compliance. The Agency is interested in comment on these issues as well as on the degree to which cost should be considered in establishing Guidance.

3. EPA has determined that adverse effects can begin to occur between 1–4 W/kg. The degree of severity depends on the sensitivity of the individual, the duration of exposure, environmental conditions, and the amount and persistence of a change in core temperature. Temperature changes of up to 1 degree Celsius that occur intermittently and for short durations are not likely to be hazardous for most people. But sustained temperature increases of this magnitude can be adverse, especially in more sensitive individuals. The onset of thermoregulatory responses appears to fall in the range of 0.4–1 W/kg; such changes are not likely to be adverse for most people. Effects below this level are presumably nonthermal in origin, and their relative adversity is not established. As noted in Section IV.D, the Agency believes RF radiation should now be treated as a noncarcinogen, and safety or uncertainty factors should be applied to derive exposure limits. With this background, the uncertainty factors applied in establishing the proposed options levels, in the resonant frequency range, are described in Table 4.

4. There are some preliminary and unconfirmed studies on RF radiation exposure and carcinogenesis. The SARs of interest fall in the range between 0.4–4 W/kg. The potential role of RF radiation exposure in carcinogenesis is not yet resolved and could affect EPA's assessment of adverse health effects levels and the treatment of RF radiation as a noncarcinogen. The Agency seeks comment on this issue.

TABLE 4. *Uncertainty factors in establishing proposed option levels in the resonant frequency range*

Option	Sar (Wk/g)	Uncertainty "Adverse Effects" 1-4 W/kg	Factors "Observed Effects" 0.4-1 W/kg
Option 1	0.04	25–100	10–25
Option 2	0.08	12.5–50	5–12.5
Option 3	0.4	2.5–10	1*–2.5
Option 4: no exposure limit		NA	NA

1*; Means no uncertainty factor applied. Because of the degree of judgement involved, the agency seeks comments on the range of uncertainty factors above and the degree of health protection afforded, considered in the context of the issues discussed in part IV.D of this notice.

5. A need for a uniform Federal guideline has been expressed to EPA, primarily by industry and other Federal agencies. EPA has no preemption authority under Federal Guidance and so uniformity cannot be enforced. It is not clear whether States, cities, or other local authorities would adopt any EPA Guidance although some jurisdictions have indirectly indicated their willingness to do so (letters placed in Central Docket). The degree of acceptance might depend on the actual level of any Guidance. To provide additional information to help resolve this question, EPA seeks specific comments on the need for a Federal guideline, its degree of acceptance at nonfederal levels of government, and whether Federal Guidance could foster uniform and consistent exposure limits nationally.

6. There are many uncertainties when assessing the health risks of RF radiation exposure. There are potential costs associated either with establishing an overly conservative limit or with establishing a too lenient guideline that must eventually be revised downward. The Agency must determine whether it is better to establish Guidance now or to delay until and if more refined scientific information becomes available, as proposed in the fourth nonregulatory option. The Agency is interested in comment on this matter.

7. EPA is proposing that Guidance, if any, should apply to the frequency range between 10 kHz and 100 GHz and that, over this range, the average-whole-body specific absorption rate (SAR) be controlled at a constant level, i.e., at 0.04, 0.08, or 0.4 W/kg depending upon the option ultimately chosen. However, it is recognized that at the lower frequencies it may also be desirable to prevent electrical shocks and RF burns which can occur because of induced currents caused by RF fields. Induced currents occur in individuals as well as in conductive structures exposed to RF fields. Both shock and RF burns can startle people, possibly leading to accidents. To help prevent shocks and burns, it is necessary to limit the electric and magnetic field strengths to levels less than might be allowed by a constant specific absorption rate. The electric field strengths proposed in Options 1, 2, and 3 are 87, 275, and 614 V/m, and the magnetic field strengths proposed are 0.23, 0.73

and 1.63 A/m, respectively. These levels approximate the different limits recommended by the International Radiation Protection Association (IRPA), the State of Massachusetts, the NCRP, and the American National Standards Institute. The IRPA applies the values 87 V/m and 0.23 A/m to frequencies below 1 MHz, and Massachusetts, NCRP, and ANSI apply their limits to frequencies below 2 MHz. Although the IRPA, Massachusetts, and NCRP general population limits are similar, the IRPA limits for low frequencies are more stringent because exposure limits should not be so high that RF shocks could occur, since it would be totally unreasonable to require this group (the general public) to take precautions to avoid shocks. (20)

EPA is soliciting comment on the values of electric and magnetic field strength to use to prevent perception, shock, and RF burns; on the frequency where these phenomena begin to predominate, i.e., 1 or 3 MHz; and on the lowest and highest frequencies to which Guidance should apply. [Low frequency fields are also discussed in Section B.2 below.]

8. EPA is interested in comment on whether Guidance should apply under all environmental conditions regardless of the air temperature, humidity, air speed, and electromagnetic energy input from sources outside the proposed frequency range. The margin of safety incorporated into Options 1 and 2 may eliminate the need to modify the Guidance for application in hot, humid environments, but this may not be so for the limits proposed in Option 3, especially for sensitive individuals.

B. Other Considerations

1. *Continuous Exposure Between 3 MHz–100 GHz:* The limits proposed in Options 1–3 for the 3 MHz–100 GHz frequency range would control the whole-body average SAR by incorporating the frequency dependence of energy absorption. This frequency dependence includes a consideration of exposure conditions which provide for maximum coupling with the electromagnetic field. Because RF radiation is not uniformly absorbed by the body tissues, specific tissue SAR values can exceed the whole-body average SAR. Depending upon frequency, the ratio of the maximum tissue SARs to whole-body average SARs may range from 3–10 for body resonant frequencies and may be larger, up to a factor 100, at nonresonant frequencies. It should be noted that although long-term local (in the body) SAR values are not explicitly stated, the recommended limits for continuous exposure under Option 1 will substantially minimize local heating effects of RF body currents by keeping the local SAR to less than 4 W/kg in anatomical areas of small cross-section. Options 2 and 3 would keep the local SAR to less than 8 and 40 W/kg, respectively. All options would permit short-term (less than six minute exposures) local SAR values greater than these values.

If EPA recommends Federal Guidance, the basic SAR limit adopted will be used to derive limits of exposure presented in units of root-mean-square (RMS) field strength, mean squared field strength, and plane-wave equivalent time-average power density to maximize convenience in implementing Guidance since commercially available instruments are typically calibrated in one of these units. The maximum continuous RMS electric and magnetic field strengths to which members of the public may be exposed for durations greater than one-tenth hour (6 minutes) in any hour will be defined and exposure limits in the corresponding units of mean squared field strengths and plane-wave equivalent time-average power densities will be given.

RF fields should be measured at least 10 centimeters (cm) away from radiating sources and from objects that act as secondary sources, in order to avoid erroneous instrument readings because of capacitive coupling to the object. For frequencies greater than 30 MHz, determination of either electric or magnetic field strength is sufficient except for near-field and multipath interference situations in which both E and H field strengths should be measured. For frequencies equal to or less than 30 MHz, both electric and magnetic field strengths must be measured.

2. *Exposures Between 10 kHz–3 MHz:* Low frequency fields can charge capacitive objects such as ungrounded vehicles, fencing, metal roofing, and any other ungrounded conductive objects including the human body, and electric shocks or RF burns are possible. Because of this additional consideration, fields in the frequency range of 10 kHz–3 MHz could be limited on the basis of the magnitude of induced RF currents. There are established methods for calculating the magnitude of such induced RF currents in different objects (54–56), and published data describe the variation with frequency of RF currents associated with perception of induced currents and shock reactions in humans (57, 58).

Shock phenomena predominate over the frequency range from 10 KHz–200 kHz. The potential for accident-causing startle reactions can be reduced by limiting the current which would flow to ground from an ungrounded individual (immersed in a low-frequency field) who touches a grounded object. For all three regulatory options proposed, the current that flows from the individual through the grounded object would be less than the value of current perceivable by most individuals (the 0.5 percentile perception level) for frequencies from 10 kHz to 200 kHz.

For frequencies above 200 kHz, current flow will be perceived through a heating reaction (RF-burn) at the point of skin contact, as opposed to shock. The NIOSH defined the induced current value of 100 mA as the RF burn threshold and assumed a skin contact area of 1 square centimeter (59). Using the techniques described in references 54–56, the RF field strengths permitted by each option proposed in this Notice would be expected to cause induced currents in a grounded individual as follows:

Option 1: 45 mA induced current at 3 MHz

Option 2: 247 mA induced current at 3 MHz

Option 3: 553 mA induced current at 3 MHz

Thus, EPA's proposed Options 2 and 3 exceed the RF-burn threshold proposed by NIOSH, but Option 1 does not.

Even when RF fields are substantially less than the levels prescribed in the various options, exposures at low frequencies can cause high values of electrically induced currents to flow from large conducting objects to a grounded individual. But, because of the very wide variety of conducting objects in the environment and the diverse opportunities for humans to contact these objects, it is impractical to specify numerical electromagnetic field intensity limits that prevent all possible shock and RF burn effects. Thus, although any Guidance would specify maximum exposure field intensities, it is recommended that in those cases where such shock and RF-burn conditions may exist action be taken to prevent their occurrence. Such action could include reducing the strength of the fields, preventing access by the public to the area or object(s) of concern, or grounding of the conducting object(s).

3. *Short-Term Exposures:* The EPA will consider establishing short-term exposure limits substantially higher than continuous exposure limits. The rationale behind permitting higher intensity exposures of limited duration is that commonplace radiation sources can produce environmental levels above the limits specified here for continuous exposure at some locations which are accessible to the public but where there is little likelihood or reason for anyone to remain in these fields for a prolonged period of time. A short-term limit introduces an element of practicality into the Guidance by allowing transient exposure to higher levels. For frequencies less than 3 MHz, the higher exposure values are not recommended since shock phenomena are unrelated to the duration of exposure.

A six minute (0.1 hour) limit has been conventionally used in the development of short-term RF exposure criteria by ANSI regardless of frequency (17). This time interval is related to consideration of the thermal response time of the human body when subjected to short-term RF exposures capable of raising the body temperature. For exposures less than 6 minutes (total) in any 1 hour, the Agency is proposing that limits be 10 times the long-term continuous exposure values permissible for all frequencies greater than 3 MHz; that is, in any hour, the amount of energy absorbed during 6 minutes will be no more than the amount absorbed in 1 hour at the levels recommended for continuous exposures.

4. *Pulsed Electromagnetic Fields:* The health significance of exposure to pulsed electromagnetic fields is not clear. The biological effects literature does not yet provide a firm basis for limiting the instantaneous peak SARs caused by pulsed fields. However, under Options 1–3, pulsed fields would be subject to the same limits on a time-average basis as non-pulsed fields.

EPA believes that establishment of accurately defined quantitative peak pulse field intensities is not possible at this time; however, EPA proposes that, in addition to any specified exposure limits, steps should be taken to preclude the occurrence of the "RF hearing" effect. Exposure levels should be limited on a case-by-case basis.

5. *Exposure Parameters:* A knowledge of the maximum values of electric and magnetic field strengths is required to fully assess the corresponding energy absorption rates in the body for near-field and reflective exposure conditions. For sufficiently short wavelengths in the vicinity of most sources, it is adequate to determine the maximum possible electric or magnetic field strength to ensure that the undetermined magnetic or electric field strength will not exceed the limitations specified in the guidance. Thus, for frequencies greater than 30 MHz under standing wave conditions where the direction of propagation of the wavefront is perpendicular to a reflective surface, the distance separating maximum electric and associated magnetic fields will not exceed 2.5 meters. In many cases, this distance is small enough to assume that measurements which determine the maximum electric or magnetic field in a region whose dimensions are approximately one-quarter of a wavelength at the exposure frequency are sufficient to specify the maximum value of the corresponding magnetic or electric field strength. This is only true, however, when it can be established that a standing wave exists by finding repeating maximum values in either of the field quantities in the region of interest. For frequencies between 10 kHz and 30 MHz, measurement of one field does not necessarily allow prediction of the other because of the longer wavelengths, and both electric and magnetic field strengths must be measured.

Under Options 1–3, EPA proposes that the RF radiation exposure limits in this Guidance should be expressed in three alternative ways: (1) Either or both RMS electric or magnetic field strength, (2) mean squared field strengths, and (3) average plane-wave equivalent power densities. These alternative measures would allow ease of implementation since existing commercial broadband instrumentation is designed to measure one or more of these field parameters. The use of power density for specifying RF radiation exposure over the entire frequency range is inappropriate and is technically incorrect for certain conditions such as reflective environments and non-planar wavefronts. Because of these considerations, any Guidance would be expressed in power density for frequencies below 30 MHz only for convenience in relating to other standards.

A significant question remains as to how close to conducting objects exposure field intensity measurements should be made. Variations in size and shape of instruments can lead to differences in measured values. These differences in measured values arise typically from capacitive coupling between the probe and nearby objects. This suggests the need for defining a minimum distance for such measurements. It is recognized that for measurements of leakage fields specified in certain consumer electronic product performance standards, shorter distances may be used if the instrument is designed for a specific device application.This is, for example, the case for microwave ovens. The ANSI has recommended a minimum 5 cm measurement distance for determining compliance with its standard (17). However, in the case of general environmental RF measurements, a minimum distance of 10 cm between the surface of conducting objects or radiating devices and the nearest part of an active element comprising a field measurement probe is preferable to reduce capacitive coupling effects between small measurement probes and the local environment (60, 61). Employment of larger distances may be advisable in the interest of further minimizing this factor.

6. *Partial-Body and Whole-Body Exposures:* In the general environment, it is impractical to distinguish between partial-body and whole-body exposures; therefore, EPA proposes that Guidance limits apply to all exposures.

7. *Mixed Frequency Fields:* For exposures to mixed frequency fields, the sum of the squares of the fractions of the field strength limits or the sum of the fractions of the power density limits, as appropriate, contributed by each frequency must not exceed unity.

8. *Exclusions:* EPA proposes to exclude from consideration occupational exposures, exposures of patients due to prescribed medical treatment or procedures using RF fields, and exposures originating from consumer electronic products. Regulating occupational exposures is within the purview of OSHA although EPA could issue occupational guidance in a separate action, if there is a need.

Environmental guidance should not apply to intentional exposure of patients. Emissions from consumer electronic products could be controlled through product performance standards. EPA, therefore, does not propose to apply any Federal Guidance for environmental exposures to such sources, but, because of increased development and use of new technologies, the Agency seeks comments and information on consumer electronic products such as portable radio communications equipment.

9. *Implementation:* If any Federal Guidance is adopted, EPA will work closely with other Federal Agencies in the development of implementation programs. The EPA considers the following issues to be important and seeks comments on matters related to the implementation of Federal Radiation Guidance, if adopted.

a. *Implementing agencies:* Federal agencies would be responsible for implementing and complying with Guidance recommended by EPA and signed by the President. EPA proposes that each agency should: (1) Take whatever actions are necessary to protect the public health, (2) ensure that RF radiation exposure of the public due to activities under their jurisdiction conforms to the specified limits, (3) implement Guidance in a timely fashion and consult with EPA on appropriate timetables, (4) rely on EPA technical expertise and advice by cooperating with EPA in the development and application of programs and techniques for evaluating RF radiation exposure in the environment, (5) apply state-of-the-art or best practical measurement technologies in compliance measurement programs, as determined by consultation with EPA, and (6) establish procedures to notify workers if their exposures in the workplace exceed public exposure limits.

b. *EPA:* To ensure efficient and effective compliance with Guidance, EPA is proposing to establish programs and develop capabilities necessary to assist Federal agencies in their implementation efforts. EPA would: (1) provide technical advice and assistance to implementing agencies to ensure cost effecive and timely compliance with exposure guidelines, (2) establish within the Office of Radiation Programs the capabilities to develop measurement techniques and instrumentation systems required to monitor environmental RF radiation exposures and to prepare to assist Federal agencies in the implementation and compliance efforts, (3) cooperate with other Federal agencies by providing review of compliance programs, (4) conduct reviews and inspections necessary to monitor compliance with Federal Guidance, (5) institute review of Guidance on at least a five-year cycle, (6) continue its environmental monitoring and assessment program to assure that data on population exposures, environmental levels, and sources is well-characterized and current for use by other agencies, (7) continue to evaluate health effects research on RF electromagnetic radiation from environmental sources to provide information to be used in the five-year review of the Guidance.

c. *Intent:* The practice of prudent radiation protection requires that sincere efforts be taken to maintain population exposures at levels as low as reasonably achieveable. Implementation programs, activities, and decisions should focus on the intent to protect public health.

VII. Estimated Impact of these Proposals

A. Introduction

As discussed in Part IX, C of this Notice, the development of Federal Radiation Protection Guidance does not require a Regulatory Impact Analysis, but the Agency has investigated the potential impact of this proposed Guidance on RF-emitting sources. The results of field studies have shown broadcast sources, particularly FM radio stations, to be the most likely sources affected by this proposed Guidance. Greatest emphasis was, thus, given to analyzing impacts on the broadcasting industry, and the results of the engineering and cost analyzes are described, respectively, in the following two reports: (1) *An Engineering Assessment of the Potential Impact of Federal Radiation Protection Guidance on the AM, FM, and TV Broadcast Services* (27), and (2) *An Estimate of the Potential Costs of Guidelines Limiting Public Exposure to Radiofrequency Radiation from Broadcast Sources* (28).

B. Economic Impacts

1. Impacts on the Broadcast Services

The estimated costs to society, to the broadcast industry, and to a hypothetical average firm associated with identifying field intensities and complying with each of the proposed regulatory options are given in Tables 4, 5, and 6 (28). Background information was not sufficient to permit development of cost estimates for the nonregulatory option, Option 4. [See also the discussion of benefits in Section 3 below.]

The cost estimates were derived by assuming that all stations will have to conduct an initial engineering survey of their emitted field intensities to determine whether they are in compliance with the Guidance. For FM and TV stations, a variety of corrective measures or mitigation strategies were used to compute costs. Fencing the area around the perimeter of an AM tower was considered as the only corrective measure to be taken by AM stations. It is possible that stations applying the same type of mitigation strategy could incur different costs because of likely

TABLE 5. *An estimate of the total present (constant dollar) value of the cost to society-at-large of guidelines limiting public exposure to radiation from FM, AM, and TV broadcast sources for the three proposed regulatory options.*

[Dollars in millions]*

	FM component			AM component			TV component			Total society cost		
	^L	^M	^H	^L	^M	^H	^L	^M	^H	^L	^M	^H
Option 1	22.2	44.7	60.4	9.4	15.0	22.0	7.1	9.8	11.0	38.7	69.5	93.4
Option 2	16.2	31.2	41.6	6.8	9.8	13.3	3.5	4.7	5.4	26.5	45.7	60.3
Option 3	7.8	12.4	16.0	6.7	9.6	12.8	1.4	1.9	2.4	15.9	23.9	31.2

^L= **Low,** ^ M= **Medium,** ^H = **High**

*[Cost couldn't be estimated for the nonregulatory option 4. See option B.3,benefits.]

variations between stations for factors such as equipment configuration, location, market, competition, power requirements, land ownership, and for AM stations, the presence and extent of fencing. Such variation was assumed in the cost analyses and is reflected in the three cost scenarios low, medium, and high shown in Tables 5, 6, and 7. Exact costs will depend on the mitigation method ultimately used by each station. It was also assumed that no station could use the posting of warning signs as the means of complying with any Guidance level.

Guidance implementation programs and procedures may ultimately not require an engineering survey or may not prohibit posting in all cases. Use of these two assumptions, therefore, means that costs of compliance may be overestimated. Allowing posting of FM stations can reduce the costs to FM broadcasters under Option 1 by as much as 20 percent. In Table 5, under the medium cost scenario for Option 1, the costs of engineering surveys account for about 25 percent of the total costs of compliance across all broadcast services. The engineering survey costs become a proportionally larger component of total costs in the less stringent Options 2 and 3.

Under the medium cost scenario, the number of sites likely to be affected under each proposed regulatory option is about:

Service	Option 1	Option 2	Option 3
AM	2,995	1,034	946
FM	1,160	752	188
TV	60	30	2
Total	4,215	1,816	1,136

It was assumed that 33 percent of AM stations already have existing fencing adequate for compliance. The figures above exclude building-mounted FM towers. In

TABLE 6. *An estimate of the present (constant dollar) value of the net after tax cost of the broadcast industry of guidelines limiting public exposure to radiofrequency radiation from FM, AM, and TV broadcast sources for three proposed regulatory options.*

[Dollars in millions]*

	FM component			AM component			TV component			Total society cost		
	^L	^M	^H	^L	^M	^H	^L	^M	^H	^L	^M	^H
Option 1	10.9	21.7	29.2	4.8	7.6	11.0	3.4	4.7	5.4	19.1	34.0	45.5
Option 2	8.0	15.2	20.3	3.6	5.2	6.9	1.7	2.3	2.7	13.4	22.7	29.9
Option 3	4.0	6.4	8.2	3.6	5.1	6.7	0.8	1.0	1.3	8.4	12.4	16.2

^L= **Low,** ^M = **Medium,** ^H = **High**

*[Cost to the industry are the combined costs of all the firms in the industry. See Table 4 for an explanation of the derivation of firm cost. Cost couldn't be estimated for the nonregulatory option, option 4. See section B.3, benefits.]

the United States, there are approximately 4,600 AM stations, 4,400 FM stations, and 1,100 TV stations. In 1984, EPA initiated an information collection request to 1,128 FM radio broadcast stations to determine the potential for public access in the immediate vicinity of antenna towers (27). The survey asked whether the antenna tower was fenced, how far fences were from towers, and for the distance to property boundaries to help us assess the feasibility of installing a fence to limit access to higher intensity fields. Installation of a fence may be one of the least costly possible mitigation measures. The response rate was approximately 52 per-

TABLE 7. *An estimate of the potential net after present value cost to the hypothetical average broadcast station of guideline limiting public exposure to radiofrequency radiation from FM, AM, and TV broadcast sources for the three proposed regulatory options.*

[Dollars in thousands]

	FM [1] component			AM [2] component			TV [3] component		
	^L	^M	^H	^L	^M	^H	^L	^M	^H
Option 1	7.5	16.1	22.0	1.4	2.0	2.6	45.6	63.7	70.3
Option 2	7.4	15.8	21.4	1.3	1.9	2.4	33.8	45.9	50.6
Option 3	6.4	13.6	18.3	1.3	1.8	2.4	23.1	30.8	34.0

^L= **Low,** ^M = **Medium,** ^H = **High**

[1] After tax present value cost to FM station based upon a hypothetical average FM station with pretax net operating income of $139,400.

[2] After tax present value cost to AM station based upon a hypothetical average AM station with pretax net operating income of $103,850.

[3] After tax present value cost to TV station based upon a hypothetical average TV station with pretax net operating income of $2,380,000.

cent. The responses indicate that, for FM stations, at least 12 percent of the FM stations that would be affected by Option 3 already have fences around their towers that limit public access. Thus, the costs of compliance are overestimated and represent the worst case situation. Also, approximately 75 percent of the FM stations potentially affected by the Option 3 control sufficient land near their towers to permit installation of fences to limit public acess. Although we have not determined the compliance cost reduction implied by this finding, it is clear that for some FM stations further cost reductions will occur over those just discussed.

2. Impacts on Nonbroadcast Sources

Estimates of the impact of proposed Federal Guidance on nonbroadcast sources were performed using a data base prepared for EPA by the Electromagnetic Compatibility Analysis Center (ECAC), a DOD installation in Annapolis, Maryland (62).

Nonbroadcast sources, such as radars and satellite communications systems, were evaluated in terms of the numbers of sources likely to be affected by the proposed Guidance. This analysis was conducted by examining theoretically calculated field intensities near U.S. government transmitting installations for which frequency assignment records are maintained by the ECAC. No cost analyses could be performed, however, because the frequency assignment records used for site identification could not be used to identify individual systems to which Guidance implementation costs could be assigned. Also, development of cost estimates would be difficult because of the diverse characteristics of the different nonbroadcast emitting sources and the unavailability of cost data for much of the sophisticated military equipment. It was estimated, however, that the number of U.S. government installations that would be affected by any of the proposed recommended exposure limits would be small in comparison to the total number of installations. The number of sites was derived by using near-field calculation techniques and conservative assumptions about side-lobe radiation properties of the transmitting antenna radiation patterns and by assuming a 100 percent duty cycle for shortwave (3–30 MHz) communication stations, i.e., they transmit continuously. At a distance of 100 meters from a source, the number of sites projected to exceed the levels under consideration in Option 1 is 164. When more realistic assumptions are made about side-lobe radiation and typical operational duty cycles for shortwave communication stations, the total number of sites predicted to exceed the Option 1 level drops to 56. The number of sites predicted to be in excess of levels under Options 2 and 3 would be smaller. The methods and results for analyses of nonbroadcast sources are discussed in the ECAC report (62).

3. Benefits

Establishing Federal Guidance to limit public exposure to RF radiation would also result in economic benefits for which EPA has not been able to assign monetary values. This information is based on review of comments and correspondence to the Agency from industry and governmental agencies at the Federal, state, and local levels. These benefits relate to a presumed reduction in costs currently incurred in the public and private sectors by, for example, litigation, inconsistent local regulations, local regulatory development and review, Environmental Impact Statement (EIS) development, and bans on installation of or modifications to communication systems. Such costs for industry are estimated to run to several million dollars per year but proprietary cost data have not been made available to EPA by industry. Similar costs may also be incurred by local governments involved in litigation, siting actions, or regulatory development. And, these costs might represent the costs to industry and society associated with not establishing Federal Guide, the fourth and nonregulatory option proposed in this Notice. It is projected that the costs of compliance with Federal Guidance will, thus, be partially offset by the savings realized by reductions in the costs just mentioned.

Various techniques and approaches could be used to bring given stations into compliance with any particular Guidance level, if adopted. These include, but are not limited to, installing new antennas, changing the design or configuration of existing antennas, limiting shared use of broadcast towers in densely populated areas, fencing, and posting. Development, sales, and application of such techniques could benefit certain sectors within the broadcasting industry (especially for antenna-related techniques) or other commercial and business interests, thereby, partially offsetting the overall costs of compliance.

Depending on the exposure limit ultimately selected, if any, compliance with Guidance could reduce the potential for "blanketing," particularly in the FM broadcast service. Blanketing refers to the delivery of intense radio signals within a region of an AM or FM broadcast station that are so strong as to cause unacceptable signal discrimination in typical radio receivers, resulting in interference with reception of stations operating at other frequencies. Blanketing is regulated by the FCC for AM stations in its *Rules and Regulations, Volume 3, Part 73, Radio Broadcast Services, Section 73.24* and for FM stations in *Section 73.318.*

VIII. Public Hearings

A public hearing will be held in Washington, D.C. for the purpose of receiving comments on these proposed recommendations. The specific date, location, and arrangements will be announced in a later Federal Register Notice.

IX. Miscellaneous Information

A. Background Reports

Development of this Notice required consideration of the biological effects of RF fields; the RF radiation environment in terms of environmental levels, public exposure, and RF emitting sources; and the potential impact, including economic impacts, that the proposed recommendations might have on affected RF sources and users of the electromagnetic spectrum. Several reports summarize our review and evaluation of these issues: *(1) The Radiofrequency Radiation Environment: Environmental Exposure Levels and RF Radiation Emitting Sources* (26). (2) *An Engineering Assessment of the Potential Impact of Federal Radiation Guidance on the AM, FM, and TV Broadcast Services* (27). (3) *An Estimate of the Potential Costs of Guidelines Limiting Public Exposure to Radiation from Broadcast Sources* (28), and (4) *Biological Effects of Radiofrequency Radiation* (25).

Information on how to obtain single copies of these reports is given under ADDRESSES in this Notice. The reports can also be purchased from the National Technical Information Service (NTIS), 5285 Port Royal Road, Springfield, Virginia 22161; requestors should cite the NTIS accession numbers given in the list of references in this Notice.

A copy of each of the background reports is available for inspection at EPAs Central Docket Section (see ADDRESSES) and at the library in each of the 10 EPA regional offices:

Region 1, JFK Federal Building, Room E-121, Boston, Massachusetts 02203, (Tel. (617) 223-5791);
Region 2, 26 Federal Plaza, Room 734, New York, New York 10278, (Tel. (212) 264-2881);
Region 3, 841 Chestnut Street, Philadelphia, Pennsylvania 19107, (Tel. (215) 597-0580);
Region 4, 345 Courtland Street, NE., Room G 6, Atlanta, Georgia 30365–2401, (Tel. (404) 881-4216);
Region 5, 230 S. Dearborn Street, Room 1670, Chicago, Illinois 60604, (Tel. (312) 353-2022);
Region 6, 1201 Elm Street, Room 2776, Dallas, Texas 75270, (Tel. (214) 767-7341);
Region 7, 726 Minnesota Avenue, Room L-10, Kansas City, Kansas 66101, (Tel. (913) 236-2828);
Region 8, Radiation Program Office (in lieu of library), 999 18th Street, Suite 215, Denver, Colorado 80202, (Tel. (303) 293-1444);
Region 9, 215 Fremont Street, 6th Floor, San Francisco, California 94105, (Tel. (415) 974-8076);
Region 10, 1200 Sixth Avenue, 12th Floor Seattle, Washington 98101, (Tel. (206) 442-1289).

B. Paperwork Reduction Act

The Paperwork Reduction Act of 1980 (Public Law 96-511) requires that the Office of Management and Budget (OMB) review reporting and record-keeping requirements that constitute "information collection" as defined. This proposed Guidance does not contain any information collection requirements subject to OMB review under the Paperwork Reduction Act of 1980 U.S.C. 3501 *et seq.*

C. Regulatory Impact Analysis

Executive Order (E.O.) 12291, requires the preparation of a Regulatory Impact Analysis for major rules, defined by the Order as those likely to result in:

1. An annual adverse effect on the economy of $100 million or more;

2. A major increase in costs or prices for consumers, individual industries, Federal, State, or local government agencies, or geographic regions; or

3. Significant adverse effects on competition, employment, investment, productivity, innovation, or on the ability of United States-based enterprises to compete with foreign-based enterprises in domestic or export markets.

EPA has determined that this proposed Guidance does not meet the definition of a major rule under E.O. 12291, and thus, a Regulatory Impact Analysis has not been prepared.

D. Regulatory Flexibility Certification

EPA recommendations to the President for radiation guidance are not subject to the requirements of the Regulatory Flexibility Act of 1980, 5 U.S.C. 605(b) for analysis of economic effects on small business or other entities; therefore, a Regulatory Flexibility Analysis is not required. Nevertheless, the Agency has examined the potential economic impact posed by each of the proposed regulatory options, as discussed in Section VII above (27, 28). The Small Business Administration defines a nonmanufacturing small business as a firm with less than 100 employees. Under this criterion, we have determined that a significant number of broadcasting stations can be considered small businesses. The information in the cost study is, thus, useful for identifying the potential impact on small business of implementation of RF radiation exposure limits for each proposed option.

Although other Federal agencies will be responsible for implementing Guidance for radiofrequency radiation and for more fully determining the economic effects of implementation on small businesses, EPA is suggesting several ways that the impact of any Guidance on small businesses could be mitigated. These include: (1) Compliance could be phased in over a five-year period, with the larger stations phased in during the earlier years. This approach is similar to that used by EPA to estimate the potential costs of compliance. (2) Passive compliance measures could be allowed for small FM and TV stations, e.g., allowing the posting of warning signs in and around areas exceeding Guidance. (3) The cost estimates discussed in Section VII-B were derived by assuming an engineering survey of emitted field intensities would be mandatory in implementation programs. Stations could first be allowed to use analytical methods and models developed by EPA to determine whether a station is in compliance or whether an engineering survey would truly be necessary.

EPA is interested in more fully determining the impact of implementing Guidance on small business or other entities and seeks comments on this subject. Information on how to provide written comments to EPA is contained in the section of this Notice entitled ADDRESSES.

E. OMB Review

This Notice of Proposed Recommendations was submitted to OMB for review as required by Executive Order 12291 and has received their concurrence for publication.

Dated: June 12, 1986.

Lee M. Thomas,

Administrator.

REFERENCES

1. NCRP (1981). Radiofrequency electromagnetic fields, properties, quantities and units, biophysical interaction, and measurements. Report No. 67. National Council on Radiation Protection and Measurements, 7910 Woodmont Ave., Bethesda, MD 20014.
2. IEEE (1977). IEEE standard dictionary of electrical and electronics terms. IEEE Std. 100–1977. Institute of Electric and Electronics Engineers, Inc., New York.
3. FCC (1982). Notice of Proposed Rule Making, FCC 82-47, in the matter of responsibility of the Federal Communications Commission to consider biological effects of radiofrequency radiation when authorizing the use of radiofrequency devices. Released February 18, 1982.
4. FCC (1984). Report and Order, FCC 85-90, in the matter of responsibility of the Federal Communications Commission to consider biological effects of radiofrequency radiation when authorizing the use of radiofrequency devices and potential effects of reduction in the allowable level of radiofrequency radiation on FCC authorized communications services and equipment, General Docket No. 79–144. Adopted February 26, 1985. Released March 14, 1985.
5. Gerber, S. and Baldwin, K. (1979). Staff report to the Portland Planning Commission on standards for microwave and radiofrequency emissions. The City of Portland, Oregon, Bureau of Planning, November 16.
6. An Ordinance amending the Zoning Ordinance regarding radio and television transmission towers (1982). Ordinance No. 330. Board of County Commissioners of Multnomah County, Oregon, July 23.
7. A local law regulating electromagnetic radiation from commercial broadcast and communication facilities (1980). Town of Onondaga, New York, local law No. 7–1980.
8. Notice of intention to amend article 175 (Radiation Control) of the New York City health code regarding environmental standards for the microwave and other radiofrequency portions of the electromagnetic spectrum (1978). City of New York, Department of Health, Bureau for Radiation Control, June 22.
9. Regulations governing fixed facilities which generate electromagnetic fields in the frequency range of 300 kHz to 100 GHz and microwave ovens (1983). 105 Code of Massachusetts Regulation (CMR) 122,000, published in Massachusetts Register, No. 379, September 1, 1983.
10. Texas (1977). Texas regulations for control of radiofrequency electromagnetic radiation. Texas Register, Vol. 2, No. 75, September 27.
11. State of New Jersey (1984). New Jersey Administrative Code, Title 7, Chapter 28, Subchapter 42.1–4, Radio Frequency Radiation. Bureau of Radiation Protection, Division of Environmental Quality, Department of Environmental Protection.
12. ANSI (1966). Safety level of electromagnetic radiation with respect to personnel. United States of America Standards Institute, C95.1–1966.
13. ANSI (1974). Safety level of electromagnetic radiation with respect to personnel. American National Standards Institute C95.1–1974.
14. OSHA (1971). Non-ionizing radiation. Occupational safety and health standards for general industry. Code of Federal Regulations, Title 29, Part 1910, Subpart G, Section 1910.97.
15. Swimline Corporation Ruling, Employee Safety and Health Guide, (CCH), February 17, 1976 and April 12, 1977.
16. Microwave News (1982). OSHA stops enforcement of RF/MW hazards. Microwave News, Vol. II, No. 3, April, p. 2.
17. ANSI (1982). Safety levels with respect to human exposure to radio frequency electromagnetic fields, 300 kHz to 100 GHz. American National Standards Institute C95.1–1982.
18. USSR State Committee on Standards of the Council of Ministers, GOST (1984). Occupational safety standards systems, electromagnetic fields of radiofrequency, permissible levels on work places and requirements for control (in Russian), GOST 12,1,006–84. Standards Publishers, Moscow.
19. NCRP (1986). Biological effects and exposure criteria for radiofrequency electromagnetic fields. Report No. 86. National Council on Radiation Protection and Measurements, 7910 Woodmont Avenue, Bethesda, MD 20814 (in press).
20. IRPA (1984). Interim guidelines on limits of exposure to radiofrequency electromagnetic fields in the frequency range from 100 kHz to 300 GHz. International Radiation Protection Association. Health Physics, Vol. 46, No. 4, pp. 975–984.

21. APL (1984). APL Health and Safety Bulletin, No. 51, October 19, 1984. Applied Physics Laboratory, The Johns Hopkins University.
22. WHO (1981). Environmental health criteria 16, Radiofrequency and microwaves. World Health Organization, Geneva.
23. NCRP (1971). Basic radiation protection criteria. Report No. 39. National Council on Radiation Protection and Measurements, 7910 Woodmont Ave., Bethesda, MD 20814.
24. ANPR (1982). Federal radiation protection guidance for public exposure to radiofrequency radiation. Advance Notice of Proposed Recommendations. Federal Register, Vol. 47, No. 247, Thursday, December 23, p. 53338.
25. EPA (1984). Biological effects of radiofrequency radiation. Ed. J.A. Elder and D.F. Cahill. EPA report, EPA 600/8–83–026F. NTIS accession number PB 85–120—-848.
26. Hankin, N.N. (1985). The radiofrequency radiation environment: environmental exposure levels and RF radiation emitting sources. EPA Technical Report, EPA 520/1–85–014.
27. Gailey, P.C. and R.A. Tell (1984). An engineering assessment of the potential impact of Federal Radiation Protection Guidance on the AM, FM and TV broadcast services. EPA Technical Report, EPA 520/6–85–011. NTIS accession number PB 85–245–868.
28. Hall, C.H. (1985). An estimate of the potential costs of guidelines limiting public exposure to radiofrequency radiation from broadcast sources. Technical report (prepared for EPA by Lawrence Livermore National Laboratory under EPA DOE interagency agreement A–89–F–2–803–0). EPA 520/1–85–025. NTIS accession number PB 86–108–826.
29. EPA (1983). Biological effects of radiofrequency radiation. Ed. J.A. Elder and D.F. Cahill. EPA report, EPA 600/8–83–026A, external review draft. NTIS accession number PB 83–262550.
30. Letter from Dr. W. Ross Adey, Associate Chief of Staff for Research and Development, Jerry L. Pettis Memorial Veterans Hospital, Veteran's Administration to the Administrator, EPA, November 1, 1983.
31. Letter from Bernard J. Wunder, Jr., Assistant Secretary for Communications and Information, National Telecommunications and Information Administration (NTIA) to Anne M. Gorsuch, Administrator, EPA, March 11, 1982.
32. Comments of the National Association of Broadcasters in response to an ANPR, February 22, 1983. Contained in Docket A–81–43.
33. Comments of Raytheon Company in response to an ANPR, February 18, 1983. Contained in Docket A–81–43.
34. Comments of the American Telephone and Telegraph Company in response to an ANPR, February 22, 1983. Contained in Docket A–81–43.
35. Comments of the GTE Service Corporation in response to an ANPR, February 12, 1983. Contained in Docket A–81–43.
36. Comments of the TV Broadcasters All Industry Committee in response to an ANPR, February 22, 1983. Contained in Docket A–81–43.
37. Tell, R.A. and E.D. Mantiply (1980). Population exposure to VHF and UHF broadcast radiation in the United States. Proc. IEEE, Vol. 68, No. 1, January, pp. 1–12.
38. Letter from Dr. Joseph M. Lary, Research Biologist. Radiation Section, Physical Agents Effects Branch, National Institute for Occupational Safety and Health to Mr. Norbert Hankin, Office of Radiation Programs, EPA, June 7, 1984.
39. Guy, A.W., et al. Effects of long-term low-level radiofrequency radiation exposure on rats, Volumes 1–8. Technical reports prepared for the U.S. Air Force School of Aerospace Medicine, Report USAFSAM-TR-83–17, -83—-18, -83–19, -83–42, -83–50, -84–2, -84–31, -85–11.
40. Balcer-Kubiczek, E.K. and G.H. Harrison (1985). Evidence for microwave carcinogenesis in vitro. Carcinogenesis, Vol. 6, No. 6, pp. 859–864.
41. Microwave News (1985). Polish epidemiology study links RF/MW exposures to cancer. Microwave News, Vol. V, No. 2, March, p. 1.
42. ONR (1984). Electromagnetic waves and neurobehavioral function: an international workshop. ONR London Conference Report, C 6–84, October 19, 1984. Office of Naval Research.
43. Kues, H.A., et al. (1985). Effects of 2.45 GHz microwaves on primate corneal endothelium. Bioelectromagnetics, Vol. 6, No. 2, pp. 177–188.
44. ACGIH (1983). Threshold limit values for chemical substances and physical agents in the work environment with intended changes for 1983–84. American Conference of Governmental Industrial Hygienist, 6500 Glenway Ave., Bldg. D 5, Cincinnati, Ohio 45211.
45. Ellis, F.P. (1972). Mortality from heat illness and heat-aggravated illness in the United States. Environmental Research, Vol. 5, pp. 1–58.

46. Nutrition Foundation (1982). A proposed food safety evaluation process. Food Safety Council, 888 7th St., N.W., Washington, DC 20006, June.
47. National Academy of Sciences (1977). Drinking water and health, part I. A report of the Safe Drinking Water Committee, Advisory Center on Toxicology, Assembly of Life Sciences, National Research Council, Washington.
48. Dourson, M.L. and J.F. Stara (1983). Regulatory history and experimental support of uncertainty (safety) factors. Regulatory Tox. and Pharm., Vol. 3, pp. 224–238.
49. EPA (1983). Guidelines for performing regulatory impact analyses. Office of Policy Analysis. EPA report, EPA 230–01–84–003, December.
50. Christian, M.S., et al., Ed. (1983). Assessment of reproductive and teratogenic hazards. Advances in Modern Environmental Toxicology, Vol. III. Princeton Scientific Publishers, Inc., Princeton, New Jersey.
51. Gandhi, O.P., et al., (1985). Likelihood of high rates of energy deposition in the human legs at the ANSI recommended 3–30 MHz RF safety limits. Proc. IEEE, Vol. 73, No. 6, June, pp. 1145–1147.
52. Berman, E., et al. (1984). Growth and development of mice offspring after irradiation in utero with 2,450 MHz microwaves. Teratology, Vol. 30, pp. 393–402.
53. EPA (1985). Radiofrequency radiation measurement survey, Honolulu, Hawaii, May 14–25, 1984. Office of Radiation Programs.
54. Deno, D.W. (1974). Calculating electrostatic effects of overhead transmission lines. IEEE Trans. Power Apparatus and Systems, Vol. PAG 3, pp. 1458–1466.
55. Banks, R.S., C.M. Kannianen, and R.D. Clark (1977). Public health and safety effects of high-voltage overhead transmission lines: An analysis for the Minnesota Environmental Quality Board, Minnesota Department of Health, Division of Environmental Health, Minneapolis, MN, October.
56. Tell, R.A., E.D. Mantiply, C.H. Durney, and H. Massoudi. Electric and magnetic field intensities and associated induced currents in man in close proximity to a 50 kW AM standard broadcast station. In Program and Abstracts, United States National Committee, International Union of Radio Science, and Bioelectromagnetics Symposium, June 18–22, 1979, Seattle, Washington, p. 360. To be submitted for publication to IEEE Transactions on Broadcasting.
57. Dalziel, C.F., E. Ogden, and C.E. Abbott (1943). Effect of frequency on let-go currents. Electrical Engineering Transactions, Vol. 62, December, pp. 745–749.
58. Dalziel, C.F. and T.H. Mansfield (1950). Effect of frequency on perception currents. AIEE Transactions, Vol. 69, pt. II, pp. 1162–1168.
59. NIOSH (1985). Radiofrequency/microwave occupational exposure standard and rationale, external review draft. National Institute for Occupational Safety and Health, U.S. Department of Health and Human Services.
60. ANSI (1973). American National Standard techniques and instrumentation for the measurements of potentially hazardous electromagnetic radiation at microwave frequencies. American National Standards Institute C95.3–1973.
61. Tell, R.A. (1983). Instrumentation for measurement of electromagnetic fields: equipment, calibrations, and selected applications. In Biological Effects and Dosimetry of Nonionizing Radiation, ed. M. Grandolfo, S.M. Michaelson, and A. Rindi. Plenum Press, New York, pp. 95–162.
62. ECAC (1982). Support to the Environmental Protection Agency nonionizing radiation source analysis. Electromagnetic Compatibility Analysis Center, Report No. ECAC–CR–82–093, September.

IRPA/INIRC GUIDELINES: PROTECTION OF THE PATIENT UNDERGOING A MAGNETIC RESONANCE EXAMINATION[†]

INTERNATIONAL NON-IONIZING RADIATION COMMITTEE OF THE INTERNATIONAL RADIATION PROTECTION ASSOCIATION

Preface

Magnetic resonance imaging (MRI) has become an established diagnostic modality. The clinical usefulness of in-vivo magnetic resonance spectroscopy (MRS) was demonstrated in several instances and is being explored further. These techniques involve exposure of the patient to static and time-varying magnetic fields and radiofrequency electromagnetic fields. In particular exposure situations, these fields may pose a health hazard.

The International Non-Ionizing Radiation Committee of the International Radiation Protection Association (IRPA/INIRC) in cooperation with the Environmental Health Division of the World Health Organization (WHO) has developed health criteria documents on magnetic fields (UNEP/WHO/IRPA 1987) and radiofrequency fields (UNEP/WHO/IRPA in press). Guidelines on limits of exposure to radiofrequency electromagnetic fields have been published by IRPA/INIRC (1988).

These publications, in conjunction with other reviews and recent literature, form the basis for this document. During its preparation, the IRPA/INIRC was composed of the following:

M. H. Repacholi, Chairman (Australia)*
H. Jammet, Chairman Emeritus (France)
J. H. Bernhardt (Federal Republic of Germany)
B. F. M. Bosnjakovic (The Netherlands)
L. A. Court (France)
P. Czerski (U.S.A.) (deceased)
M. Grandolfo (Italy)
B. Knave (Sweden)
A. F. McKinlay (United Kingdom)
M. G. Shandala (U.S.S.R.)
D. H. Sliney (U.S.A.)
J. A. J. Stolwijk (U.S.A.)
M. A. Stuchly (Canada)
L. D. Szabo (Hungary)
*Scientific Secretary: A. S. Duchêne.***

[†]Health Physics Vol. 61, No. 6 (December), pp. 923—928, 1991. Printed in the U.S.A.
[*] Royal Adelaide Hospital, Australia.
[**]Rue Grambetta 92260 fontenay-aux-Roses, France.

The IRPA Associate Societies, as well as a number of competent institutions and individual experts, were consulted in the preparation of this document. Their cooperation is gratefully acknowledged.

Purpose And Scope

The purpose of this document is to provide information on levels of exposure and health effects from magnetic and radiofrequency electromagnetic fields associated with MR diagnostic devices, and on precautions to be taken to minimize health hazards to patients undergoing MR examinations.

The present document does not apply to the occupational safety of the operator or to the safety of the general public. Guidelines on occupational and general public exposure limits to radiofrequency electromagnetic fields have been published (IRPA/INIRC 1988). Guidance on occupational and public exposure limits to static magnetic fields is in preparation. This document is intended for use by international or national medical device regulatory authorities, MR users and health professionals, and those involved in the design and manufacture of MR equipment for clinical applications. Contraindications, warnings, precautions, and safety considerations for the patients are given.

Rationale

A review of the biological effects from exposure to magnetic fields is contained in UNEP/WHO/IRPA (1987). Additional data and references can be found in Budinger (1981), Mansfield and Morris (1982), Saunders and Orr (1983), Budinger and Lauterbur (1984), Tenforde and Budinger (1985), Bernhardt (1986, 1988), Grandolfo (1987), Mathur-De Vre (1987a, 1987b), Podo (1987), and Czerski (1988). Recommendations for radiofrequency exposure levels are based on the data contained in reports by the EPA (1984), NCRP (1986), UNEP/WHO/IRPA (in press), and on the rationale appended to IRPA/INIRC (1988).

Following is a brief summary of conclusions drawn from the review of scientific literature.

Static magnetic fields

The scientific literature does not indicate adverse effects from exposure of the whole body to 2 T and of the extremities to 5 T. For whole-body exposure at 5 T, magnetoelectrodynamic interactions with blood flow may lead to effects on the cardiocirculatory system (Tenforde and Budinger 1985; UNEP/WHO/IRPA 1987). Volunteers who were exposed to 10 T without adverse effects reported discomfort (Beischer 1962). Animals exposed to the same flux density also did not show adverse effects but exhibited behavioral modifications (UNEP/WHO/IRPA 1987). Theoretical analyses indicate that at 24 T, direct interference with ionic conduction current is likely. Some predictions indicate the possibility of interaction at lower levels with conduction loops within the central nervous system. Hence, the recommendation is to monitor patients for symptoms referable to the nervous system at levels above 2 T.

Time-varying magnetic fields

Recommendations on limiting the exposure to time-varying magnetic fields were based primarily on effects of induced currents on excitable cell membranes in the nervous system and muscles, and to a certain extent on more subtle effects in other cells (Tenforde and Budinger 1985; Bernhardt 1986; Czerski and Athey 1987; Reilly 1987; UNEP/WHO/IRPA 1987; Athey and Czerski 1988).

In the absence of adverse health effects, it may be assumed that current densities on the order of 1–10 mA m^{-2} induced by continuous sinusoidal magnetic fields are of no concern. Current densities of 10–100 mA m^{-2} can have effects that are strongly dependent on the frequency but are not considered adverse. For example, at 10–50 Hz and at fields of more than 5 mT, sensations of light flashes in the eyes (magnetophosphenes) have been observed; 100–1000 mA m^{-2} is the range where stimulation of excitable cell membranes is observed and where health hazards are possible. A current density of more than 1 A m^{-2} in the vicinity of the heart or an electric field strength exceeding 5 V m^{-1} in tissue may cause ventricular fibrillation (UNEP/WHO/IRPA 1987).

It is difficult to correlate the induced body currents with the magnetic flux change of the different magnetic field gradients occurring in pulse sequences from MR equipment. When wave shapes deviate from sinusoidal, it is difficult to predict the biological effectiveness in causing stimulation. As a result, in case of non-sinusoidal currents, each specific situation must be evaluated on the basis of the shape and frequency of the wave.

It can be estimated that a magnetic flux change of 3 T s^{-1} induces a maximum current density of 30 to 60 mA m^{-2} in the head or trunk, respectively (Budinger 1981). A flux change of 20 T s^{-1} induces a maximum current density of 400 mA m^{-2} at the periphery of the trunk inside MRI equipment. For a single pulse, under worst-case assumptions, Reilly (1987) calculated that this current density remains below the threshold for peripheral nerve stimulation by a factor of at least 3. As the pulse duration of dB/dt is shortened to less than 0.1 ms, higher flux change rates can be permitted. In the MR environment, peripheral nerve stimulation occurs before effects on the function of the heart are induced (McRobbie and Foster 1984, 1985) and can be used as a primary criterion for the assessment of MR safety (Czerski and Athey 1987). Because of the smaller induction loops in magnets used for MR examinations of limbs, the values for exposure of limbs alone can be increased compared with the trunk.

Radiofrequency fields

Limitations on radiofrequency energy deposition are intended to eliminate the elevation of temperature to levels at which local thermal injury or systemic thermal overload may occur. They are based on experimental and human data, including experimental, clinical, and modelling studies on thermal effects of MR exposure (Borup and Gandhi 1984; Spiegel 1984; Bottomley et al. 1985; Adair and Berglund 1986; Shellock et al. 1986; Shellock and Crues 1987; Athey and Czerski 1988; Grandolfo et al. 1990). Thus, the primary criterion for radiofrequency exposure is based on elevation of temperature in the skin, body core, or in spatially limited volumes of tissues where local temperature increases ("hot spots") may occur under conditions of MR exposure. Nonuniformities in RF energy deposition, particularly in vascular or hypovascular structures characterized by a higher radiofrequency absorption and lower heat dissipation, such as the eyes, brain ventricles, hydrocephalus, tumors, and hemorrhagic foci (De Ford et al. 1983; Athey 1989; Shellock and Crues 1988), were considered in the recommendations that follow. The values for the specific absorption rates and total energy absorption over time indicated below were derived under worst-case assumptions and represent conservative approximations.

Caution about the exposure of pregnant women, particularly during the first trimester, is based on questions on the efficacy of fetus imaging and on its thermal vulnerability (Tenforde and Budinger 1985; UNEP/WHO/IRPA 1987). Safety of MR examinations during pregnancy has not been established.

There is virtually no information about any delayed effects that may result from long or repeated exposure, and no guidance can be derived in this area other than the benefits to the patients.

General Recommendations

Until now, most MRI or MRS examinations have been made using static magnetic fields up to 2 T; however, higher magnetic flux densities offer potential diagnostic advantages, particularly for MRS. From the review of the biological effects of magnetic fields, it can be concluded that no adverse health effects are to be expected from short-term (hours) exposure to static fields up to 2 T (UNEP/WHO/IRPA 1987). Also, there are many gaps in our knowledge of biological effects and interaction mechanisms of static magnetic fields with tissues. The Committee emphasizes that in the application of MR, the following issues deserve special attention:

(1) Magnetic resonance (MR) in-vivo examinations should be performed only when there is a potential clinical advantage to the patient.

(2) An assessment of risks and benefits of the MR examinations should be made, and the decision to proceed must be based on the relationship between the patient and the physician.

(3) Consideration should be given to the clinical advantages and disadvantages of MR compared with other diagnostic techniques.

(4) Where MR examinations form part of a research project, the project should be guided by rules of human ethics; informed consent of the patient should be obtained.

(5) MR equipment users must be adequately trained in the principles and operation of the equipment, indications and contraindications for use, recordkeeping requirements, safety aspects, and precautions.

(6) Manufacturers should supply complete documentation about patient exposure levels for their equipment, and these safety guidelines should be considered in the design of equipment and facility layout so that exposures to magnetic and radiofrequency fields are within the levels recommended for patients.

Recommendations About Exposure Levels

Clinical experience currently indicates that adequate diagnostic information can be obtained while examining a patient for periods ranging from 15 min to 1 h and may be repeated several times over the course of the disease. The exposure levels below refer to patient studies from 15 min to less than 1 h, and where none of the contraindications listed below exist. Exposure levels are stated in SI quantities and units (IRPA/INIRC 1985).

Static magnetic fields

No adverse health effects are expected from exposures of the head and/or trunk to magnetic flux densities up to 2 T, or from exposure of the limbs to magnetic flux densities up to 5 T.

Exposures of the head and trunk to magnetic flux densities above 2 T require an assessment of the potential adverse effects vs. the likely benefit to the patient. Short-term whole-body exposures to fields of 5 T may pose health hazards, particularly for people with cardiovascular diseases, including high blood pressure. Therefore, monitoring the patient's cardiovascular function must be undertaken whenever exposures are above 2 T for the head or trunk, and above 5 T for limbs. Experimental data above 5 T are sparse; until further information is available, magnetic flux densities above 10 T should not be used.

Time-varying magnetic fields

Clinical experience indicates that no adverse health effects are to be expected when the rate of change of magnetic flux density does not exceed 6 T s^{-1}. However, patients with changes in the electrocardiogram (ECG) indicative of abnormalities in conduction may be particularly susceptible to exposure to magnetic fields. Therefore, an assessment of cardiac function (i.e., an ECG) should be made when exposures above 6 T s^{-1} are contemplated, and the patient's cardiovascular function should be monitored during exposure above 6 T s^{-1}. There is no wide-spread clinical experience above 6 T s^{-1}; theoretical calculations (Czerski and

Athey 1987; Reilly 1989) indicate that above 20 T s^{-1} peripheral nerve stimulation could occur. Therefore, 20 T s^{-1} should not be exceeded.

Radiofrequency fields

Radiofrequency energy at frequencies between 10 and 100 MHz deposited in the body during an MR examination will be converted to heat, which will be distributed largely by convective heat transfer through blood flow. As the body temperature increases, there will be an increase in blood flow and cardiac output, as well as an increase in sweat secretion and evaporation.

For whole-body exposures or exposures to the head and trunk, no adverse health effects are expected if the increase in body temperature does not exceed 1°C. In the case of infants, pregnant women, and persons with cardiocirculatory impairment, it is desirable to limit temperature increases to 0.5°C.

In practice, due to its thermal capacity, no tissue will increase in temperature at a rate more than 1°C h^{-1} for each W kg^{-1} of power deposition. In persons (infants, aged persons, patients with local or systemic cardiovascular impairment) in whom the thermoregulatory mechanisms are less efficient than in a healthy human adult, signs of distress may appear at a whole-body average SAR of 2 W kg^{-1} after 10 min of exposure (Budinger et al. 1985). Considering the modifying effects of blood flow and environmental heat exchange, no adverse health effects are to be expected in persons without cardiovascular abnormalities exposed to 2 W kg^{-1} for 1 h. In persons with cardiovascular abnormalities, 1 W kg^{-1} for 1 h is an acceptable level, provided proper monitoring is instituted.

In MR exposures up to 1 h, the total body exposure should be limited to a total energy deposition of 120 W min kg^{-1} (7.2 J g^{-1}) in order not to overload the thermoregulatory system. To avoid overheating any local area, the product of time and local SAR should not exceed:

60 W min kg^{-1} (3.6 J g^{-1}) averaged over the head, or

120 W min kg^{-1} (7.2 J g^{-1}) averaged over the trunk, or

180 W min kg^{-1} (10.8 J g^{-1}) averaged over the extremities, provided that the instantaneous SAR does not exceed:

4 W kg^{-1} averaged over the head, or

8 W kg^{-1} averaged over the trunk, or

12 W kg^{-1} averaged over the extremities.

To protect poorly perfused tissues, the eyes for example, such tissues should not be exposed to a local SAR of more than 10 W kg^{-1}, averaged over 0.01 kg (0.1 W/10 g) for more than 10 min.

For exposures of infants, pregnant women, or persons with cardiocirculatory and/or cerebral vascular impairment, a reduction of these values by a factor of two is recommended. For an RF-emitting surface coil, the average should be taken over the volume affected by the coil.

Users of diagnostic magnetic resonance devices usually do not have adequate resources to determine energy deposition within the patient's body. Such information should be supplied by the manufacturer, and it is recommended that the user request reliable and detailed data from the manufacturer.

Contraindications

Examinations of patients who have electrically, magnetically, or mechanically activated implants (e.g., cardiac pacemakers), or who rely on electrically, magnetically, or mechanically activated life-support systems, are contraindicated. Examinations of patients with ferromagnetic aneurysm clips or metallic implants (e.g., intrauterine contraceptive devices, prostheses) are also contraindicated.

Warnings And Safety Considerations

Exposure during pregnancy

There is no firm evidence that mammalian embryos are sensitive to the magnetic fields encountered in magnetic resonance systems. However, pending the accumulation of more data regarding MR in pregnancy, it is recommended that elective examination of pregnant women should be postponed until after the first trimester. Because ultrasound is the modality of choice for fetal and uterine examination during pregnancy, an MR examination should be limited to cases in which unique diagnostic information can be obtained. Exposure duration should be reduced to the minimum, consistent with obtaining useful diagnostic information (Weinreb et al. 1985; NIH 1988).

Other safety considerations related to patient's condition

Communication with the patient or monitoring of the anesthetized patient must be assured throughout the examination.

Certain patients may experience claustrophobia. Claustrophobic reactions should be explored before an examination is undertaken.

Because some individuals may exhibit hypersensitivity to heating, it is advisable to ascertain if the patient's history comprises incidents indicative of hypersensitivity to heat and, if necessary, limit the duration of the examination.

Metallic exclusions

Ferromagnetic objects are attracted by magnetic fields. Depending on size, composition, and location of metallic implants or inclusions, serious injuries may result because of motions and displacement of such objects. Large metallic objects, such as hip prostheses, may become heated because of preferential radiofrequency absorption, leading to local thermal injury. Moreover, the presence of such objects results in artifacts in diagnostic information because of magnetic distortion.

The presence or absence of such objects in the body has to be ascertained and the consequences evaluated before an examination is undertaken.

Collision hazards and electromagnetic interference

The field near the magnet may be strong enough to attract ferromagnetic objects and to cause them to fly towards the magnet. Thus, metallic objects, particularly with sharp edges, may become dangerous projectiles. All such objects have to be eliminated from the examination room and proper warning signs must be posted. Such hazards may arise also during installation or transport of magnets. Proper precautions should be taken, with warning signs posted in the area and placed on crates and packages during transport.

The manufacturer should provide information regarding the extent of the zone in which collision hazards and danger of uncontrolled movements of objects exist (e.g., uncontrolled movement of hospital carts, trolleys, loose tools, medical instruments, etc.).

Various medical and non-medical equipment and magnetic data carriers may be affected by magnetic fields. X-ray imaging equipment may be affected at magnetic flux densities above 0.05 mT, and cathode-ray devices and tubes affected at 0.2 mT. Patient monitoring equipment and emergency equipment may be affected at magnetic flux densities of 0.2 mT and above. Electronic implants, such as cardiac pacemakers, may be affected above 0.5 mT. Computers and magnetic storage media may be affected above 0.5 mT, and credit cards and analog watches affected at fields above 1 mT. The extent of zones in which such fields exist must be determined, and proper warning signs must be posted.

Quench

For MR facilities using superconducting magnets, there is a rare possibility that the liquid helium will suddenly become gaseous. This can occur if the superconductor becomes "normal," resulting in the dissipation of heat and evaporation of cryogens. An appropriate exhaust system should be attached to the magnet so that in the event of a quench, the gases will be vented to the outside and the helium does not become an asphyxiation hazard. If this system fails, the patient must be removed very quickly. An emergency procedure should be established to remove the patient from the examination room in the event of a quench.

Patient monitoring

Special requirements apply to the equipment and methods used for the monitoring of the patient under MR exposure conditions. Cardiorespiratory function may be monitored using non-ferromagnetic transducers to register the heart beat rate, blood pressure, and respiratory rate. The ECG is subject to distortion because of electrodynamic interactions and does not yield useful information. Non-perturbing fiber-optic probes for measurement of temperature are available. Under MR exposure conditions, oral temperature and the temperature of the skin of exposed body parts, possibly supplemented by rectal temperature measurement, are suitable for patient monitoring. Detailed information on body temperature measurements may be found in the review by Togawa (1985).

Resuscitation and emergency procedures

In view of the problems associated with collision hazards and electromagnetic interference, it may be impractical to institute resuscitation procedures and intensive care for the patient in the examining room. All necessary equipment should be assembled and tested in an adjoining room, outside the zone of interference. Speedy transport of the patient to an emergency area must be readily available.

Recordkeeping and patient follow-up

Examination records should be kept and patients should be monitored according to standard requirements of good medical practice. It is recommended that follow-up studies be carried out on children born following magnetic resonance examination in utero, or who were examined during early childhood. Observations on adverse reactions should be collected, reported according to national requirements, and published in the medical literature.

Acknowledgments

The International Non-Ionizing Radiation Committee is funded by the International Radiation Protection Association. The support of the World Health Organization, the United Nations Environment Programme, the International Labour Office, and the Commission of the European Communities is gratefully acknowledged.

REFERENCES

Adair, E.R., Berglund, L.G. On the thermoregulatory consequences of NMR imaging. Magnetic Resonance Imaging 4:321–333;1986.

Athey, T.W. A model of the temperature rise in the head due to magnetic resonance imaging procedures. Magnetic Resonance in Med. 9:177–184;1989.

Athey, T.W., Czerski, P. Safety of magnetic resonance in vivo diagnostic examinations. In: Proceedings of the 10th Annual Conference of the IEEE Engineering in Medicine and Biology Society; Piscataway, NJ: IEEE;Vol. 10:892–893;1988.

Beischer, D.E. Human tolerance to magnetic fields. Astronautics 42:24–25;1962.

Bernhardt, J.H. Evaluation of human exposures to low frequency fields. Medizin Verlag, Munich; BGA Schriften 3/86;1986.

Bernhardt, J.H. The establishment of frequency dependent limits for electric and magnetic fields and evaluation of indirect effects. Radiat. Environ. Biophys. 27:1–27;1988.

Borup, D.T., Gandhi, O.P. Fast Fourier transform method for calculation of SAR distribution in finely discretized inhomogenous models of biological bodies. IEEE Trans. on Microwave Theory and Techniques MTT-32:355–360;1984.

Bottomley, P.A., Redington, R.W., Edelstein, W.A., Schenck, J.F. Estimating radiofrequency power deposition in body NMR imaging. Magnetic Resonance in Med. 2:336–349;1985.

Budinger, T.F. Nuclear magnetic resonance (NMR) in vivo studies: Known thresholds for effects. J. Comput. Assist. Tomogr. 5:800–811;1981.

Budinger, T.F., Lauterbur, P.C. Nuclear magnetic resonance technology for medical studies. Science 226:288–298;1984.

Budinger, T.F., Pavlicek, W., Faul, D.D., Guy, A.W. RF heating at 1.5 tesla and above in proton imaging. In: Abstracts of the Fourth Meeting of Magnetic Resonance in Medicine, Berkeley, CA; Society of Magnetic Resonance in Medicine;1985:916–917.

Czerski, P. Extremely low frequency magnetic fields: Biological effects and health risk assessment. In: Repacholi, M.H., ed. Non-ionizing radiations. Physical characteristics, biological effects and health hazards assessment. Proceedings of an INIR Workshop, Melbourne, Australia;1988:291 301. Available from: Australian Radiation Laboratory, Yallambie, Victoria. Australia, 3085.

Czerski P., Athey, T.W. Safety of magnetic resonance in vivo diagnostic examinations: Theoretical and clinical considerations. Rockville, MD: Food and Drug Administration, Docket Management Branch: Magnetic resonance diagnostic device panel recommendation and report on petitions for MR reclassification. Docket 87P–0214;1987.

De Ford, J.F., Gandhi, O.P., Hagmann, M.J. Moment-method solutions and SAR calculations for inhomogenous models of man with large number of cells. IEEE Trans. Microwave Theory and Technology MTT-31:848–851;1983.

Environmental Protection Agency. Biological effects of radiofrequency radiation. Research Triangle Park, NC: U.S. Environmental Protection Agency, EPA 600/8–83–026 F;1984.

Grandolfo, M. Radiofrequency power deposition in medical NMR equipment. In: Schmidt, K.H., ed. Safety assessment of NMR clinical equipment. Stuttgart and New York: George Thieme Verlag;1987:50–60.

Grandolfo, M., Vecchia, P., Gandhi, O.P. Magnetic resonance imaging: Calculation of rates of energy absorption by a human-torso model. Bioelectromagnetics 11:117–128;1990.

International Non-Ionizing Radiation Committee of the International Radiation Protection Association (IRPA/INIRC). Review of concepts, quantities, units, and terminology for non-ionizing radiation protection. Health Phys. 49:1329–1362;1985.

International Non-Ionizing Radiation Committee of the International Radiation Protection Association (IRPA/INIRC). Guidelines on limits of exposure to radiofrequency electromagnetic fields in the frequency range from 100 kHz to 300 GHz. Health Phys. 54:115–123;1988.

Mansfield, P., Morris, P.G. Biomagnetic effects. In: NMR imaging in biomedicine. New York: Academic Press;1982:297–332.

Mathur-De Vre, R. Safety aspects of magnetic resonance imaging and magnetic resonance spectroscopy applications in medicine and biology: I. Biomagnetic effects. Arch. B. Med. Soc. Hyg. Med. Tr. Med. Leg. 45:394–424;1987a.

Mathur-De Vre, R. Safety aspects of magnetic resonance imaging and magnetic resonance spectroscopy applications in medicine and biology: II. Biomagnetic effects. Arch. B. Med. Soc. Hyg. Med. Tr. Med. Leg. 45:425–438;1987b.

McRobbie, D., Foster, M.A. Thresholds for biological effects of time varying magnetic fields. Clin. Phys. Physiol. Meas. 5:67–78;1984.

McRobbie, D., Foster, M.A. Cardiac response to pulsed magnetic fields with regard to safety in NMR imaging. Phys. Med. Biol. 30:695–702;1985.

National Council on Radiation Protection and Measurements (NCRP). Biological effects and exposure criteria for radiofrequency electromagnetic fields. Washington, D.C.: NCRP, NCRP Report No. 86;1986.

National Institutes of Health. Magnetic resonance imaging. In: Report of a NIH Consensus Development Conference, 26–28 October 1987, Bethesda, MD; Washington, D.C.: National Institutes of Health;1988.

National Radiological Protection Board (NRPB). Exposure to nuclear magnetic resonance clinical imaging. Radiology 47:258–260;1981.

National Radiological Protection Board (NRPB). Revised guidance on acceptable limits of exposure during nuclear magnetic resonance clinical imaging. Br. J. Radiol. 56:974–977;1983.

Podo, F. Introduction to the concerted action's programme in the safety assessment of NMR clinical equipment. In: Schmidt, K.H., ed. Safety assessment of NMR clinical equipment. Stuttgart and New York: Georg Thieme Verlag;1987:2–5.

Reilly, J.P. Peripheral stimulation by pulsatile currents: Applications to time varying magnetic field exposure. Rockville, MD: Food and Drug Administration, Center for Devices and Radiological Health, TM 87–100;1987.

Reilly, J.P. Peripheral nerve stimulation by induced electric currents: Exposure to time-varying magnetic fields. Med. Biol. Eng. Comp. 23:101–110;1989.

Saunders, R.D., Orr, J.S. Biological effects of NMR. In: Partain, C.L., ed. Nuclear magnetic resonance (NMR) imaging. Philadelphia: W.B. Saunders;1983:383–396.

Shellock, F.G., Crues, J.V. Temperature, heart rate, and blood pressure changes associated with clinical MR imaging at 1.5 T. Radiology 163:259–262;1987.

Shellock, F.G., Crues, J.V. Temperature changes caused by MR imaging of the brain with a head coil. Am. J. Neuroradiol. 9:287–291;1988.

Shellock, F.G., Schaefer, D.J., Gordon, C.J. Effect of a static magnetic field on body temperature of man. Magnetic Resonance in Med. 3:644–647;1986.

Spiegel, R.J. A review of numerical models for predicting the energy deposition and resultant thermal response of humans exposed to electromagnetic fields. IEEE Trans. on Microwave Theory and Technology. MTT-3:730–746;1984.

Tenforde, T.S., Budinger, T.F. Biological effects and physical safety aspects of NMR imaging and in vivo spectroscopy. In: Thomas, S.R., Dickson, R.L. eds. NMR in medicine. New York: American Association of Physicists in Medicine;1985.

Togawa, T. Body temperature measurement. Clin. Phys. Physiol. Meas. 6:83–108;1985.

United Nations Environment Programme/World Health Organization/International Radiation Protection Association (UNEP/WHO/IRPA). Environmental Health Criteria No. 69. Magnetic fields. Geneva: WHO;1987.

United Nations Environment Programme/World Health Organization/International Radiation Protection Association (UNEP/WHO/IRPA). Environmental health criteria for electromagnetic fields in the range of 300 Hz to 300 GHz. Geneva: WHO;(in press).

Weinreb, J.C., Lowe, T., Cohen, J.M., Kutler, M. Human fetal anatomy: MR imaging. Radiology 157:715–720;1985.

Appendix III

SMRI REPORT: POLICIES, GUIDELINES, AND RECOMMENDATIONS FOR MR IMAGING SAFETY AND PATIENT MANAGEMENT[1]

Frank G. Shellock, Ph.D[2], Emanuel Kanal, M.D.[2] and the SMRI Safety Committee[3]

The following are policies, guidelines, and recommendations from the Safety Committee of the Society for Magnetic Resonance Imaging (SMRI) concerning various issues related to magnetic resonance (MR) imaging safety and patient management. These policies, guidelines, and recommendations were developed to provide standardized and consistent information for use by health practitioners involved in clinical MR imaging.

Index terms: Artifacts; Biological effects; Psychological effects; Quality assurance; Safety

---

[1]From the Section of MRI, Cedars-Sinai Medical Center and University of California Los Angeles School of Medicine, 8700 Beverly Blvd, Los Angeles, CA 90048 (F.G.S.); University of Pittsburgh School of Medicine, and the Pittsburgh NMR Institute Pittsburgh (E.K.). Received May 4, 1990; revision requested August 15; revision received September 21; accepted September 24. Address reprint requests to F.G.S.

[2]Co-chairman of the SMRI Safety Committee.

[3]G. Jerome Beers, MD, College of Physicians and Surgeons of Columbia University, New York, NY; Michael J. Bronskill, PhD, Ontario Cancer Institute, Toronto; Joel Gray, PhD, Mayo Clinic Foundation, Rochester, Minn; Elaine Keeler, PhD, Picker International, Highland Heights, Ohio; Larry Kroger, PhD, GE Medical Systems, Milwaukee; John LaFiore, MD, MSPH, Berlex Laboratories, Cedar Knolls, NJ: Andre Lutten, MS, Phillips Medical Systems, Eindhoven, The Netherlands; Richard Magin, PhD, University of Illinois, Urbana, Ill: William Pavlicek, PhD, Mayo Clinic Foundation, Rochester, Minn; Frank Prato, PhD, St Joseph's Health Centre, London, Ont; Allen Ruszkowski, Resonex, Inc, Sunnyvale, Calif; Richard Sano, Philips Medical Systems and National Electrical Manufacturers Association, Shelton, Conn; Javad Seyedzadeh, Toshiba America Medical Systems, Tustin, Calif; Reuven Schreiber, MD, Elscint, Inc, Boston; Ralph Shuping, ScD, Center for Devices and Radiological Health, Food and Drug Administration, Rockville, Md, and American Association of Physicists in Medicine; and Jeffrey Weinreb, MD, New York University, New York, NY.

JMRI 1991;1:97–101.

Abbreviation: FDA = U.S. Food and Drug Administration.

The information for this report is based on data compiled from the currently available literature and on the experience and consensus of the Society for Magnetic Resonance Imaging (SMRI) Safety Committee. The SMRI Safety Committee comprises an international panel of scientists and physicians who are actively involved in MR imaging and who have special interest and expertise in MR imaging safety and patient management issues. Included in this panel are representatives from the U.S. Food and Drug Administration (FDA), the National Electrical Manufacturers Association (NEMA), various commercial manufacturers of MR imaging systems, and manufacturers of MR imaging contrast agents. In addition to the SMRI Safety Committee, the Board of Directors of the SMRI reviewed and accepted this report.

In the future, additional policies, guidelines, and recommendations will be developed on other topics related to MR imaging safety and patient management. Furthermore, the existing policies, guidelines, or recommendations will be revised as new information becomes available on the individual topics.

MR IMAGING AND PATIENTS WITH ELECTRICALLY, MAGNETICALLY, OR MECHANICALLY ACTIVATED OR ELECTRICALLY CONDUCTIVE DEVICES

The FDA requires labeling of MR imagers to indicate that the device is contraindicated for patients who have electrically, magnetically, or mechanically activated implants because the magnetic and electromagnetic fields produced by MR systems may interfere with the operation of these devices (1). Therefore, patients with internal or external cardiac pacemakers, implantable cardioverter defibrillators, cochlear implants, neurostimulators, bone-growth stimulators, implantable drug-infusion pumps, and similar devices that could be adversely affected by the electromagnetic fields used in MR imaging should not be examined with this modality (2,3).

The risks associated with MR imaging of patients with cardiac pacemakers are related to the possibility of movement of the device, reed switch closure or damage, programming changes, inhibition or reversion to an asynchronous mode of operation, electromagnetic interference, and induced currents in lead wires or other conducting materials of the device (2–8).

A letter to an editor recently indicated that a patient who was not dependent on a pacemaker underwent MR imaging after his pacemaker was "disabled" during the procedure (9). Although this patient experienced no apparent discomfort and the pacemaker was not damaged, it is inadvisable to perform this type of maneuver in patients with pacemakers because of the potential to encounter any combination of the aforementioned hazards (3). Of particular concern is the possibility that the pacemaker lead wire(s) or other similar intracardiac wire configuration could act as an antenna in which the gradient and/or radio-frequency electromagnetic fields may induce sufficient current to cause fibrillation, thermal injury, or other potentially dangerous event (2,3,8,10–12). Because of this theoretically deleterious and unpredictable effect, potential risks are associated with MR imaging in patients with residual external pacing wires, temporary pacing wires, thermodilution Swan-Ganz catheters, and/or any other type of internally or externally positioned conductive wire or similar device (2,10,11,13).

All unnecessary and/or unused electrically conductive materials should be removed from the MR system before the onset of imaging. For example, unused surface coils or gating leads should not be left within the MR system even if disconnected from the system (11). Special care should be taken to ensure that no unnecessary loops are created in any electrically conductive materials within the MR system (11). Furthermore, surface coils, electrically activated gating equipment, and similar devices should be inspected and tested routinely to identify damaged or improperly operating equipment that could be hazardous to the patient undergoing MR imaging.

In some types of cochlear implants, a relatively high-field-strength cobalt-samarium magnet is used in conjunction with an external magnet to align and retain a radio-frequency transmitter coil on the patient's head, while other types of cochlear implants are electronically activated (2,3). Consequently, MR imaging is strictly contraindicated in patients with these implants because of the probability of injuring the patient or altering the operation of the cochlear implant.

Since there is a potential to demagnetize and/or move implants that involve magnets (e.g., dental implants, magnetic sphincters, magnetic stoma plugs, magnetic ocular implants, tissue expanders with magnetic ports, magnetic prosthetic appliances, etc.), these implants should be removed from the patient before MR imaging, if possible. Otherwise, MR imaging in patients with magnetically activated implants should be performed only in light of the relative risks involved (14,15). The fact that a patient has previously undergone MR imaging safely does not preclude the possibility of injury by a different type of MR system. It is the responsibility of the clinician to determine whether MR imaging is critical in the management of an individual patient and to assess the potential benefits versus the potential risks of MR imaging in these cases.

A patient with any other similar electrically, magnetically, or mechanically activated or electrically conductive device should be excluded from MR imaging unless the particular device has been previously shown to be unaffected by the magnetic and electromagnetic fields used for clinical MR imaging and there is no possibility of injuring the patient.

THE USE OF MR IMAGING IN PREGNANT PATIENTS

The current FDA guideline require labeling of MR systems to indicate that the safety of MR when used to image the fetus and the infant "has not been established" (1). In Great Britain, the acceptable limits of exposure for clinical MR imaging recommended by the National Radiological Protection Board specify that "it might be prudent to exclude pregnant women during the first 3 months of pregnancy"(16).

Although MR imaging is not considered hazardous to the fetus, only a few investigations have examined the teratogenic potential of this imaging modality (17–27). A number of mechanisms exist that could conceivably cause adverse biologic effects with respect to the interaction between the electromagnetic fields used for MR imaging and the developed fetus (28–29). Futhermore, it is well known that cells undergoing division, as in the case of the developing fetus during the first trimester, are more susceptible to damage from a variety of physical agents. Therefore, although no definitive association has been demonstrated between MR imaging and any deleterious effects on the developing fetus, and in view of the currently available limited evidence and experience in this area, a cautious approach to the use of MR imaging during pregnancy is recommended until additional investigations provide more information regarding safely in this patient population.

MR imaging may be used in pregnant women if other nonionizing forms of diagnostic imaging are inadequate or if the examination provides important information that would otherwise require exposure to ionizing radiation (e.g., fluoroscopy, CT, etc.) (3,13). It is recommended that pregnant patients be informed that, to date, there has been no indication that the use of clinical MR imaging during pregnancy has produced deleterious effects. However, as noted by the FDA, the safety of MR imaging during pregnancy has not been proved (1).

It should be noted that there is a high spontaneous abortion rate during the first trimester of pregnancy in the general population (>30%). Therefore, because of the associated potential medicolegal implications related to spontaneous abortions, particular caution should be exercised in the use of MR imaging in patients who are in the first trimester of pregnancy. Patients who are pregnant or suspect that they might be pregnant should be identified before undergoing MR imaging in order to assess the relative risks versus the benefits of the examination.

SCREENING PATIENTS FOR SUSPECTED METALLIC FOREIGN BODIES BEFORE MR IMAGING

Patients may come for MR imaging with a history of metallic foreign bodies such as bullets, shrapnel, or other types of metallic fragments. The relative risk of imaging these patients depends on multiple factors, including the ferromagnetic properties of the object, the geometry and dimensions of the object, the strength with which the object is embedded in the tissue, the strength of the static and gradient magnetic fields of the MR system, and whether the object is in or adjacent to a potentially hazardous site, such as a vital neural, vascular, or soft-tissue structure (3,13,36,37).

A patient who encounters the static and gradient magnetic fields of the MR system with an intraocular ferromagnetic foreign body is at risk for significant eye damage. To our knowledge, the single confirmed case of a patient who experienced an MR imaging-related injury resulting in blindness involved imaging on a 0.35-T MR system. The patient sustained a vitreous hemorrhage due to movement of an intraocular ferromagnetic metal fragment that was 2.0 × 3.5 mm (36). This underscores the importance of adequately screening patients with suspected intraocular ferromagnetic metallic foreign bodies before MR imaging.

A recent study demonstrated that intraocular metallic fragments as small as 0.1 × 0.1 × 0.1 mm were detected with standard plain radiographs (38). In addition, metallic fragments of various sizes and dimensions ranging from 0.1 × 0.1 × 0.1 to 3.0 × 1.0 × 1.0 mm were examined in this study to determine if they were moved or dislodged from the eyes of laboratory animals during exposure to a 2.0-T MR system. Only the 3.0 × 1.0 × 1.0-mm fragment moved (it rotated but did not cause any discernible clinical damage) (38). This report indicated that if a patient with a suspected intraocular ferromagnetic foreign body has no symptoms and a series of plain radiographs of the orbits does not demonstrate a radiopaque foreign body, MR imaging may be performed safely (38). Therefore, the use of plain radiography is considered to be an acceptable technique for identifying or excluding an intraocular metallic foreign body that represents a potential hazard to the patient about to undergo MR imaging.

Each imaging site should develop a standardized policy for screening patients with suspected metallic foreign bodies; the policy should include guidelines as to which patients require radiographic and/or CT examinations and the specific radiographic or CT technique(s) to be used (e.g., number of views, position of the anatomy to be examined, etc). Each case should be considered individually on the basis of the relative risk of imaging this type of patient.

The above precautions should be taken with regard to patients referred for MR imaging in any MR system regardless of the field strength, magnet type, and presence or absence of magnetic shielding.

MR IMAGING OF PATIENTS WITH HALO VESTS OR OTHER SIMILAR EXTERNALLY APPLIED DEVICES

The potential risks and problems associated with MR imaging in patients with metallic implants or when other metallic materials are present are related to movement or dislodgment of the object, induction of electrical current, heating, and the artifacts that either severely distort the image rendering it diagnostically unacceptable or that may be misinterpreted as an abnormality (3,39,40). The use of MR imaging to assess cervical spine trauma in patients who require stabilization of the spine with a halo vest or similar device is usually not possible because most of these devices are composed of metallic materials that may present risks and produce mild to severe artifacts (3,41–43). This is unfortunate because MR imaging frequently provides a useful diagnostic evaluation of the spinal cord and associated soft-tissue structures that is not obtainable with other imaging techniques.

Investigators who evaluated the effect of various halo vests on image quality reported that these devices caused image distortion that depended on the type of material used to construct the halo rings and support uprights. Halo vests made from stainless steel resulted in the poorest image quality, followed by those made from aluminum, titanium, and graphite (41). This study did not directly assess deflection forces, heating, or induced currents, all of which potentially represent hazards to the patient if the halo vest is primarily composed of ferromagnetic and/or conductive materials.

Although some commercially available halo devices are composed of nonferromagnetic materials, there is still the theoretical hazard of inducing electric current in the ring portion of any halo device made from electrically conductive materials according to Faraday's law of electromagnetic induction, which states that a current can be induced in a closed-loop conductor as it moves through a magnetic field (41,42). The current within such a loop is of additional concern because of eddy current induction and potential image degradation effects (44). Furthermore, there is a potential for the patient to be involved in part of this current loop, so that there would be the concern of a possible burn or electrical injury to the patient.

Specially designed, commercially available halo vests have been developed recently that are made from nonferromagnetic and nonconductive materials that have little or no interaction with the electromagnetic fields used for MR imaging (42,43) and are therefore not associated with safety-related problems or imaging artifacts. The advantages of using a nonferromagnetic, nonconductive halo device include (a) no associated deflection forces, (b) little or no heating, (c) no artifacts that distort the imaging area of interest, and (d) no likelihood of induction of current (42). To our knowledge, there have been no reports of injuries associated with MR imaging of patients with halo devices (although one incident of "electrical arcing" without injury was reported in the 1988 SMRI Safety Survey, Phase I Study; Kanal E, personal oral communication, 1988).

Because of the known theoretical hazards associated with MR imaging in patients with halo vests or similar devices, it would be prudent, from both safety and image artifact standpoints, to image only patients with halo vests and similar externally applied devices that are composed of materials that are both nonferromagnetic and nonconductive, especially since these devices are currently available from several commercial manufacturers.

POTENTIAL RISK ASSOCIATED WITH ACOUSTIC NOISE PRODUCED DURING MR IMAGING

Another potential risk of MR imaging is related to acoustic noise produced during operation of the imager. Acoustic noise is associated with the activation and deactivation of electric current within the gradient coils and is enhanced with higher static magnetic field strengths, stronger gradient duty cycles, and faster pulse repetition frequencies (45,46). A recently published report indicated that gradient magnetic field-related noise levels measured on several commercial MR imagers were considered to be within the recommended safety guidelines (46). However, acoustic noise generated during MR imaging has also been demonstrated to cause patient annoyance, interference with oral communication, and reversible hearing loss in patients who do not wear ear protection (3,46–48). Furthermore, the possibility exists that significant gradient coil-induced noise may produce permanent hearing impairment in certain patients who are particularly susceptible to the damaging effects of relatively loud noises (13,49).

The safest and least expensive means of preventing problems associated with acoustic noise during clinical MR imaging is to encourage the routine use of disposable earplugs or similar noise reduction devices (3,13,45). The use of earplugs has been demonstrated to successfully prevent temporary hearing loss that can be associated with clinical MR imaging examinations (47). An acceptable alternative strategy for reducing noise levels during MR imaging is to use an "antinoise" or destructive interference technique that not only effectively reduces noise but also permits better patient communication (13,50). Although these techniques have not been widely applied to clinical MR systems, they have considerable potential for minimizing acoustic noise and its associated problems.

MR IMAGING AND PATIENTS WITH CLAUSTROPHOBIA, ANXIETY, OR EMOTIONAL DISTRESS

Claustrophobia and a variety of other psychological reactions, including anxiety and panic disorders, may occur in patients before or during MR imaging (13,48,51–54). These reactions are due to several factors, including the restrictive dimensions of the interior of the imager, the duration of the examination, the gradient coil-induced noises, and the ambient condition within the imager bore (3,13,48,51–56). Certain MR systems that use a vertical magnetic field offer a more open design that might reduce the frequency of psychological problems associated with MR imaging.

Fortunately, adverse psychological responses to MR imaging are usually transient. However, there has been a report of two patients with no previous history of claustrophobia who tolerated MR imaging with great difficulty and developed persistent claustrophobia that required long-term psychiatric treatment (52). Because adverse psychological responses to MR imaging typically delay or require cancellation of the examination, several techniques have been developed and may be used to avert these problems (13,53–56). These include (a) briefing the patient concerning specific aspects of MR imaging (the level of gradient coil-induced noise to expect, the internal dimensions of the imager, etc.), (b) allowing an appropriately screened relative or friend to remain with the patient during the procedure, (c) maintaining physical or verbal contact with the patient throughout the examination, (d) placing the patient in a prone position to alleviate the "closed-in" feelings and/or introducing the patient feetfirst versus headfirst into the imager, (e) using imager-mounted mirrors or mirror or prism glasses within the imager to allow the patient to see out, (f) using a blindfold so that the patient is not as aware of the close surroundings, (g) using relaxation strategies such as controlled breathing and mental imagery, and (h) using psychological "desensitization" techniques.

The aforementioned procedures used either individually or in combination will have various degrees of success. if all else fails, short-acting sedation or anesthesia may be required to successfully accomplish MR imaging in patients experiencing claustrophobia, anxiety, or emotional distress.

REFERENCES

1. U.S. Food and Drug Administration. Magnetic resonance diagnostic device: panel recommendation and report on petitions for MR reclassification. Federal Register 1988;53:7575–7579.
2. Persson BRR, Stahlberg F. Health and safety of clinical NMR examinations. Boca Raton, Fla; CRC, 1989.
3. Shellock FG. Biological effects and safety aspects of magnetic resonance imaging. Magn Reson Q 1989;5:243–261.
4. Erlebacher JA, Cahill PT, Pannizzo F, Knowles RJR. Effect of magnetic resonance imaging on DDD pacemakers. Am J Cardiol 1986;57:437–440.
5. Fetter J, Abram G, Holmes D, Gray JE, Hayes DL. The effects of nuclear magnetic resonance imager on external and implanted pulse generators. PACE 1984;7:720–727.
6. Hayes DL, Holmes DR, Gray JE. Effect of 1.5 T nuclear magnetic resonance imaging on implanted permanent pacemakers. J Am Coll Cardiol 1987;10:782–786.
7. Holmes D, Hayes D, Gray J, Merideth J. The effects of magnetic resonance imaging on implantable pulse generators. PACE 1986;9:360–370.
8. Zimmerman BH, Faul DD. Artifacts and hazards in NMR imaging due to metal implants and cardiac pacemakers. Diagn Imaging Clin Med 1984;53:53–56.
9. Alagona P Jr, Toole JC, Maniscalco BS, et al. Nuclear magnetic resonance imaging in a patient with a DDD pacemaker (letter). PACE 1989;12:619.
10. A new MRI complication? ECRI Health Devices Alerts, May 27, 1988:1.
11. Kanal E, Shellock FG. Burns associated with clinical MR examinations (letter). Radiology 1990;175:585.
12. Pavlicek W, Geisinger M, Castle L, et al. The effects of magnetic resonance on patients with cardiac pacemakers. Radiology 1983;147:149–153.
13. Kanal E, Shellock FG, Talagala L. Safety considerations in MR imaging. Radiology 1990; 176:593–606.
14. Shellock FG. Ex vivo assessment of deflection forces and artifacts associated with high-field MRI of "mini-magnet" dental prostheses. Magn Reson Imaging 1989; 7(suppl 1):P38.
15. Liang MD, Narayanan K, Kanal E. Magnetic ports in tissue expanders: a caution for MRI. Magn Reson Imaging 1989;7:541–542.
16. National Radiological Protection Board. Revised guidance on acceptable limits of exposure during nuclear magnetic clinical imaging. Br J Radiol 1983;56:974–977.
17. Cooke P, Morris PG. The effects of NMR exposure on living organisms. II. A genetic study of human lymphocytes. Br J Radiol 1981; 54:622–625.
18. Geard CR, Osmak RS, Hall EJ, et al. Magnetic resonance and ionizing radiation: a comparative evaluation in vitro of oncogenic and genotoxic potential. Radiology 1984; 152:199–202.
19. Heinrichs WL, Fong P, Flannery M, et al. Midgestational exposure of pregant balb/c mice to magnetic resonance imaging. Magn Reson Imaging 1988; 6:305–313.
20. Kay HH, Herfkens RJ, Kay BK. Effect of magnetic resonance imaging on *Xenopus laevis* embryogenesis. Magn Reson Imaging 1988; 6:501–506.
21. McRobbie D, Foster MA. Pulsed magnetic field exposure during pregnancy and implications for NMR foetal imaging: a study with mice. Magn Reson Imaging 1985; 3:231–234.
22. Osbakken M, Griffith J, Taczanowsky P. A gross morphologic, histologic, hematologic, and blood chemistry study of adult and neonatal mice chronically exposed to high magnetic fields. Magn Reson Med 1986; 3:502–517.
23. Prasad N, Bushong SC, Thornby JL, Bryan RN, Hazelwood CF, Harrell JE. Effect of nuclear magnetic resonance on chromosomes of mouse bone marrow cells. Magn Reson Imaging 1984; 2:37–39.

24. Prasad N, Wright DA, Forster JD. Effect of nuclear magnetic resonance on early stages of amphibian development. Magn Reson Imaging 1982; 1:35–38.
25. Prasad N, Wright DA, Ford JJ, Thornby JI. Safety of 4–T MR imaging: study of effects on developing frog embryos. Radiology 1990; 174:251–253.
26. Schwartz JL, Crooks LE. NMR imaging produces no observable mutations or cytotoxicity in mammalian cells. AJR 1982; 139:583–585.
27. Wolf S, Crooks LE, Brown P, Howard R, Painter RB. Tests for DNA and chromosomal damage induced by nuclear magnetic resonance imaging. Radiology 1980; 136:707–710.
28. Adey WR. Tissue interactions with nonionizing electromagnetic fields. Physiol Rev 1981; 61:435–514.
29. Barnothy M. Biological effects of magnetic fields. New York: Plenum, 1969.
30. Gordon CJ. Biological effects of radiofrequency radiation. EPA–600/8–83–026A. Washington, DC: Environmental Protection Agency, 1984; 4–1 4–28.
31. Michaelson SM, Lin JV. Biological effects and health implications of radiofrequency radiation. New York: Plenum, 1987.
32. Biological effects and exposure criteria for radiofrequency electromagnetic fields. NCRP report no. 86. Bethesda, Md: National Council for Radiation Protection and Measurements, 1986.
33. O'Conner ME. Mammalian teratogenesis and radio-frequency fields. Proc IEEE 1980; 68:56–60.
34. Sheppard AR, Eisenbud M. Biological effects of electric and magnetic fields of extremely low frequency. New York: New York University Press, 1977.
35. Tofani S, Agnesod G, Ossola P. Effects of low-level exposure to radiofrequency radiation on intrauterine development in rats. Health Phys 1986; 51:489–499.
36. Kelly WM, Pagie PG, Pearson A, San Diego AG, Solomon MA. Ferromagnetism of intraocular foreign body causes unilteral blindness after MR study. AJNR 1986; 7:243–245.
37. Teitelbaum GP, Yee CA, Van Horn DD, Kim HS, Colletti PM. Metallic ballistic fragments: MR imaging safety and artifacts. Radiology 1990; 175:855–859.
38. Williams S, Char DH, Dillon WP, Lincoff N, Moseley M. Ferrous intraocular foreign bodies and magnetic resonance imaging. Am J Ophthalmol 1988; 105:398–401.
39. Pusey E, Lufkin RB, Brown RKJ, et al. Magnetic resonance imaging artifacts: mechanisms and clinical significance. RadioGraphics 1986; 6:891–911.
40. Shellock FG. MR imaging of metallic implants and materials: a compilation of the literature. AJR 1988; 151:811–814.
41. Ballock RT, Hajek PC, Byrne TP, Garfin SR. The quality of magnetic resonance imaging, as affected by the composition of the halo orthosis. J Bone Joint Surg (Am) 1989; 71:431–434.
42. Shellock FG, Slimp G. MRI-compatible halo vest for cervical spine fixation. AJR 1990; 154:631–632.
43. Clayman DA, Murakami ME, Vines FS. Compatibility of cervical spine braces with MR imaging: a study of nine nonferrous devices. AJNR 1990; 11:385–390.
44. Malko JA, Hoffman JC, Jarrett PJ. Eddy-current-induced artifacts caused by an MR-compatible halo device. Radiology 1989; 173:563–564.
45. Gangarosa RE, Minnis JE, Nobbe J, Praschan D, Genberg RW. Operational safety issues in MRI. Magn Reson Imaging 1987; 5:287–292.
46. Hurwitz R, Lane SR, Bell RA, Brandt-Zawadzki MN. Acoustic analysis of gradient-coil noise in MR imaging. Radiology 1989; 173:545–548.
47. Brummet RE, Talbot JM, Charuhas P. Potential hearing loss resulting from MR imaging. Radiology 1988; 169:539–540.
48. Quirk ME, Letendre AJ, Clottone RA, Lingley JF. Anxiety in patients undergoing MR imaging. Radiology 1989; 170:463–466.
49. Kanal E, Shellock FG, Sonnenblick D. MRI clinical site safety survey: phase I results and preliminary data (abstr). Magn Reson Imaging 1988; 7(suppl 1):106.
50. Goldman AM, Grossman WE, Friedlander PC. Reduction of sound levels with antinoise in MR imaging. Radiology 1989;173:549–550.
51. Flaherty JA, Hoskinson K. Emotional distress during magnetic resonance imaging. N Engl J Med 1989; 320:467–468.
52. Fishbain DA, Goldberg M, Labbe E, Zacher D, Steele-Rosomoff R, Rosomoff H. Long-term claustrophobia following magnetic resonance imaging. Am J Psychiatry 1988; 145:1038–1039.
53. Klonoff EA, Janata JW, Kaufman B. The use of systematic desensitization to overcome resistance to magnetic resonance imaging (MRI) scanning. J Behav Ther Exp Psychiatry 1986; 17:189–192.

54. Weinreb J, Maravilla KR, Peshock R, Payne J. Magnetic resonance imaging: improving patient tolerance and safety. AJR 1984; 143:1285–1287.
55. Hricak H, Amparo EG. Body MRI: alleviation of claustrophobia by prone positioning. Radiology 1984; 152:819.
56. Quirk ME, Letendre AJ, Clottone RA, Lingley JF. Evaluation of three psychological interventions to reduce anxiety during MR imaging. Radiology 1989; 173:759–762.

PART II[1]

This is the second of a series of such policy statements developed by the SMRI Safety Committee (1). In the future, additional policies, guidelines, and recommendations will be developed on other topics related to MR imaging safety and patient management. Furthermore, the existing policies, guidelines, or recommendations will be revised as new information becomes available on the individual topics.

Index terms: Biological effects; Patient monitoring; Quality assurance; Safety.

PATIENT MONITORING DURING MR EXAMINATIONS

It is good practice for all patients undergoing MR examinations to be visually and/or verbally monitored (2–24). All patients who are sedated, anesthetized, or, for whatever reason, unable to communicate readily with the imager operator and/or accompanying personnel should be physiologically monitored by appropriate means. The specific type(s) of monitoring should be determined by the site. Suggestions include physiologic monitoring of respiration, heart rate, blood pressure, and/or electrocardiographic output, as clinically indicated.

If this monitoring is to be achieved by electrical and/or mechanical devices, it is important that MR compatibility (patient safety and performance of the device and the MR system)[2] be demonstrated by prior testing, manufacturer declaration, and/or clearance by a recognized authorizing body such as the Food and Drug Administration[3] (25).

---

[1]JMRI 1992: 2:247–248.

[2]There exists a small but finite chance that use of monitoring devices during MR examinations can result in adverse reactions such as burns, even though MR compatibility has been demonstrated. This risk can be decreased by following the manufacturer's installation and operating instructions.

[3]For a manufacturer to market a device as "MR compatibile" in the United States, the FDA has stated that the device should have undergone the scrutiny of a premarket notification (510[k]). To determine that a 510(k) has been cleared, the user can request a copy of the clearance letter from the manufacturer. Such information can also be obtained from the Freedom of Information Office Center for Devices and Radiological Health, FDA.

REFERENCES

1. Shellock FG, Kanal E, SMRI Safety Committee. Policies, guidelines, and recommendations for MR imaging safety and patient management. JMRI 1991;1:97–101.
2. Barnett GH, Ropper AH, Johnson KA. Physiological support and monitoring of critically ill patients during magnetic resonance imaging. J Neurosurg 1988;68:246–250.
3. Dimick RN, Hedlund LW, Herfkens RF, Fram EK, Utz J. Optimizing electrocardiographic electrode placement for cardiac-gated magnetic resonance imaging. Invest Radiol 1987;22:17–22.
4. ECRI. A new MRI complication? Health Devices Alert 1988;May 27:1.
5. ECRI. Thermal injuries and patient monitoring during MRI studies. Health Devices Alert 1991;20:362–363.
6. Edelman R, Shellock FG, Ahladis J. Practical MRI for the technologist and imaging specialist. In: Edelman R, Hesselink J, eds. Magnetic resonance clinical applications/advanced techniques. Philadelphia: Saunders Co., 1990;39–73.
7. Legrendre JP, Misner R, Frester GV, Geoffrion Y. A simple fiber-optic monitor of cardiac and respiratory activity for biomedical magnetic resonance applications. Magn Reson Med 1986;3:953–957.
8. Kanal E, Shellock FG. Burns associated with clinical MR examinations (letter). Radiology 1990;175:585.
9. Karlik SJ, Heatherley T, Pavan F, et al. Patient anesthesia and monitoring at a 1.5 T MRI Installation. Magn Reson Med 1988;7:210–221.
10. McArdle CB, Nicholas DA, Richardson CJ, Amparo EG. Monitoring of the neonate undergoing MR imaging: technical considerations. Radiology 1986;159:223–226.
11. Rejger VS, Cohn BF, Vielvoye GJ, de-Raadt FB. A simple anesthetic and monitoring system for magnetic resonance imaging. Eur J Anesthesiol 1989;6:373–378.
12. Roos CF, Carol FE. Fiber-optic pressure transducer for use near MR magnetic fields. Radiology 1985;156:548.
13. Roth JL, Nugent M, Gray JE, et al. Patient monitoring during magnetic resonance imaging. Anesthesiology 1985;62:80–83.
14. Selden H, De Chateau P, Ekman G, Linder B, Saaf J, Wahlund LO. Circulatory monitoring of children during anesthesia in low-field magnetic resonance imaging. Acta Anesthesiol Scand 1990;34:41–43.
15. Shellock FG. Monitoring sedated patients during MR imaging (letter). Radiology 1990;177:586.
16. Shellock FG. Monitoring during MRI: an evaluation of the effect of high-field MRI on various patient monitors. Med Electronics 1986;September:93–97.
17. Shellock FG. Monitoring vital signs in conscious and sedated patients during magnetic resonance imaging: experience with commercially available equipment (abstr). In: Book of abstracts: Society of Magnetic Resonance in Medicine 1986, Berkeley, Calif: Society of Magnetic Resonance in Medicine, 1986;1030–1031.
18. Shellock FG. Biological effects and safety aspects of MRI. In: Stark DD, Bradley WG, eds. Magnetic resonance imaging: a comprehensive text. 2nd ed. St Louis: Mosby, 1992;522–545.
19. Shellock FG, Schaefer DJ, Crues JV. Evaluation of skin blood flow, body and skin temperatures in man during MR imaging at high levels of RF energy (abstr). Magn Reson Imaging 1989;7(suppl 1):335.
20. Shellock FG. MRI-compatible monitoring systems (abstr). In: Bioelectromagnetics Society, 12th Annual Meeting abstracts. Gaithersburg, Md: Bioelectromagnetics Society, 1990;44.
21. Shellock FG, Kimble K, Myers S. Monitoring heart rate and oxygen saturation during MRI with a fiber-optic pulse oximeter. AJR (in press).
22. Shellock FG, Slimp G. Severe burn of the finger caused by using a pulse oximeter during MRI (letter). AJR 1989;153:1105.
23. Wendt RE, Rokey R, Vick GW, Johnston DL. Electrocardiographic gating and monitoring during NMR imaging. Magn Reson Imaging 1988;6:8995.
24. Wickersheim KA, Sun MH. Fluoroptic thermometry. Med Electronics 1987;February:84–91.

PART III SCREENING PATIENTS BEFORE MR PROCEDURES[1]

Frank G. Shellock, Ph.D[2], Emanuel Kanal, M.D.[2] and SMRI Safety Committee[3]

This is the third of a series of such policy statements developed by the Safety Committee of the SMRI (1,2). In the future, additional guidelines and recommendations will be developed on other topics related to biologic effects and the safety and management of patients undergoing MR procedures. Furthermore, the existing guidelines and recommendations will be revised as new information becomes available on the individual topics.

Index terms: Biological effects; Patient monitoring; Quality assurance; Safety.

SCREENING PATIENTS BEFORE MR PROCEDURES

All individuals, including patients, volunteer subjects, family members, and visitors must be thoroughly screened by qualified personnel before being exposed to the static, gradient, or radio-frequency electromagnetic fields of the MR system. Conducting a careful screening procedure is crucial to ensure the safety of everyone entering the area containing the MR system.

An important component of the screening process involves completion of a

---

[1]From Tower Imaging, Ste 106, 444 S San Vicente Blvd, Los Angeles, CA 90048 (F.G.S.); the Department of Radiological Sciences, UCLA School of Medicine, Los Angeles, CA (F.G.S.); the Department of Imaging, St John's Hospital and Health Center, Santa Monica, CA (F.G.S.); and the University of Pittsburgh and the Pittsburgh NMR Institute, Pittsburgh, PA (E.K.). Received September 20, 1993; accepted March 17, 1994. Address reprint requests to F.G.S.

[2]Co-Chairmen of the SMRI Safety Committee.

[3]G. Jerome Beers, MD, Shields Health Care Group, Inc, Brockton, Mass; Michael J. Bronskill, PhD, Sunnybrook Health Science Center, Ontario; D. Lawrence Burk, Jr. MD, Duke University Medical Center, Durham, NC; Dick J. Drost, PhD, St Joseph's Health Center of London, Ontario; J.M.L. Engels, MD, Philips Medical Systems, Best, The Netherlands; Joel Felmlee, PhD, Mayo Clinic, Rochester, Minn; Lawrence Gifford, MD, Berlex Laboratories, Wayne, NJ; Steven E. Harms, MD, Baylor University Medical Center, Dallas, Tex; Elaine Keeler, PhD, Picker International, Highland Heights, Ohio; Richard Magin, PhD, University of Illinois, Urbana, Ill; William Maloney, U.S. Food and Drug Administration, Rockville, Md; William Pavlicek, PhD, Mayo Clinic, Scottsdale, Ariz; J. Thomas Payne, PhD, Abbott Northwestern Hospital, Minneapolis, Minn; James Rogers, Hitachi Medical Systems of America, Twinsburg, Ohio; Allen Ruszkowski, Resonex, Sunnyvale, Calif; Richard Sano, Philips Medical Systems, Shelton, Conn, National Electrical Manufacturers Association (NEMA), Washington, D.C., International Electrotechnical Commission (IEC), Geneva, Switzerland; Daniel J. Schaefer, PhD, GE Medical Systems, Milwaukee, Wis; Reuven Schreiber, MD, Sunnyvale, Calif; Javad Seyedzacieh, Toshiba America Medical Systems, San Francisco, Calif; Ralph Shuping, ScD, U.S. Food and Drug Administration, Rockville, Md; Melinda Vasila, BSRT, Ohio State University Hospitals, Columbus, Ohio; Jeffrey Weinreb, MD, New York University Medical Center, New York, NY.

JMRI 1994;4:749–751.

MR PROCEDURE SCREENING FORM

Date ____________________
Name ____
Sex ________ Age ______ Physician ____________________ Patient No. __________
Date of Birth ______________ Height ____________ Weight ______________
Procedure ______________________________ Outpatient ____Inpatient ______
Diagnosis ____
Clinical History ____

	YES	NO
Have you ever had a surgical procedure or operation of any kind?........................	___	___
If yes, please list all prior surgeries and approximate dates: ______________		
Have you ever been injured by any metallic foreign body (e.g., bullet, BB, shrapnel, etc.)?........................	___	___
Please describe: ______________		
Have you ever had an injury to the eye involving a metallic object (e.g., metallic slivers, shavings, foreign body, etc.)?........................	___	___
Please describe: ______________		
Do you have anemia or diseases that affect your blood?........................	___	___
Do you have a history of renal disease, seizure, asthma, or allergic respiratory disease?........................	___	___
Do you have any drug allergies?........................	___	___
If yes, please list: ______________		
Have you ever had a reaction to a contrast medium used for MRI or CT?.............	___	___
Are you pregnant or do you suspect that you are pregnant?........................	___	___
Are you breast feeding?........................	___	___
Last menstrual period: ______________ Post-menopausal?...........	___	___
Are you taking oral contraceptives or receiving hormone treatment?.....................	___	___

PERTINENT PREVIOUS STUDIES:

	BODY PART	DATE
X-rays	______________	_____
Computed tomography	______________	_____
Ultrasound	______________	_____
Nuclear Medicine	______________	_____
MRI	______________	_____

We STRONGLY recommend using the ear plugs or headphones we supply for your MRI examination since some patients may find the noise levels unacceptable and the noise levels may temporarily affect your hearing.

Continued on other side.

Page 1

FIG. 1A. The screening form (front).

THE FOLLOWING ITEMS MAY BE HAZARDOUS OR MAY INTERFERE WITH THE MRI EXAMINATION BY PRODUCING AN ARTIFACT.

PLEASE INDICATE IF YOU HAVE ANY OF THE FOLLOWING:

Please mark on this drawing the location of any metal inside your body.

Right

Left

YES	NO	
___	___	Cardiac pacemaker
___	___	Aneurysm clip(s)
___	___	Implanted cardiac defibrillator
___	___	Neurostimulator
___	___	Any type of biostimulator
		Type: ___________________
		Any type of internal electrode(s), including:
___	___	Pacing wires
___	___	Cochlear implant
___	___	Other: ___________________
___	___	Implanted insulin pump
___	___	Swan-Ganz catheter
___	___	Halo vest or metallic cervical fixation device
___	___	Any type of electronic, mechanical, or magnetic implant
		Type: ___________________
___	___	Hearing aid
___	___	Any type of intravascular coil, filter, or stent (e.g., Gianturco coil,Gunther IVC filter, Palmaz stent, etc.)
___	___	Implanted drug infusion device
___	___	Any type of foreign body, shrapnel, or bullet
___	___	Heart valve prosthesis
___	___	Any type of ear implant
___	___	Penile prosthesis
___	___	Orbital/eye prosthesis
___	___	Any type of implant held in place by a magnet
___	___	Any type of surgical clip or staple(s)
___	___	Vascular access port
___	___	Intraventricular shunt
___	___	Artificial limb or joint
___	___	Dentures
___	___	Diaphragm
___	___	IUD
___	___	Pessary
___	___	Wire mesh
___	___	Any implanted orthopedic item(s) (i.e., pins, rods, screws, nails, clips, plates, wire, etc.)
		Type: ___________________
___	___	Any other implanted item
		Type: ___________________
___	___	Tattooed eyeliner*

* A SMALL PERCENTAGE OF PATIENTS WITH TATTOOED EYELINER HAVE EXPERIENCED TRANSIENT SKIN IRRITATION IN ASSOCIATION WITH MRI. THEREFORE, YOU MUST DECIDE IF THIS SLIGHT RISK WARRANTS UNDERGOING YOUR EXAMINATION. YOU MAY WANT TO DISCUSS THIS MATTER WITH YOUR REFERRING PHYSICIAN.

I attest that the above information is correct to the best of my knowledge. I have read and understand the entire contents of this form and I have had the opportunity to ask questions regarding the information on this form.

Patient's signature ______________________________

MD / RN / RT signature ______________________________ Date __________

Print MD / RN / RT name ______________________________

page 2

FIG. 1B. The screening form (back).

questionnaire designed primarily to determine if there is any reason an individual may experience an adverse reaction to the electromagnetic fields used for MR procedures. In consideration of this, the Safety Committee of the SMRI developed a standardized screening form for use in the clinical MR setting (Fig. 1).

This questionnaire includes queries concerning previous surgery (which are important for determining the presence of any metallic object) and previous injury from a metallic foreign body (especially with regard to an eye injury), and asks whether the individual is pregnant (1,2).

Questions are posed to determine if the patient has any underlying conditions that may affect the decision to use contrast media. Also, there are questions related to the phase of the menstrual cycle and the use of oral contraceptives and/or hormone treatment that are relevant to patients undergoing MR studies for suspected gynecologic abnormalities.

The screening questionnaire helps determine if the individual has any of the various implants, materials, and devices that are contraindications for the MR procedure (3,4). This includes any object that is electrically, magnetically, or mechanically activated (3). Other items are included on the questionnaire to help the clinician determine if a metallic object is present that may produce an artifact that can either interfere with the MR imaging examination or be misinterpreted as an abnormal finding (5,6). A diagram of the human body is provided on the questionnaire so that the individual being screened can indicate the location of any object that may be potentially hazardous or interfere with the MR procedure.

This questionnaire also asks if the patient has tattooed eyeliner, because of the associated imaging artifacts and, more important, because a small number of patients with tattooed eyeliner have experienced transient skin irritation or cutaneous swelling associated with MR procedures (7,8). Apparently, certain ferrous pigments used in the tattooing process can interact with the electromagnetic fields used for MR procedures, resulting in these minor-to-moderate problems (7,8). Therefore, it is necessary to inform individuals with tattooed eyeliner about these possible hazards so that they can decide if the risk versus benefit of undergoing an MR procedure is acceptable to them and/or their referring physicians.

Any individual undergoing an MR procedure must remove all metallic personal belongings and devices (i.e., analog watches, jewelry, etc.) and clothing items with metallic fasteners, loose metallic components, or metallic threads. The easiest means of accomplishing the above is to require that the individual wear a patient gown during the MR procedure.

REFERENCES

1. Shellock FG, Kanal E. Policies, guidelines, and recommendations for MR imaging safety and patient management. *J Magn Reson Imaging* 1991;1:97–101.

2. Kanal E, Shellock FG. Policies, guidelines, and recommendations for MR imaging safety and patient management. *J Magn Reson Imaging* 1992;2:247–248.
3. Shellock FG, Kanal E. *Magnetic resonance: bioeffects, safety, and patient management.* New York, NY: Raven, 1994.
4. Shellock FG, Morisoli S, Kanal E. MR procedures and biomedical implants, materials, and devices: 1993 update. *Radiology* 1993;189:587–599.
5. Bellon EM, Haacke EM, Coleman PE, Sacco DC, Steiger DA, Gangarosa RE. MR artifacts: a review. *Magn Reson Imaging* 1984;2:41–52.
6. Pusey E, Lufkin RB, Brown RKJ, et al. Magnetic resonance imaging artifacts: mechanisms and clinical significance. *RadioGraphics* 1986;6:891–911.
7. Jackson JG, Acker JD. Permanent eyeliner and MR imaging (letter). *AJR Am J Roentgenol* 1987;49:1080.
8. Lund G, Nelson JD, Wirtschafter JD, Williams PA. Tatooing of eyelids: magnetic resonance imaging artifacts. *Ophthalmol Surg* 1986;17:550–553.

Appendix IV

SUMMARY OF MAGNETIC RESONANCE BIOEFFECTS RESEARCH

Study description	Results	Reference
1.5 T —simulated imaging conditions —human subjects —studied RF power levels equivalent to an SAR of 3 W/kg for 20 min	"Examinations on patients without thermoregulatory impairment can be carried out safely up to at least this SAR level (3 W/kg)".	Abart et al. (1)
—mathematic modeling of thermoregulatory responses	"Assuming a criterion elevation in deep body temperature of 0.6 degrees C, Ta = 20 degrees C and v = 0.8 m/sec, a 70 kg patient could undergo an NMR exposure of infinite duration at SAR $\leq$ 5 W/kg".	Adair et al. (2)
—mathematic modeling of thermoregulatory responses with an emphasis on cardiovascular impairment	"Under conditions that are desirable in the clinic (Ta = 20 degrees C, 50% RH, still air), moderate restrictions (up to 67%) of SkBF yield tolerable increases in core temperature (TCO $\leq$ 1 degree C) during NMR exposures (SAR $\leq$ 4 W/kg of 40 min or less".	Adair et al. (3)
2.0 T —clinical imaging conditions —rats studied effect of MRI on blood-brain barrier permeability	"no MRI-induced difference was detected"	Adzamil et al. (4)

APPENDIX IV. *Continued.*

Study description	Results	Reference
—mathematic modeling of thermoregulatory responses	"The model suggests that current practices in MR imaging will not cause a temperature rise in the center of small unperfused regions such as the eye of more than 1 degrees C".	Athey (5)
1.5 T —exposure to RF radiation in excess of clinical imaging conditions —sheep —studied RF radiation induced heating	"For exposure periods in excess of standard clinical imaging protocols the temperature increase was insufficient to cause adverse thermal effects."	Barber et al. (6)
0.5 and 1.5 T —clinical imaging conditions —human subjects —studied effect of MRI on the EEG and evaluated neuropsychological status	"no measurable influence of MRI on cognitive functions"	Bartels et al. (7)
0.04 T —clinical imaging conditions —human subjects —studied effects of MRI on cognition	"MRI did not cause any cognitive deterioration"	Besson et al. (8)
1.6 T —quenched magnet —pig —studied effect of quenching a magnet	"our findings, which in the circumstances of this experiment, suggested that the risks are small"	Bore et al. (9)
MRI gradient induced electric fields —dogs —studied bioeffects at high MRI gradient-induced fields	"as the strength of MRI gradient-induced fields increases, biological effects in order of increasing field and severity include stimulation of peripheral nerves, nerves of respiration and finally, the heart"	Bourland et al. (10)
1.5 T —clinical imaging conditions —human subjects —studied memory loss	"No gross or subtle memory changes could be attributed to MR imaging, because control groups showed similar patterns of memory loss."	Brockway and Beam (11)
0.38 T —static magnetic field only —deoxygenated erythrocytes —studied orientation of sickle erythrocytes	"further studies are needed to assess possible hazards of MRI of sickle cell disease"	Brody et al. (12)

APPENDIX IV. *Continued.*

Study description	Results	Reference
0.35 and 1.5 T —clinical imaging conditions —human subjects with sickle cell disease —studied effects of MRI on patients with sickle cell disease	"no change in sickle cell blood flow during MR imaging in vivo"	Brody et al. (13)
0.35 T —clinical imaging conditions —human subjects —studied effects of noise during MRI on hearing	"noise generated by MR imaging may cause temporary hearing loss, and earplugs can prevent this"	Brummet et al. (14)
—varying gradient fields —humans —studied neural stimulation threshold with varying oscillations and gradient field strength	"the threshold decreases with the number of oscillations and increases with frequency. The repeatable threshold of 63 T/s (1270 Hz) remains constant from 32 oscillations (25.6 ms) to 128 oscillations (102.4 ms)"	Budinger et al. (15)
60 T/s for 1.2-kHz sinusoids	"Assuming a 0.03-m radius current loop in the heart, 1,600 T/s corresponds to an induced electric field of 24 V/m. This field is approximately four times greater than that expected to cause perceptible sensation in the human torso".	Budinger et al. (16)
0.15 T —stimulated imaging conditions —HL60 promyelocytic cells —studied effect of MRI of Ca^{++}	"results demonstrate that time-varying magnetic fields associated with MRI procedures increase Ca^{++}"	Carson et al. (17)
—gradient magnetic fields up to 66 T/s in dogs and 61 T/s in humans —dogs —human subjects studied physiologic responses to large amplitude time-varying magnetic fields	dogs—"no motion, twitch, or ECG abnormalities" humans—"brief minimal muscular twitches observed on various parts of the body due to magnetic stimulation"	Cohen et al. (18)
0.5 and 1.0 T —simulated imaging conditions —cultured human blood cells —studied effect of static magnetic fields and line scan imaging on human blood cells	"neither treatment had any significant effect on any of the parameters measured"	Cooke and Morris (19)

APPENDIX IV. *Continued.*

Study description	Results	Reference
4.7 T —exposures to static and RF electromagnetic fields only —isolated rabbit hearts —studied effects on cardiac excitability and vulnerability	no measurable effect on strength interval relationship or ventricular vulnerability	Doherty et al. (20)
—gradient magnetic fields only —sinusoidal gradients at a frequency of 1.25 kHz with amplitudes up to 40 mT/min for a z coil and 25 mT/min for an x coil —human subjects studied physiologic effects, physiologic responses	observed peripheral muscle stimulation, no extrasystoles or arrhythmias	Fischer (21)
0.3, 0.5, 1.5 T —stimulated imaging conditions and static/RF and gradient fields separately —rats —studied blood-brain barrier permeability	"increased brain mannitol associated with gradient fluid flux may reflect increased blood-brain barrier permeability or blood volume in brain"	Garber et al. (22)
2.2 to 2.7 T —simulated imaging conditions —mouse cells —studied oncogenic and genotoxic effects of MRI	"data clearly mitigate against an association between exposure to MR imaging modalities and both carcinogenic and genotoxic effects"	Geard et al. (23)
60 T/s —gradient magnetic fields only —human subjects —studied effects of gradient magnetic fields on cardiac and respiratory function	"no changes were observed"	Gore et al. (24)
—mathematic modeling of rates of RF energy absorption	"fair to good agreement was found between SAR and those predicted by simple phenomenological models"	Grandolfo et al. (25)
0.1 to 1.5 T —static magnetic field only —human subjects —studied effects of static magnetic fields on temperature	temperatures increased or decreased depending on field strength of magnet	Gremmel et al. (26)

APPENDIX IV. *Continued.*

Study description	Results	Reference
2.11 T —static magnetic field only —isolated rat hearts —studied effect of static magnetic field on cardiac muscle contraction	"static magnetic fields used in NMR imaging do not constitute any hazard in terms of cardiac contractility"	Gulch and Lutz (27)
2.0 T —RF at 90 MHz —simulated imaging conditions —phantom —Caphuchin monkey —studied temperature changes in phantom and monkey brain during high RF power exposures	"blood flowing through the brain used the body as a heat sink"	Hammer et al. (28)
0.35 T —simulated imaging conditions —mice —studied teratogenic effects of MRI	"prolonged midgestional exposure failed to reveal any overt embryotoxicity or teratogenicity" "slight but significant reduction in fetal crown-rump length after prolonged exposure justifies further study of higher MRI energy levels"	Heinrichs et al. (29)
1.5 T —static magnetic field only —human subjects —studied effect of static magnetic field on somato-sensory evoked potentials	"short-term exposure to 1.5 T static magnetic field does not effect SEPs in human subjects"	Hong and Shellock (30)
0.15 T —simulated imaging conditions —rats —studied effects on cognitive processes	"MRI procedure has no significant effect on spatial memory processes in rats"	Innis et al. (31)
2.0 T —static magnetic field only —human subjects —studied effect of static magnetic field on cardiac rhythm	cardiac cycle length was significantly increased but this is probably harmless in normal subjects, safety in dysrrhythmic patients remains to be determined	Jehenson et al. (32)

APPENDIX IV. *Continued.*

Study description	Results	Reference
—survey of thermal injuries/ incidents related to MR procedures	"The increasing incidence of such clinical MR-related reports of patient burns in conjunction with the ever-increasing number of MR sites, examinations, and applications (e.g., MRA) strongly indicate the need for increased physician awareness and education concerning this rare, but real, MR-related potential hazard"	Kanal et al. (33)
1.5 T —simulated imaging conditions —frog embryo —studied effect of MRI on embryogenesis	"no adverse effects of MRI components on development of this vertebrate (Xenopus laevis)"	Kay et al. (34)
2.3, 4.7, & 10 T —static magnetic fields only —physiologic solutions (2.3 & 4.7 T) and mathematic modeling (10 T) —studied hydrostatic pressure and electrical potentials across vessels in presence of static magnetic fields	"A 10-T magnetic field changes vascular pressure in a model of the human vasculature by less than 0.2%"	Keltner et al. (35)
1.5 T —clinical imaging conditions —human subjects —studied physiologic changes during high field strength MRI	"temperature changes and other physiologic changes were small and of no clinical concern"	Kido et al. (36)
1.5 T —simulated imaging conditions —rats —studied effects of MRI on receptor-mediated activation of pineal gland indole biosynthesis	"strong magnetic fields and/or radiofrequency pulsing used in MRI inhibited beta-adrenergic activation of the gland"	LaPorte et al. (37)
1.0 and 1.5 T —clinical imaging conditions —human subjects —studied acoustic noise	". . . many sequences produce noise levels above the safe levels defined by Department of Health and the Health and Safety Executive."	McJury (38)

APPENDIX IV. *Continued.*

Study description	Results	Reference
1.5 T —clinical imaging conditions —human subjects —studied acoustic noise	". . . for certain protocols, the exposure to acoustic noise falls outside safety guidelines unless ear protection is used."	McJury et al. (39)
3.5 to 12 kT/s —gradient magnetic fields only —mice —studied effect of gradient magnetic fields on pregnancy and post-natal development	"no significant difference between the litter numbers and growth rates of the exposed litters compared with controls"	McRobbie and Foster (40)
—various strong magnetic field —gradient magnetic fields only anesthetized rats —studied cardiac response to gradient magnetic fields	"the types of pulsed magnetic magnetic fields used in the present study did not affect the cardiac cycle of anesthetized rats"	McRobbie and Foster (41)
1.89 T —simulated imaging sequence —rats —studied taste aversion in rats to evaluate possible toxic effects of MRI	"rats exposed to MRI did not display any aversion to the saccharin solution"	Messmer et al. (42)
1.89 T —simulated imaging sequence —mouse spleen cells —studied possible interaction between ionizing radiation and MRI on damage to normal tissue	"for the normal tissues studied, MR imaging neither increases radiation damage nor inhibits repair"	Montour et al. (43)
0 to 2.0 T —clinical imaging conditions —human subjects —studied the extent of changes of the brainstem evoked potentials with MRI	"routine MRI examinations do not produce pathological changes in auditory evoked potentials"	Muller et al. (44)
1.5 T —simulated imaging condition —in vitro —studied the amalgam-related mercury release for typical MRI conditions	"in vitro study demonstrated no evidence of an elevated mercury dissolution . . ."	Muller-Miny et al. (45)

APPENDIX IV. *Continued.*

Study description	Results	Reference
0.75 T —static magnetic field only —hamster cells —studied effect of static magnetic field on DNA synthesis and survival of mammalian cells irradiated with fast neutrons	"presence of the magnetic field either during or subsequent to fast-neutron irradiation does not effect the neutron-induced radiation damage or its repair"	Ngo et al. (46)
1.5 T —simulated imaging conditions —human subjects —studied effect of MRI on somatosensory and brainstem auditory evoked potentials	"it may be assumed that MRI causes no lasting changes"	Niemann et al. (47)
1.89 T —static magnetic field only —mice —studied effects of long term exposure to a static magnetic field	"no consistent differences found in gross and microscopic morphology, hematocrit and WBCs, plasma creatine phosphokinase, lactic dehydrogenase, cholesterol, triglyceride, or protein concentrations in magnet groups compared to two control groups"	Osbakken et al. (48)
0.15 T —simulated imaging conditions —rats —studied effects of MRI on behavior of rats	"results fail to provide any evidence for short or long term behavioral changes in animals exposed to MRI"	Ossenkopp et al. (49)
0.15 T —simulated imaging conditions —rats —studied effect of MRI on murine opiate analgesia levels	"NMRI procedure alter both day and night time responses to morphine"	Ossenkopp et al. (50)
1.0 T —static magnetic field only —mice —studied effect of static magnetic field on in vivo bone growth	"results suggest that exposure to intense magnetic fields does not alter physiological mechanisms of bone mineralization"	Papatheofanis and Papathefanis (51)

APPENDIX IV. *Continued.*

Study description	Results	Reference
2.35 T —static and gradient magnetic fields only —nematodes —studied toxic effects of static and gradient magnetic fields	"static magnetic fields have no effect on fitness of test animals" "time-varying magnetic fields cause inhibition of growth and maturation" "combination of pulsed magnetic field gradients in a static uniform magnetic field also has a detrimental effect on the fitness of the test animals"	Peeling et al. (52)
0.7 T —simulated imaging conditions —frog spermatazoa, fertilized eggs, and embryos, —studied effects of MRI on development	"NMR exposure, at the dose used does not cause detectable adverse effects in this amphibian"	Prasad et al. (53)
0.7 T —simulated imaging conditions —mouse bone marrow cells —studied the cytogenic effects of MRI	"NMR exposure causes no adverse cytogenic effects"	Prasad et al. (54)
2.35 T —simulated imaging conditions —mice —studied the effect of MRI on tumor development	"immune response may be enhanced following MRI exposure, as indicated by the longer latency and smaller sizes of tumors in animals receiving MRI exposure"	Prasad et al. (55)
4.5 T —simulated imaging conditions —mice —studied the effects of high field strength MR imaging on mouse testes epididymes	"little, if any, damage to male reproductive tissues from . . . high intensity MRI exposure"	Prasad et al. (56)
2.35 T —simulated imaging conditions —human peripheral blood mononuclear cells (PBMC) —studied effect of MRI on natural killer cell toxicity of PBMC with and without interleukin-2	"in neither case was cytotoxicity affected by prior exposure to MR imaging"	Prasad et al. (57)

APPENDIX IV. *Continued.*

Study description	Results	Reference
0.15 T —simulated imaging conditions —mice —studied effects of MRI on immune system	"MR exposure has no adverse effect on the immune system, as evidenced by natural killer cell activity"	Prasad et al. (58)
0.15 and 4.0 T —simulated imaging conditions —fertilized frog eggs studied effect of MRI on developing embryos	"no adverse effect early development"	Prasad et al. (59)
0.15 T —exposed separately to static, gradient and RF electromagnetic fields —mice —studied separate effects of static, gradient and RF electromagnetic fields on morphine induced analgesia in mice	"time-varying, and to a lesser extent the RF, fields associated with the MRI procedure inhibit morphine-induced analgesia in mice"	Prato et al. (60)
4.7 T —clinical imaging conditions —human subjects —studied bioeffects of 4.7 T scanner	"mild vertigo" "headaches, nausea" "magnetophosphenes" "metallic taste in mouth"	Redington et al. (61)
0.04 T —clinical imaging conditions —human subjects —follow-up study	"average follow-up time was 6 months . . . none of the 35 deaths recorded was unexpected" "using the magnetic field and radiofrequency levels currently in operation . . . we believe NMRI to be a safe, non-invasive method of whole-body imaging	Reid et al. (62)
1.5 T —simulated imaging conditions —fetal mice —studied combined effect of exposure to gadopentetate dimeglumine and MR imaging on the developing embryo	". . . MR exposure with and without gadopentetate dimeglumine had no adverse effect on the end points analyzed."	Rofsky et al. (63)

APPENDIX IV. *Continued.*

Study description	Results	Reference
4.0 T —RF at 8 MHz to 170 MHz —no gradient magnetic fields —human subjects —studied response of human auditory system to RF-pulses	"in accordance with the used RF modulation envelope three distinct chirps per sequence could be resolved" "RF induced auditory noise is usually completely masked by noise from simultaneously switched gradient fields"	Roschmann et al. (64)
2.7 T —simulated imaging conditions —rats —studied effects of MRI on ocular tissues	"there were no discernible effects on the rat eye"	Sacks et al. (65)
1.5 T —clinical imaging conditions —human subjects —studied effect of electromagnetic fields on melatonin levels	"MR imaging at high field strengths . . . did not suppress melatonin levels in human subjects."	Schiffman et al. (66)
0.35 T —simulated imaging conditions —hamster ovary cells —studied effects of MRI on observable mutations and cytotoxicity	"NMR imaging caused no detectable genetic damage and does not affect cell viability"	Schwartz and Crooks (67)
1.5 T —static magnetic field only —human subjects —studied effect of static magnetic field on body temperature	"no effect on body temperature of normal human subjects"	Shellock et al. (68)
1.5 T —clinical imaging conditions —human subjects —studied thermal effects of MRI of the spine	"no surface "hot spots" "temperature effects were well-below known thresholds for adverse effects"	Shellock et al. (69)
1.5 T —clinical imaging conditions —human subjects —studied possible hypothalamic heating produced by MRI of the head	"there was probably no direct hypothalamic heating produced by clinical MRI of the head"	Shellock et al. (70)

APPENDIX IV. *Continued.*

Study description	Results	Reference
1.5 T —clinical imaging conditions —human subjects —studied effect of MRI on corneal temperatures	"MR imaging . . . causes relatively minor increases in corneal temperature that do not appear to pose any thermal hazard to ocular tissue"	Shellock and Crues (71)
1.5 T —clinical imaging conditions —human subjects —studied temperature, heart rate, and blood pressure changes associated with MRI	"MR imaging . . . not associated with any temperature or hemodynamic related deleterious effects"	Shellock and Crues (72)
1.5 T —clinical imaging conditions —human subjects —studied temperature changes associated with MRI of the brain	"no significant increases in average body temperature" "observed elevations in skin temperatures were physiologically inconsequential"	Shellock and Crues (73)
1.5 T —static magnetic field only —human subjects —studied effects of static magnetic field on body and skin temperatures	"there were no statistically significant changes in body or any of the skin temperatures recorded"	Shellock et al. (74)
1.5 T —clinical imaging conditions —human subjects —studied effect of MRI performed at high SAR levels	"recommended exposure to RF radiation during MR imaging of the body for patients with normal thermoregulatory function may be too conservative"	Shellock et al. (75)
1.5 T —clinical imaging conditions —human subjects —studied effect of MRI on scrotal skin temperature	"absolute temperature is below threshold known to affect testicular function"	Shellock et al. (76)
1.5 T —clinical imaging conditions —phantom —studied acoustic noise	"MR imaging performed with the worst-case pulse sequences did not produce noise levels that exceeded federal guidelines"	Shellock et al. (77)
0.15 T —simulated imaging conditions —anesthetized rats —studied effect of MRI on blood-brain barrier permeability	"these findings raise the possibility that exposure to clinical MRI procedures may also temporarily alter the central blood-brain permeability in human subjects"	Shivers et al. (78)

APPENDIX IV. *Continued.*

Study description	Results	Reference
1.5 T —simulated imaging conditions —anesthetized dogs —studied effect of MRI performed at high SAR levels	"these findings argue for continued caution in the design and operation of imagers capable of high specific absorption rates"	Shuman et al. (79)
0.4 to 8.0 T —static magnetic field only —mice —studied effect of static magnetic field on temperature	"observed a field-induced increase in temperature"	Sperber et al. (80)
0.4 to 1.0 T —static magnetic field only —human subjects —studied the effects of static magnetic fields on tissue perfusion	"neither at the skin of the thumb nor at the forearm were the changes in local blood flow attributable to the magnetic fields applied"	Stick et al. (81)
0.4 T —static magnetic field only —human subjects —studied magnetic field induced changes in auditory evoked potentials	"strong steady magnetic fields induce changes in human auditory evoked potentials"	Stojan et al. (82)
0.15 T —clinical imaging conditions —human subjects —studied effect of MRI on cognitive functions	"no significant effect upon cognitive functions assessed"	Sweetland et al. (83)
0.6 T/sec —gradient magnetic field only —mice —studied effect of gradient magnetic fields on the analgesic properties of specific opiate antagonists	"results indicate that the time-varying fields associated with MRI have significant inhibitory effects on analgesic effects of specific my-opiate-directed ligands"	Teskey et al. (84)
0.15 T —simulated imaging conditions —rats —studied effects of MRI on survivability and long-term stress reactivity levels	"results fail to provide any evidence for changes in survivability and long-term reactivity levels in rats exposed to MRI"	Teskey et al. (85)

APPENDIX IV. *Continued.*

Study description	Results	Reference
0.01 and 1.0 T —simulated imaging conditions and static magnetic field only —Echerichia coli —studied effect of MRI and static magnetic field on various properties of E. coli	"no mutations or lethal effects observed"	Thomas and Morris (86)
1.5 T —simulated imaging conditions —mice —studied tthe potential effects of MRI fields on eye development	"these data suggest a potential for MRI teratogenicity in a strain of mouse predisposed to eye malformations"	Tyndall (87)
1.5 T —simulated imaging conditions —C57BL/6J mouse —studied combined effects of MRI and X-irradiation on the developing eye of the mouse	"results . . . suggested that the MRI techniques employed for this investigation did not enhance teratogenicity of X-irradiation on eye malformations produced in the C657BL/6J mouse"	Tyndall and Sulik (88)
0.35 and 1.5 T —clinical imaging conditions —human subjects —studied effects of MRI on temperature	"no significant changes in central or peripheral temperatures resulting from the application of static or dynamic or radiofrequency"	Vogl et al. (89)
0.35 T —static magnetic field only —human subjects —studied effect of static magnetic field on auditory evoked potentials	"magnetically induced shift may be explained by changes in electric capacities of the magnetically exposed biological system"	Von Klitzing (90)
0.2 T —static magnetic field only —human subjects —studied effect of static magnetic field on power intensity of EEG	"the increased control values following on inverted magnetic flux vector point to a reversible alteration of brain function induced by a static magnetic field"	Von Klitzing (91)
0.2 T —static magnetic field only —human subjects studied —studied encephalomagnetic fields during exposure to static magnetic field	"exposure to static magnetic fields as used in NMR-equipment generates a new encephalomagnetic field in the human brain"	Von Klitzing (92)

APPENDIX IV. *Continued.*

Study description	Results	Reference
1.5 and 4.0 T —static magnetic fields only —rats —studied effect of magnetic field on behavior	"at 4 T . . . in 97% of the trials the rats would not enter the magnet"	Weiss et al. (93)
0.16 T —static and gradient magnetic fields only —anesthetized rats and guinea pigs —studied effects of static and gradient magnetic fields on cardiac function of rats and guinea pigs	"no change in blood pressure, heart rate, or ECG"	Willis and Brooks (94)
0.3 T —static magnetic field only —mouse sperm cell —studied effect of static magnetic field on spermatogenesis	"acute and subacute exposure to static magnetic fields associated with diagnostic MR imaging devices is unlikely to have any significant adverse effect on spermatogesis"	Withers et al. (95)
0.35 T —simulated imaging conditions —hamster ovary cells —studied effect of MRI on DNA and chromosomes	"the conditions used for NMR imaging do not cause genetic damage which is detectable by any of these methods"	Wolff et al. (96)
—varying gradient fields —human subjects —studied the effects of time-varying gradient fields on peripheral nerve stimulation using trapezoidal and sinusoidal pulse trains	"the thresholds of trapezoidal pulses were higher than those of sinusoidal pulses by 11% and 30% respectively, at equivalent power level"	Yamagata et al. (97)
1.5 T —simulated imaging conditions —chick embryos —studied teratogenicity of magnetic resonance field exposure	". . . exposed embryos . . . showed a trend toward higher abnormality and mortality rates than their controls."	Yip et al. (98)
1.5 T —simulated imaging conditions —chick embryos —studied effect of magnetic resonance exposure on proliferation and migration of motoneurons	". . . birth rates, migration, and proliferation of lateral motoneurons were unaffected compared to their controls."	Yip et al. (99)

APPENDIX IV. *Continued.*

Study description	Results	Reference
1.5 T —simulated imaging conditions —chick embryos —studied effects of magnetic resonance exposure on the rate and specificity of sympathetic preganglionic axonal outgrowth	". . . MR exposure conditions used in this study do not affect axonal growth in the sympathetic nervous system of the chick."	Yip et al. (100)
0.5 and 1.5 Tesla —static and gradient magnetic field —human subject —studied magnetic field effects on phantom limb pain	"The painful symptoms mimicked those experienced in the presence of the imagers".	Yuh et al. (101)

REFERENCES

1. Abart J, Brinker G, Irlbacher W, Grebmeier J. Temperature and heart rate changes in MRI at SAR levels of up to 3 W/kg. In: *Book of Abstracts, Society of Magnetic Resonance in Medicine.* Berkeley, CA: Society of Magnetic Resonance in Medicine;1991;2:683.
2. Adair ER, Berglund LG. On the thermoregulatory consequences of NMR imaging. *Magn Reson Imag* 1986;4:321–333.
3. Adair ER, Berglund LG. Thermoregulatory consequences of cardiovascular impairment during NMR imaging in warm/humid environments. *Magn Reson Imag* 1989;7:25–37.
4. Adzamli IK, Jolesz FA, Blau M. An assessment of blood–brain barrier integrity under MRI conditions: brain uptake of radiolabeled Gd-DTPA and In-DTPA-IgG. *J Nucl Med* 1989;30: 839.
5. Athey TW. A model of the temperature rise in the head due to magnetic resonance imaging procedures. *Magn Reson Med* 1989;9:177–184.
6. Barber BJ, Schaefer DJ, Gordon CJ, et al. Thermal effects of MR imaging: worst-case studies in sheep. *AJR Am J Roentgenol* 1990;155:1105–1110.
7. Bartels MV, Mann K, Matejcek M, et al. Magnetresonanztomographie und Sicherheit: Elektroenzephalographische und neuropsychologische Befunde vor und nach MR–Untersuchungen des Gehirns. *Fortschr Rontgenstr* 1986;145: 383–385.
8. Besson J, Foreman EI, Eastwood LM, et al. Cognitive evaluation following NMR imaging of the brain. *J Neurol Neurosurg Psychiatry* 1984;47:314–316.
9. Bore PJ, Galloway GJ, Styles P, et al. Are quenches dangerous? *Magn Reson Imag* 1986;3: 112–117.
10. Bourland JD, Nyenhuis JA, Mouchawar GA, et al. Physiologic indicators of high MRI gradient-induced fields. In: *Book of Abstracts, Society of Magnetic Resonance in Medicine.* Berkeley, CA: Society of Magnetic Resonance in Medicine; 1990; 1276.
11. Brockway JP, Bream PR. Does memory loss occur after MR imaging? *J Magn Reson Imag* 1992;2:721–728.
12. Brody AS, Sorette MP, Gooding CA, et al. Induced alignment of flowing sickle erythrocytes in a magnetic field. A preliminary report. *Invest Radiol* 1985;20:560–566.
13. Brody AS, Embury SH, Mentzer WC, et al. Preservation of sickle cell blood flow patterns during MR imaging. An in vivo study. *AJR Am J Roentgenol* 1988;151:139–141.

14. Brummett RE, Talbot JM, Charuhas P. Potential hearing loss resulting from MR imaging. *Radiology* 1988;169:539–540.
15. Budinger TF, Fischer H, Hentschel D, et al. Physiological effects of fast oscillating magnetic field gradients. *J Comput Assist Tomogr* 1991;15:909–914.
16. Budinger TF, Brennan KN, Gilbert JC, et al. Excitation of the heart by rapidly oscillating magnetic fields. *Radiology* 1991;181(P):191.
17. Carson JJL, Prato FS, Drost DJ, et al. Time-varying fields increase cytosolic free Ca^{2+} in HL-60 cells. *Am J Physiol* 1990;259:C687-C692.
18. Cohen MS, Weisskoff R, Rzedzian R, et al. Sensory stimulation by time-varying magnetic fields. *Magn Reson Med* 1990;14:409–414.
19. Cooke P, Morris PG. The effects of NMR exposure on living organisms. II. A genetic study of human lymphocytes. *Br J Radiol* 1981;54:622–625.
20. Doherty JU, Whitman GJR, Robinson MD, et al. Changes in cardiac excitability and vulnerability in NMR fields. *Invest Radiol* 1985;20:129–135.
21. Fischer H. Physiological effects of fast oscillating magnetic field gradients. *Radiology* 1989;173:(P)382.
22. Garber HJ, Oldendorf WH, Braun LD, et al. MRI gradient fields increase brain mannitol space. *Magn Reson Imag* 1989;7:605–610.
23. Geard CR, Osmak RS, Hall EJ, et al. Magnetic resonance and ionizing radiation: a comparative evaluation in vitro of oncongenic and genotoxic potential. *Radiology* 1984;152:199–202.
24. Gore JC, McDonnell MJ, Pennock JM, et al. An assessment of the safety of rapidly changing magnetic fields in the rabbit: implications for NMR imaging. *Magn Reson Imag* 1982;1:191–195.
25. Grandolfo M, Vecchia P, Gandhi OP. Magnetic resonance imaging: calculation of rates of energy absorption by a human-torso model. *Bioelectromagnetics* 1990;11:117–128.
26. Gremmel H, Wendhausen H, Wunsch F. Biologische Effekte statischef Magnetfelder bei NMR-Tomographie am Menschen. Wiss, Radiologische, Klinik, Christian-Albrechts-Universitat zu Kiel, 1983.
27. Gulch RW, and Lutz O. Influence of strong static magnetic fields on heart muscle contraction. *Phys Med Biol* 1986;31:763–769.
28. Hammer BE, Wadon S, Mirer SD, et al. In vivo measurement of RF heating in Capuchin monkey brain. In: *Book of Abstracts, Society of Magnetic Resonance in Medicine.* Berkeley, CA: Society of Magnetic Resonance in Medicine; 1991;3:1278.
29. Heinrichs WL, Fong P, Flannery M, et al. Midgestational exposure of pregnant balb/c mice to magnetic resonance imaging. *Magn Reson Imag* 1988;6:305–313.
30. Hong CZ, Shellock FG. Short-term exposure to a 1.5 Tesla static magnetic field does not effect somato-sensory evoked potentials in man. *Magn Reson Imag* 1989;8: 65–69.
31. Innis NK, Ossenkopp KP, Prato FS, et al. Behavioral effects of exposure to nuclear magnetic resonance imaging: II. Spatial memory tests. *Magn Reson Imag* 1986;4:281–284.
32. Jehenson P, Duboc D, Lavergne T, et al. Change in human cardiac rhythm by a 2 Tesla static magnetic field. *Radiology* 1988;166:227–230.
33. Kanal E, Applegate GR. Thermal injuries/incidents associated with MR imaging devices in the US: a compilation and review of the presently available data. In: *Book of Abstracts, Society of Magnetic Resonance in Medicine.* Berkeley, CA: Society of Magnetic Resonance in Medicine; 1990;1:274.
34. Kay HH, Herfkens RJ, Kay BK. Effect of Magnetic resonance imaging on Xenopus laevis embryogenesis. *Magn Reson Imag* 1988;6:501–506.
35. Keltner JR, Roos MS, Brakeman PR, et al. Magnetohydrodynamics of blood flow. *Magn Reson Med* 1990;16:139–149.
36. Kido DK, Morris TW, Erickson JL, et al. Physiologic changes during high field strength MR imaging. *AJNR Am J Neuroradiol* 1987;8:263–266.
37. LaPorte R, Kus L, Wisniewski RA, et al. Magnetic resonance imaging (MRI) effects on rat pineal neuroendocrine function. *Brain Res* 1990;506:294–296.
38. McJury MJ. Acoustic noise levels generated during high field MR imaging. *Clin Radiol* 1995: 50:331–334.
39. McJury M, Blug A, Joerger C, Condon B, Wyper D. Acoustic noise levels during magnetic resonance imaging scanning at 1.5 T. *Br J Radiol* 1994;413–415.

40. McRobbie D, Foster MA. Cardiac response to pulsed magnetic fields with regard to safety in NMR imaging. *Phys Med Biol* 1985;30: 695–702.
41. McRobbie D, Foster MA. Pulsed magnetic field exposure during pregnancy and implications for NMR foetal imaging: a study with mice. *Magn Reson Imag* 1985;3:231–234.
42. Messmer JM, Porter JH, Fatouros P, et al. Exposure to magnetic resonance imaging does not produce taste aversion in rats. *Physiol Behav* 1987;40:259–261.
43. Montour JL, Fatouros PP, Prasad UR. Effect of MR imaging on spleen colony formation following gamma radiation. *Radiology* 1988;168:259–260.
44. Muller S, Hotz M. Human brainstem auditory evoked potentials (BAEP) before and after MR examinations. *Magn Reson Med* 1990;16:476–480.
45. Muller-Miny H, Erber D, Moller H, Muller-Miny B, Bongartz G. Is there a hazard to health by mercury exposure from amalgam due to MRI? *J Magn Reson Imag* 1996;1:258–260.
46. Ngo FQH, Blue JW, Roberts WK. The effects of a static magnetic field on DNA synthesis and survival of mammalian cells irradiated with fast neutrons. *Magn Reson Med* 1987;5:307–317.
47. Niemann G, Schroth G, Klose U, et al. Influence of magnetic resonance imaging on somatosensory potential in man. *J Neurol* 1988;235:462–465.
48. Osbakken M, Griffith J, Taczanowsky P. A gross morphologic, histologic, hematologic, and blood chemistry study of adult and neonatal mice chronically exposed to high magnetic fields. *Magn Reson Med* 1986;3:502–517.
49. Ossenkopp KP, Kavaliers M, Prato FS, et al. Exposure to nuclear magnetic imaging procedure attenuates morphine-induced analgesia in mice. *Life Sci* 1985;37:1507–1514.
50. Ossenkopp KP, Innis NK, Prato FS, et al. Behavioral effects of exposure to nuclear magnetic resonance imaging: I. Open-field behavior and passive avoidance learning in rats. *Magn Reson Imag* 1986;4:275–280.
51. Papatheofanis FJ, Papthefanis BJ. Short-term effect of exposure to intense magnetic fields on hematologic indices of bone metabolism. *Invest Radiol* 1989;24:221–223.
52. Peeling J, Lewis JS, Samoiloff MR, et al. Biological effects of magnetic fields on the nematode *Panagrellus redivivus. Magn Reson Imag* 1988;6:655–660.
53. Prasad N, Wright DA, Ford JJ, Thornby JI. Effect of nuclear magnetic resonance on early stages of amphibian development. *Magn Reson Imag* 1982;1:35–38.
54. Prasad N, Bushong SC, Thornby JI, et al. Effect of nuclear resonance on chromosomes of mouse bone marrow cells. *Magn Reson Imag* 1984;2:37–39.
55. Prasad N, Kosnik LT, Taber KH, et al. Delayed tumor onset following MR imaging exposure. In: *Book of Abstracts, Society of Magnetic Resonance in Medicine.* Berkeley, CA: Society of Magnetic Resonance in Medicine; 1990; 1:275.
56. Prasad N, Prasad R, Bushong SC, et al. Effects of 4.5 T MRI exposure on mouse testes and epididymes. In: *Book of Abstracts, Society of Magnetic Resonance in Medicine.* Berkeley, CA: Society of Magnetic Resonance in Medicine; 1990;2:606.
57. Prasad N, Lotzova E, Thornby JI, et al. Effects of MR imaging on murine natural killer cell cytotoxicity. *AJR Am J Roentgenol* 1987;148:415–417.
58. Prasad N, Lotzova E, Thornby JI, et al. The effect of 2.35-T MR imaging on natural killer cell cytotoxicity with and without interleukin-2. *Radiology* 1990;175:251–263.
59. Prasad N, Wright DA, Ford JJ, et al. Safety of 4-T MR imaging: A study of effects of developing frog embryos. *Radiology* 1990;174:251–253.
60. Prato FS, Ossenkopp KP, Kavaliers M, et al. Attenuation of morphine-induced analgesia in mice by exposure to magnetic resonance imaging: Separate effects of the static, radiofrequency and time-varying magnetic fields. *Magn Reson Imag* 1987;5:9–14.
61. Redington RW, Dumoulin CL, Schenck JL, et al. MR imaging and bio-effects in a whole body 4.0 Tesla imaging system. In: *Book of Abstracts, Society of Magnetic Resonance Imaging.* Berkeley, CA: Society of Magnetic Resonance Imaging; 1988;1:20.
62. Reid A, Smith FW, Hutchison JMS. Nuclear magnetic resonance imaging and its safety implications: follow-up of 181 patients. *Br J Radiol* 1982;55:784–786.
63. Rofsky NM, Pizzarello DJ, Weinreb JC, Ambrosino MM, Rosenberg C. Effect on fetal mouse development of exposure to MR imaging and gadopentetate dimeglumine. *J Magn Reson Imag* 1994;805–807.
64. Roschmann P. Human auditory system response to pulsed radiofrequency energy in RF coils for magnetic resonance at 2.4 to 170 MHz. *Magn Reson Med* 1991;21:197–215.

65. Sacks E, Worgul BV, Merriam GR, et al. The effects of nuclear magnetic resonance imaging on ocular tissues. *Arch Ophthalmol* 1986;104:890–893.
66. Schiffman SJ, Lash, HM, Rollag MD, Flanders AE, Brainard GC, Burk DL. Effect of MR imaging on the normal human pineal body: measurement of plasma melatonin levels. *J Magn Reson Imag* 1994;4:7–11.
67. Schwartz JL, Crooks LE. NMR imaging produces no observable mutations or cytotoxicity in mammalian cells. *AJR Am J Roentgenol* 1982;139:583–585.
68. Shellock FG, Schaefer DJ, Gordon CJ. Effect of a 1.5 T static magnetic field on body temperature of man. *Magn Reson Med* 1986;3:644–647.
69. Shellock FG, Crues JV. Temperature, heart rate, and blood pressure changes associated with clinical MR imaging at 1.5 T. *Radiology* 1987;163:259–262.
70. Shellock FG, Schaefer DJ, Grundfest W, et al. Thermal effects of high-field (1.5 Tesla) magnetic resonance imaging of the spine: clinical experience above a specific absorption rate of 0.4 W/kg. *Acta Radiol Suppl* 1986;369:514–516.
71. Shellock FG, Gordon CJ, Schaefer DJ. Thermoregulatory responses to clinical magnetic resonance imaging of the head at 1.5 Tesla: lack of evidence for direct effects on the hypothalamus. *Acta Radiola Suppl* 1986;369:512–513.
72. Shellock FG, Crues JV. Corneal temperature changes associated with high-field MR imaging using a head coil. *Radiology* 1986;167:809–811.
73. Shellock FG, Crues JV. Temperature changes caused by clinical MR imaging of the brain at 1.5 Tesla using a head coil. *AJNR Am J Neuroradiol* 1988;9:287–291.
74. Shellock FG, Schaefer DJ, Crues JV. Effect of a 1.5 Tesla static magnetic field on body and skin temperatures of man. *Magn Reson Med* 1989;11:371–375.
75. Shellock FG, Schaefer DJ, Crues JV. Alterations in body and skin temperatures caused by MR imaging: is the recommended exposure for radiofrequency radiation too conservative? *Br J Radiol* 1989;62:904–909.
76. Shellock FG, Rothman B, Sarti D. Heating of the scrotum by high-field–strength MR imaging. *AJR Am J Roentgenol* 1990;154:1229–1232.
77. Shellock FG, Morisoli SM, Ziarati M. Measurement of acoustic noise during MR imaging: evaluation of six "worst-case" pulse sequences. *Radiology* 1994;191:91–93.
78. Shivers RR, Kavaliers M, Tesky CJ, et al. Magnetic resonance imaging temporarily alters blood–brain barrier permeability in the rat. *Neurosci Lett* 1987;76:25–31.
79. Shuman WP, Haynor DR, Guy AW, et al. Superficial and deep-tissue increases in anesthetized dogs during exposure to high specific absorption rates in a 1.5-T MR imager. *Radiology* 1988;167:551–554.
80. Sperber D, Oldenbourg R, Dransfeld K. Magnetic field–induced temperature change in mice. *Naturwissenschaften* 1984;71:100–101.
81. Stick VC, Hinkelmann ZK, Eggert P, et al. Beeinflussen starke statische magnetfelder in der NMR-Tomographie die gewebedurchblutung? (Strong static magnetic fields of NMR: do they affect tissue perfusion?). *Fortschr Rontgenstr* 1991;154:326–331.
82. Stojan L, Sperber D, Dransfeld K. Magnetic-field–induced changes in the human auditory evoked potentials. *Naturwissenschaften* 1988;75:622–623.
83. Sweetland J, Kertesz A, Prato FS, et al. The effect of magnetic resonance imaging on human congnition. *Magn Reson Imag* 1987;5:129–135.
84. Teskey GC, Prato FS, Ossenkopp KP, et al. Exposure to time varying magnetic fields associated with magnetic resonance imaging reduces fentanyl-induced analgesia in mice. *Bioelectromagnetics* 1988;9:167–174.
85. Tesky GC, Ossenkopp KP, Prato FS, et al. Survivability and long-term stress reactivity levels following repeated exposure to nuclear magnetic resonance imaging procedures in rats. *Physiol Chem Phys Med NMR* 1987;19:43–49.
86. Thomas A, Morris PG. The effects of NMR exposure on living organisms. I. A microbial assay. *Br J Radiol* 1981;54:615–621.
87. Tyndall DA, Sulik KK. Effects of magnetic resonance imaging on eye development in the C57BL/6J mouse. *Teratology* 1991;43:263–275.
88. Tyndall DA. MRI effects on the tertogenicity of X-irradiation in the C57BL/6J mouse. *Magn Reson Imag* 1990;8:423–433.
89. Vogl T, Krimmel K, Fuchs A, et al. Influence of magnetic resonance imaging on human body core and intravascular temperature. *Med Phys* 1988;15:562–566.

90. Von Klitzing L. Do static magnetic fields of NMR influence biological signals. *Clin Phys Physiol Measurement (Bristol)* 1986;7(2): 157–160.
91. Von Klitzing L. Static magnetic fields increase the power intensity of EEG of man. *Brain Res* 1989;483:201–203.
92. Von Klitzing L. A new encephalomagnetic effect in human brain generated by static magnetic fields. *Brain Res* 1991;540:295–296.
93. Weiss J, Herrick RC, Taber KH, et al. Bio-effects of high magnetic fields: a study using a simple animal model. *Magn Reson Imag* 1990;8(S1):166.
94. Willis RJ, Brooks WM. Potential hazards of NMR imaging. No evidence of the possible effects of static and changing magnetic fields on cardiac function of the rat and guinea pig. *Magn Reson Imag* 1984;2:89–95.
95. Withers HR, Mason KA, Davis CA. MR effect on murine spermatogenesis. *Radiology* 1985;156:741–742.
96. Wolff S, Crooks LE, Brown P, et al. Tests for DNA and chromosomal damage induced by nuclear magnetic resonance imaging. *Radiology* 1980;136:707–710.
97. Yamagata H, Kuhara S, Eso Y, et al. Evaluation of dB/dt thresholds for nerve stimulation elicited by trapezoidal and sinusoidal gradient fields in echo-planar imaging. In: *Book of Abstracts, Society of Magnetic Resonance in Medicine.* Berkeley, CA: Society of Magnetic Resonance in Medicine; 1991;3:1277.
98. Yip YP, Capriotti C, Talagala SL, Yip JW. Effects of MR exposure at 1.5 T on early embryonic development of the chick. *J Magn Reson Imag* 1994;4:742–748.
99. Yip YP, Capriotti C, Norbash SG, Talagala SL, Yip JW. Effects of MR exposure on cell proliferation and migration of chick motoneurons. *J Magn Reson Imag* 1994;4:799–804.
100. Yip YP, Capriotti C, Yip JW. Effects of MR exposure on axonal outgrowth in the sympathetic nervous system of the chick. *J Magn Reson Imag* 1995;4:457–462.
101. Yuh WTC, Fisher DJ, Shields RK, et al. Phantom limb pain induced in amputee by strong magnetic fields. *J Magn Reson Imag* 1992;2:221–223.

Appendix V

International Magnetic Resonance Safety Central Web Site Information

WEB SITE ADDRESS:

http://kanal.arad.upmc.edu/mrsafety.html

Discuss issues or ask questions on:

- Static magnetic field (Bo): biologic effects
- Static magnetic field (Bo): mechanical effects
- RF power deposition/heating effects and burns
- RF biologic effects (nonthermal)
- dB/dt (gradient switching) effects (e.g., EPI)
- Cryogen safety issues
- Contrast agent safety issues
- Psychological/anxiety/claustrophobia issues
- MR and pregnancy
- MR and pacemakers
- MR screening
- Other miscellaneous issues

Subject Index

Subject Index

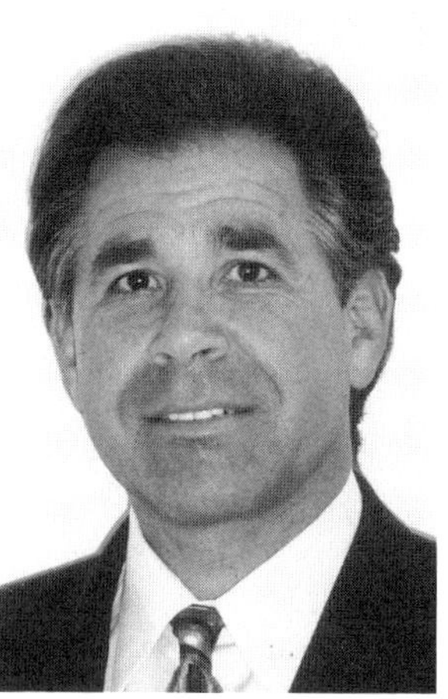

Frank G. Shellock, Ph.D., is a Clinical Professor of Radiology at the University of Southern California, School of Medicine, and the Director of Research and Development for RadNet Management, Inc., and Future Diagnostics, Inc., in Los Angeles, California. He is a member of the Safety Committees for the International Society for Magnetic Resonance in Medicine and American College of Radiology and a former member of the Board of Directors of the Society for Magnetic Resonance Imaging. Dr. Shellock is a Fellow of the American College of Cardiology and American College of Sportsmedicine. He has published two textbooks, more than 40 book chapters, and more than 100 peer-reviewed articles. Dr. Shellock's current research interests include the evaluation of electromagnetic field–related bioeffects and the development of new MR imaging applications. At Future Diagnostics, Inc., he is involved in physician credentialing, quality assurance procedures, and the development of practice guidelines for diagnostic imaging.

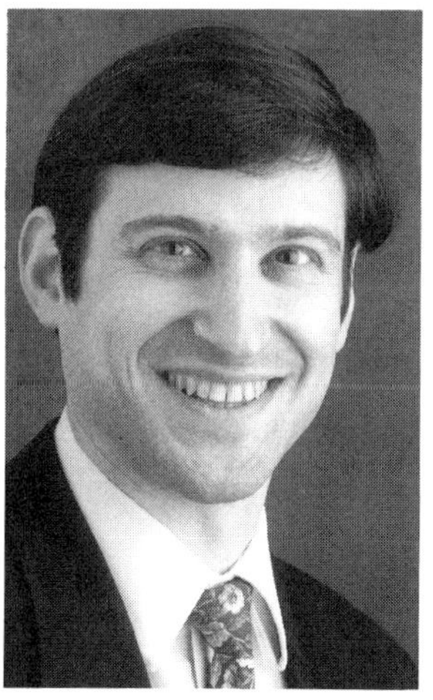

Emanuel Kanal, M.D., is an Associate Professor of Radiology and the Director of Clinical and Educational MR at the University of Pittsburgh Medical Center in Pittsburgh, Pennsylvania. He is a member of the Safety Committees for the International Society for Magnetic Resonance in Medicine and American College of Radiology and a former co-chairman of the Safety Committee for the Society of Magnetic Resonance Imaging. He is the creator of the Kanal's MR Tutor, a popular software program that teaches basic and advanced aspects of MRI and the originator of the International MR Safety Web Site, devoted to providing rapid and timely access to MR safety information to all MR users. Dr. Kanal has published two textbooks and numerous book chapters and scientific articles on a variety of MR imaging, angiography, and safety related topics.